DECEIT AND DENIAL

The Deadly Politics of Industrial Pollution

GERALD MARKOWITZ AND DAVID ROSNER

University of California Press

BERKELEY   LOS ANGELES   LONDON

The Milbank Memorial Fund

NEW YORK

The Milbank Memorial Fund is an endowed national foundation that engages in nonpartisan analysis, study, research, and communication on significant issues in health policy. In the Fund's own publications, in reports or books it publishes with other organizations, and in articles it commissions for publication by other organizations, the Fund endeavors to maintain the highest standards for accuracy and fairness. Statements by individual authors, however, do not necessarily reflect opinions or factual determinations of the Fund.

University of California Press
Berkeley and Los Angeles, California

University of California Press, Ltd.
London, England

Library of Congress Cataloging-in-Publication Data

Markowitz, Gerald E.
    Deceit and denial : the deadly politics of industrial pollution /
David Rosner.
        p.   cm.
    Includes bibliographical references and index.
    ISBN 0-520-21749-7 (alk. paper).
    1. Environmental health.   2. Environmental health—Social aspects.
3. Factory and trade waste—Environmental aspects.   4. Pollution—
Health aspects.   I. Rosner, David, 1947–   II. Title.

RA566 .M265   2002
615.9'02—dc21   2001058515

Manufactured in the United States of America
10   09   08   07   06   05   04   03   02
10   9   8   7   6   5   4   3   2   1

The paper used in this publication meets the minimum requirements of
ANSI/NISO Z39.48-1992(R 1997) (*Permanence of Paper*).∞

For Andrea and Kathy

Contents

FOREWORD

The Milbank Memorial Fund is an endowed national foundation that engages in nonpartisan analysis, study, research, and communication on significant issues in health policy. The Fund makes available the results of its work in meetings with decision makers, reports, articles, and books.

This is the sixth of the California/Milbank Books on Health and the Public. The publishing partnership between the Fund and the Press seeks to encourage the synthesis and communication of findings from research that could contribute to more effective health policy.

Gerald Markowitz and David Rosner demonstrate the significance for policy of the methods and findings of historical scholarship. On the basis of research that has been reviewed by experts in history, biomedical science, and policy, they describe decisions by executives of corporations that produce lead products and plastics to withhold information about the health hazards of their products and production processes from their employees and regulators. These decisions contributed to the severe illness and death of many employees of these corporations as well as of persons who lived in the wrong place at the wrong time.

The authors' findings are both dismaying and encouraging. On the one hand, executives of major corporations systematically compromised the health of many people. On the other hand, the independence of the American judiciary and the attentiveness of many legislators to the concerns of their constituents brought dangerous situations and their consequences to public attention. This attention yielded compensation for victims and their families and new policy to prevent health hazards in workplaces and communities.

Daniel M. Fox, President
Samuel L. Milbank, Chairman
Milbank Memorial Fund

PREFACE

A number of years ago, just after we had completed *Deadly Dust,* our book on the history of an occupational lung disease called silicosis, we had the opportunity to visit one of the communities that had been devastated by this affliction. Picher, Oklahoma is a tiny town that once was the center of a huge lead-mining belt. Including parts of Oklahoma, Missouri, and Kansas, it was the biggest lead-producing area in the world from 1900 to1935. The Tri-State region intensely concerned government, the public health community, and a range of industrial hygienists, occupational physicians, and even the general public. The whole country learned of the "Street of Walking Death," the phrase used to describe the main street of one of the mining villages that dotted this 2,000-square-mile area. Thousands of miners were said to have been killed or seriously injured by silicosis, a disease produced by the inhalation of fine silica dust created while pulverizing rock or by shooting sand at metallic objects in a variety of trades from foundry work to building construction.

Our trip to Picher was like a trip back in time. The town had been a symbol of one of the worst public health disasters of the Depression era, when lead miners had organized to protest the deaths and disability caused by industrial disease. Not much had changed. Bypassed by all major highways, connected to more populated areas only by pitted asphalt roads, and seemingly untouched by the past fifty years of population mobility or technological change lay a wasteland of dilapidated houses surrounded by huge piles of waste materials from nearly a half century of mining. Huge "chat" piles, thousands of tons of silica flint that had been ripped from the earth, dotted the town of a couple of thousand people who, by reason of chance, dedication, or family had not abandoned what was becoming a ghost town. The only new buildings we saw were a 1960ish red brick funeral parlor and a 1970ish yellow brick school.

Many people in the town, even some children, seemed to have chronic lung obstructions that they, if not the physicians, called silicosis. Winds brushing the chat piles surrounding the community, we were told, constantly blew finely ground crystals into every crack and crevice of every home. Many children had spent afternoons sliding down the hills of silica sand on makeshift sleds of cardboard or rolling and tumbling down the mounds, which circled many of the homes. Every time the wind blew, especially in the fall, when the winds would build up over the plains, dust was everywhere. Coming into the town, we had noticed a distinct "beach" smell that we had always associated with the ocean but soon suspected was related to silica sand.

We had startling discussions with former miners and their wives that forced us to confront the assumptions underlying our previous work on occupational disease. The residents told us that our focus on workers alone was wrong: that what happened to people in the mines was only half the equation of the problem with industrial disease. The other half was the impact of disease on a community, what happened when toxins and knowledge about them leaked out of the workplace. Our questions then were only partly formed, but they would become the central issues that would form the basis of this book: Why were community perceptions of the problem of industrial disease so completely different from those of the expert? How did these differing perceptions get resolved at different historical moments? How did changing public perceptions about disease affect the sciences and the scientists who were given the authority by public bodies to define these conditions? Where did "real" science fit into contentious issues of blame and responsibility? Who had the right to define the real nature of the health problem? Where was the public in public health?

Visiting Picher and talking with people there led us to see that the notion of "social construction" or "framing" of disease that we had used in *Deadly Dust* was extremely limited. We had been so consumed by the subject of silicosis in the Tri-State area that we had failed even to note what was staring at us from beneath those chat piles and destroyed lives: that the same toxins that caused occupational disease also become environmental problems. In *Deadly Dust*, we viewed silicosis as part of history. It was an occupational disease that once had caused enormous pain and suffering but was now under control—since the 1940s—as a result of the combined actions of the industrial hygiene, engineering, and medical communities. After all, we had dug deeply into the literature and had found that many in the entire public health and medical communities agreed that silicosis, while "epidemic" in the 1930s, was essentially a thing of the past by the

1940s. We had analyzed the way in which the public perception of this disease was manipulated and had clearly raised the question whether a chronic disease whose symptoms appeared decades after exposure could possibly be "controlled" in the short span of a decade. But we had believed it was, in large measure, a disease of the past, because the medical community and the professional literature had virtually stopped talking about it by the late 1940s. If the disease was out of sight and out of mind today, it must no longer be a problem.

Yet almost immediately after the publication of the book some public health professionals invited us to speak at a two-day forum scheduled to follow the American Public Health Association meetings in San Francisco that year. Of course, we were happy to address professionals, yet we wondered why so many people would be interested in a historical account of silicosis, a disease long dead. In short, it appeared silicosis was not a dead issue. We learned that a new epidemic of the disease had swept through the Louisiana shipbuilding industries and was now striking many Mexican American oil field workers in Odessa and Midland, Texas, and elsewhere. In a short time, our book became a principal reference in numerous lawsuits and federal government actions leading to the National Conference to Eliminate Silicosis in 1997.

A number of law firms asked us to serve as expert witnesses on behalf of workers suffering from silicosis. The defendants had argued that there was no way for companies to have known that silicosis was a problem in their industry. We presented evidence from our book that showed the long and tragic history of this disease. In 1993 Diane Dwight, one of the attorneys who retained us, had asked if we would be willing to evaluate a warehouse of material that Billy Baggett Jr., a lawyer at another firm in Louisiana, had accumulated in another case. The case, unrelated to silica, involved a number of workers dying, apparently of angiosarcoma of the liver, a rare cancer of the linings of that organ's blood vessels. It was known that this disease was caused by exposure to vinyl chloride monomer (VCM), a chlorinated hydrocarbon that was the fundamental building block in a widely used plastic, polyvinyl chloride (PVC). Through discovery proceedings the law firm in Louisiana had accumulated hundreds of thousands of documents that it believed showed that the chemical industry had long known of the dangers of this material but had failed to protect its workers from exposure, leading to unnecessary deaths. Dwight's firm asked for our help in evaluating the evidence so it could decide whether to go forward with the case. We were asked to determine the answer to standard legal questions: When did the vinyl industry know it had exposed workers to VCM? What did they know about the relationship between vinyl and cancer at the time? What did they do about it? Billy Baggett Jr. was the only person who had ever systematically examined these materials.

Over the next three years we studied these papers, becoming ever more incredulous about their contents. We produced a 300-page timeline and a detailed summary of the critical documents. Since then this timeline has been shared with the chemical companies, newspaper reporters, and television journalists such as Bill Moyers. In the fall of 1996 Daniel M. Fox, president of the Milbank Memorial Fund, approached us with the offer of support for a book to be copublished by the Fund and the University of California Press that would examine the history of occupational and environmental disease through the lens of case studies of specific toxins. This support was crucial, particularly in the first three years of our research. More recently, we have benefited from the support of the National Science Foundation.

Lawyers have an incredible tool for historical research available to them: the power to ask private industries for a wide variety of materials from company files and the right to depose individuals whom they expect to have information relevant to their case. As Bill Moyers noted in his television special *Trade Secrets*, the papers we found were a gold mine, containing the kind of information found in the tobacco papers, the trove of tobacco company documents that became the basis for the lawsuits by smokers and various states.

Early in 1998 an article we had written in 1985 on the maneuvering by General Motors, Standard Oil, DuPont, and Ethyl Corporation over the introduction of tetraethyl lead into gasoline in the 1920s led to our involvement in a lead suit then being developed by the city of New York against the lead industry—specifically those companies (and their trade association) that manufactured lead pigments and lead paint. This opened up to us yet another trove of company documents never before reviewed by scholars unaffiliated with the lead industry. At least two others, Peter C. English and John Heitmann, hired by the lead industry's lawyers, have reviewed these documents and written affidavits supporting the lead industry's positions. Like the vinyl materials, these documents were both overwhelming in their breadth and eye-opening in what they illustrated about the inner workings of a major industry.

These records of the lead and plastics industries shed a bright light on historical questions about how groups in our society define disease and what causes ill health, as well as questions regarding the laboratory, the means of assessing danger, the methods for documenting industrial health problems, and ideas about appropriate cures and even treatment of conditions. These legal records gave us a window into a world historians (and certainly the general public) are rarely allowed to enter: the world of corporate meetings, where corporate officials shape our ideas about their products and make decisions about the production and marketing of products that may pose a danger for workers and the consuming public. As was true of silica, the story of vinyl chloride is one in which a seemingly benign material was found to have a profound impact on workers' health. But something more seemed to go on with vinyl chloride than with silica. Not only did vinyl chloride pose a risk to workers, but also its products subjected everyone who used or disposed them to problems that are still only barely understood today. If we worried about chronic disease in the 1930s and cancers in the 1970s and 1980s, today we worry about subtler but potentially more devastating effects involving endocrine disruption, genetic damage, and behavioral change. During the 1930s the focus of the medical and public health community shifted from infectious and acute illness to chronic disease. Today we are concerned as well about the subclinical effects of environmental toxins. The histories of lead and vinyl chloride demonstrate how we arrived at this point.

Acknowledgments

During the time we have been working on this book numerous people have helped in ways both big and small. Of course we must begin by thanking the Milbank Memorial Fund, whose president, Daniel M. Fox, was instrumental in prodding us to undertake this effort and to provide us with funds that enabled us to collect early in this project the huge amount of primary materials in Louisiana, the National Archives, and elsewhere. Dan Fox's patience, encouragement, and intellectual support should be a model for other foundations and funding agencies. Gail Cambridge at the Fund was always helpful in facilitating the arrangements necessary in our travels around the country. Toward the end of the project the National Science Foundation provided funds necessary to free us from many of our responsibilities at our respective universities so that we could complete the research and prepare a first draft of the book. We thank Michael Sokal, Bruce Seely, and John Perhonis of the National Science Foundation for their encouragement and help.

A unique aspect of the Milbank and University of California Press process was the intellectual support provided. They brought together scholars and practitioners whose expertise in a variety of aspects of our project provided us with valuable perspectives on the issues that we raise and detail in the book. In an intellectually vibrant meeting in Berkeley, Milbank and the Press brought together historians, industrial hygienists and physicians, public health practitioners, and former government officials for a cross-disciplinary discussion. We received astute commentaries on our writing from Elizabeth Blackmar of Columbia University; Blanche Wiesen Cook of John Jay College and the City University of New York Graduate Center; Ruth Heifetz of the University of California, San Diego; David Kotelchuck of Hunter College; John Rosen of Montifiore Medical Center;

Paul Templet of Louisiana State University; Arthur Upton, former director of the National Cancer Institute; and Christian Warren of the New York Academy of Medicine.

We were extremely fortunate to have been asked by a number of law firms to evaluate an enormous store of primary documents about lead and vinyl that had been collected over the course of many years through extensive discovery proceedings in conjunction with a number of lawsuits. While providing these firms with our expert opinion, we were given unfettered access to a range of materials never before viewed by historians unaffiliated with industry and with no restrictions about what we would be able to publish about these materials. William (Billy) Baggett Jr. of Baggett, McCall, Burgess, and Watson of Lake Charles, Louisiana, made available a virtual warehouse of documents detailing the activities of the Manufacturing Chemists' Association and its member companies in the postwar decades. The New York City Law Department, especially John Low-Beer, Yair Goldstein, and Alan Kleiman, provided access to another store of documents concerning the Lead Industries Association and its member companies during the twentieth century. Adele Oltman and Nina Kushner of Columbia University provided critical research assistance in our efforts to sort through such a vast wealth of material. While we were in Louisiana, Robert Kuehn, director of Tulane University's Environmental Law Clinic, was extremely generous with his time and also allowed us to sort through the clinic's files on environmental pollution in Louisiana and the efforts by community residents to challenge the chemical industry. Mary Lee Orr of the Louisiana Environmental Action Network (LEAN) also generously opened up the organization's files to us. We are also grateful to Gloria Roberts and Emelda West, residents of Convent, Louisiana, who gave us a tour of their community and invited us into their homes. Beth Zilbert, an organizer for Greenpeace in Lake Charles, Louisiana, spent many hours with us touring the community, introducing us to residents and providing us with leaflets and other materials used in the organizing drives in Lake Charles. Barbara Dudley, former director of Greenpeace, USA, and Monique Harden, staff attorney at Greenpeace in Washington, were also helpful in providing material about Greenpeace's campaign against polyvinyl chloride and environmental racism. Robert Knox, director of the Office of Civil Rights of the Environmental Protection Agency (EPA), Peter Infante and Loretta Schuman of the Occupational Safety and Health Administration (OSHA), and Matt Gillen and Lore Jackson Lee of the National Institute of Occupational Safety and Health (NIOSH) all were generous with their time. At the National Archives, Bill Creech and Marjorie Ciarlante were always available and provided expert guidance to the wealth of material in the EPA, OSHA, and NIOSH files. David Michaels, then assistant secretary in the Department of Energy, sent us files of material he had collected as a graduate student. Tony Mazzocchi, former vice president of the Oil, Chemical and Atomic Workers International Union, gave us access to his files.

This project has attracted the interest of the broader public as well as scholars. In March 2001 Bill Moyers produced an excellent documentary, *Trade Secrets,* that was based in part on the vinyl chloride documents. In 2002 Judith Helfand and Dan Gold produced another award-winning documentary, *Blue Vinyl,* which also examines the relationship between the hazards of vinyl chloride and polyvinyl chloride and on which we were pleased to consult. Tom Engelhardt and Jonathan Cobb are two friends and editors who have given us constant feedback and support.

A number of colleagues both at Columbia and the City University of New York have been extremely helpful. Ezra Susser, the chair of the Department of Epidemiology at Columbia's Mailman School of Public Health, and Gerald Oppenheimer of Brooklyn College closely read sections of the book that addressed science and public policy. Jeanne Stellman provided us with critical documents and constant support and suggestions.

Our colleagues at Columbia's Mailman School of Public Health, particularly the Center for the History and Ethics of Public Health and the Department of Sociomedical Sciences, have been extremely supportive. We thank Amy Fairchild, Martina Lynch, Ron Bayer, David Rothman, Sheila Rothman, Paul Edelson, and Barron Lerner. James Colgrove, Nick Turse, Whitney Bryant, and Rochelle Frounfelker provided invaluable research assistance. We want to particularly thank Elizabeth Robilotti for her extraordinary dedication to our project and her cheerful and always efficient help. Cheryl Heaton, Nancy Devanter, and Richard Parker, successive chairs of the department, and Dean Allan Rosenfield were always supportive. Alan Brinkley, Eric Foner, Elizabeth Blackmar, Kenneth Jackson, Alice Kessler-Harris, and Nancy Stepan of Columbia's History Department were wonderful colleagues.

Our colleagues at John Jay College's Thematic Studies Program and History Department and the City University of New York Graduate Program provided an extraordinary community of scholars and teachers. They are Michael Blitz, Blanche Wiesen Cook, Kojo Dei, Geoff Fairweather, Josh Freeman, Betsy Gitter, Don Goodman, Carol Groneman, David Nasaw, Jim Oakes, Carol Quirke, Shirley Sarna, Dennis Sherman, and Abby Stein. President Gerald W. Lynch, Provost Basil Wilson, and Vice President Roger

Witherspoon have made working at John Jay a pleasure. As the book neared completion, Ed Cohen added his fine editorial skill and Leon Unruh copy-edited the manuscript with care.

It is no exaggeration to say that this book could not have been written without the extraordinary editorial skills and perceptive reading of Kathlyn Conway. She read draft after draft and forced us to sharpen our argument. We are extremely grateful for the enormous amount of time, effort, and love that she put into this book.

Finally, we want to thank our families: Andrea, Billy, Toby, Elena, Steve, Isa, Anton, and Mason and Kathy, Zach, and Molly. You are great joys to us!

INTRODUCTION
Industry's Child

In the depths of the Depression, with millions of workers unemployed, Annie Lou Emmers, a mother of eleven children, wrote to President Franklin Delano Roosevelt because of his "interest and sympathy for cripples." Mrs. Emmers's husband, Frank, was an employee of a pesticide subsidiary of the DuPont Company in Gary, Indiana, and had been lead poisoned on the job and laid off by the company. While Mrs. Emmers accepted this terrible fate for her husband, she could not abide the fact that one of her children, Mary Jane, had been born with extensive physical disabilities and severe mental retardation. Mrs. Emmers suspected that her husband had inadvertently brought the lead into their house on his clothing and that the child's development had been affected in utero. Her little girl, now three years old, was unable to raise her head, feed herself, or speak.

Mrs. Emmers called her daughter "industry's child" and was willing to take her before the public if it would help shock industry and the government into taking action to prevent lead poisoning. Was there anything the government could do to help her support her family or to get the industry to clean up its plant, she asked. "I've heard of similar babies—in the pottery works at Crooksville, Ohio—in the lead mines' 'smelters,' of Colorado and Wyoming—in the large fruit orchards where arsenate of lead is used in powerful spraying machines, and among garage workers, handling tetraethyl, and I recently heard of another one in the chemical industry. How many more are there unheard of? How many babies are crippled each year—by lead?"[1]

Frustrated New Deal administrators told Mrs. Emmers there was absolutely nothing the federal, state, or local government could do except write on her behalf to a local voluntary agency to ask them to help her. Charity, not the regulatory power of the state, was all they could offer.

Since Mrs. Emmers's appeal to President Roosevelt, the arena in which questions regarding industrial pollution and responsibility are considered has broadened. No longer is lead poisoning the problem of one family with no recourse but to write a letter to the president and no outcome but a polite reply saying nothing could be done. Today lead poisoning is the subject of intense concern in state legislatures considering regulation, in a variety of lawsuits brought by individual plaintiffs, in municipalities concerned with recovering costs for housing rehabilitation, in Medicaid reimbursement for damaged children, and in special educational costs for lead-poisoned children. Other substances like tobacco, asbestos, silica, and gasoline additives are also the subject of legislative and legal battles. In many instances those with grievances are getting much more of a response than Mrs. Emmers did—in the form of ordinances, lead poisoning prevention programs, educational programs, and successful lawsuits sometimes resulting in restitution to the tune of millions of dollars from industry.

The question so humbly expressed by Mrs. Emmers—Was there anything government could do to help her support her family or to get the industry to clean up?—has been magnified a hundredfold, with consumer groups, political activists, law firms, and even governments addressing these issues. As was evidenced in the November 1999 protests against the World Trade Organization in Seattle, the demonstrations in Geneva at the G-8 summit in July 2001, and the protests at the New York World Economic Forum in February 2002, the campaign to protect consumers and ordinary citizens is waged not by individuals but by a coalition of groups—unions, environmental activists, and consumer organizations—that had previously worked separately and sometimes at cross-purposes. This campaign is no longer even focused on a particular industry but on international economic and social policy.

Such protests raise important and difficult questions. How can the physical environment be protected from the actions of huge multinational corporations whose activities have, until recently, gone virtually unchallenged and unregulated? How can people separated by language, politics, nationality, and culture come together to challenge corporations whose power transcends national boundaries? How can the poor and disenfranchised have their voices heard when they express outrage at the unequal share of the burden of industrial pollution their countries and communities have had to bear?

Although these large questions of corporate responsibility sound rather new, in fact they are the result of a century-long conflict over the costs of industrial progress and the responsibilities of industry to the general population. How much should government regulate private companies to ensure that they act responsibly and in accord with the broader public interest? How can government and industry create incentives for responsible corporate behavior? Industry has long responded to calls for corporate responsibility by arguing that voluntary compliance was sufficient to ensure that it acted responsibly. But there have always been those inside and outside of government who believed that voluntary compliance on the part of industry is not sufficient to safeguard the public's health for the reason that industry's financial interests often prevent it from doing what would be socially responsible.

As early as 1905, federal action was taken to protect the consumer and the environment from the irresponsible actions of industry. That year Theodore Roosevelt and other conservationists established the principle of federal protection of national forests. In 1906 Congress passed the Pure Food and Drug Act that extended its authority to inspect and test for adulterated consumer products. In 1970 the federal government established the Environmental Protection Agency and the Occupational Safety and Health Administration to protect the environment and the workforce. Unfortunately, these measures have not always been adequate. At times, the federal government, under pressure from industry lobbyists and legal challenges, has exercised its regulatory powers selectively or without sufficient resolve.

It is a tenet of democracy that citizens should have full access to information so they can make informed decisions about policies that affect their lives. In the case of industrial toxins, such information has been regularly denied to workers and the general public. As a result, factory workers have been assailed by noxious fumes and dangerous chemicals even while beseeching industry for information and protection. Over time these toxins have been vented into the air, spilled into waterways, and dumped onto the land, both legally and illegally, making industrial pollution an issue of widespread public concern. But the general public, like workers before them, has not been given sufficient information to understand the danger that exists all around them. It has taken catastrophes like Love Canal in Niagara Falls, New York, Times Beach, Missouri, and Bhopal, India, to bring home to people the danger industry poses to their lives and the environment and the public's need to have free access to information about toxic substances in the environment. Despite all this, industry has continued to hide and obfuscate information it had about the toxic characteristics of some of its products and, in the wake of the attack on the World Trade Center, the Bush administration has further undermined the Freedom of

Information Act. As a result, people have been denied information about the toxins they have been ingesting and inhaling every day.

Nonetheless, a great deal has happened outside of industry (often in spite of industry manipulation) to educate the public about the dangers of pollution and to begin to confront industry's negligence. In 1962 Rachel Carson published *Silent Spring,* which publicized the harm pesticides caused the environment. Ralph Nader began his crusade as a consumer advocate by exposing the willingness of General Motors to sacrifice human beings for profit, as exemplified in its promotion of the dangerously designed Corvair. Paul Brodeur and Barry Castleman dramatized the duplicity of the asbestos industry's willingness to expose workers and entire communities to asbestos, despite the known risk of cancer and lung diseases. By the 1970s questions were raised about the safety of a host of products: DES growth hormone, red dye No. 2, phosphates, Firestone radial tires, the Ford Pinto, tampons, Dalkon Shields, cyclamates, and saccharine. The Three Mile Island disaster led to widespread skepticism about the safety of the nuclear power industry.

By the 1980s, civil rights groups developed the concept of "environmental racism" to describe the tendency of industry to situate polluting plants and toxic waste dumps primarily in poor and minority communities. Environmental activists made "environmental justice" a rallying cry when demanding that industry redress the race and class bias in many industry decisions. In the 1990s citizens became aware of perhaps the most serious breach of the social contract with corporations: major players in the tobacco industry, after decades of denying that cigarettes were addictive and carcinogenic, were finally forced to admit that they had manipulated the nicotine content of their products for the specific purpose of keeping smokers addicted and that they had falsified scientific research, thereby lying to the public about the deadly effects of smoking tobacco. Companies like Johns Manville, which mined and processed asbestos, and Philip Morris, which grew and marketed tobacco products, were notorious for their willingness to hide information about the dangers of their products. Although it might be maintained that these were rogue corporations acting outside the norms of industrial practice, the history of industry points to a different conclusion. In the case of lead and vinyl, entire industries have banded together to deny and suppress information about the toxic nature of their products and to call into question results by outside researchers that indicated their products pose a danger to the health of individuals.

In addition to withholding information, some industries, including lead and vinyl, have reassured the public that their products are benign by controlling research and manipulating science. Throughout much of the twentieth century, most scientific studies of the health effects of toxic substances have been done by researchers in the employ of industry or in universities with financial ties to members of that industry. At times their results were subject to review by industry; if the results indicated a problem, the information was suppressed. At times the independence of the academy has been undermined by industry's influence through grants and other support for research. As Marcia Angell, editor of the *New England Journal of Medicine,* has argued, "When the boundaries between industry and academic medicine become as blurred as they now are, the business goals of industry influence the mission of the medical schools in multiple ways."[2] Dr. Linda Rosenstock, head of the National Institute for Occupational Safety and Health (NIOSH) in the Clinton administration, observed that "efforts of powerful constituencies to manipulate researchers and scientific organizations may constrain vital research on health risks."[3] A recent study of corporate funding of academic research revealed that "more than half of the university scientists who received gifts from drug or biotechnology companies admitted that the donor expected to exert influence over their work."[4] The concern about corporate corruption of science is so widespread that many scientific journals, including the prestigious *New England Journal of Medicine,* now require that the source of support for the investigator's research be clearly identified. Even NIOSH's own "scientific work continues to be attacked by special interests on an issue by issue basis," Rosenstock asserted, such that "in many cases of public health science, politics is winning out over research because of the carefully executed tactics of special interest groups."[5]

Since the establishment of the Occupational Safety and Health Administration (OSHA), NIOSH, and the Environmental Protection Agency (EPA) in 1970 and of independent foundations working with university researchers and public interest groups, a new generation of scientists not employed by industry is highlighting the risks and discounting industry's assurances about their products and production processes. They are providing research for the public and the public health community to consider. Newspaper articles, television specials, and presentations in other media bring home the personal toll that industry practices take on people's lives. Increased knowledge has become a powerful weapon in the battle to hold corporations accountable for their impact on public health.

At the heart of the current struggle is the very difficult question of how industry or the government decides what is safe. Industry has always taken the position that there is no reason to hold up production of useful products if no danger has been proven. But the history of the twentieth century is riddled with disasters resulting from industry's moving forward with products whose danger only became apparent over time. Lead, asbestos, tobacco, and radioactive materials became widely used because scientific studies could not *prove* with certainty that these substances caused harm. In the realm of environmental health, it is extremely difficult to say that a particular substance causes a particular health problem; usually only after decades of observation can a statistically significant correlation be made between exposure to a chemical and increased death and disease in a large population. Even then it may not be possible to establish a connection conclusively and to the satisfaction of the entire scientific community.

As a result, the battle being waged today by public health advocates is to establish a different method for deciding how and when industry should proceed with the introduction of new substances or products. Many argue for the *precautionary principle,* according to which suspect substances must be held off the market until their potential dangers are more clearly understood and their safety is better established. Public health officials and some politicians are increasingly aware that the threats from dioxins, chlorinated hydrocarbons, and greenhouse gases in the environment are so high that social policy demands regulatory action—even before the existing data absolutely prove danger. Many argue that we should protect our citizens and not wait for "objective studies" to prove further danger.

The lead and plastics industries have been central to the expansion of the American economy throughout the twentieth century. For the first half of the century, lead was critical to every industry involved in the building of the urban infrastructure, the modern suburb, and the expanded agricultural system. After World War II the plastics industry came to dominate American consumer society; plastics were used in vinyl siding, linoleum, tabletops, rugs, clothing, phonograph records, computers, and thousands of other products. Because evidence about danger from these products or the chemicals that went into them began appearing, a struggle developed over the fate of these two substances. In many ways, these struggles are paradigmatic of a broader struggle that continues to this day over the responsibilities of industry and government to protect public health.

Industry was well aware of the dangers of lead throughout the nineteenth century. In the early twentieth century reformers such as Dr. Alice Hamilton, often considered the founder of industrial hygiene in America, documented the extent of lead poisoning among the workforce and sought to clean up paint factories, battery manufacturing plants, potteries, and other industries where workers were being poisoned by lead. Despite this understanding of the toxic nature of lead, the automobile and gasoline industries decided in the 1920s to proceed with the introduction of tetraethyl lead into gasoline. Alarmed public health officials warned about the possible long-range effects of putting so much lead into the streets of cities all over the country, but industry successfully argued that in the absence of absolute proof of tetraethyl lead's dangers to consumers, such a tremendously useful product must not be banned or restricted. Industry learned valuable lessons from the tetraethyl lead crisis in the early 1920s, when workers died in factories producing this gasoline additive and municipalities, fearing widespread contamination of urban streets, banned its sale. Industry's successful effort to end the ban of its product taught it about the need to keep knowledge about harm out of the public eye or to find ways to argue that while these constituent materials might be toxic, the products produced from them were not.

The story of lead paint illustrates industry's efforts to keep information about dangers hidden. As children were identified as suffering from lead poisoning, industry sought to forestall a threat to its product's popularity. In many ways the story of lead in paint is that of a guerrilla war fought by small groups of individuals—mostly doctors and a few public health officials—against the giant lead corporations. As evidence of lead's dangers emerged, first in the factory, then among children, then in the environment, the industry attempted to frustrate the efforts of any people or organizations who warned of the dangers of lead or called for lead regulation in consumer products. Industry also controlled the damage to its image by funding the research conducted about the toxic effects of lead.

The most cynical response of the lead industry to reports of danger was a fifty-year advertising campaign to convince people that lead was safe, and most insidiously, to target its marketing campaign specifically to children. Not until the 1950s was there a significant challenge to the lead industry's dominance over lead research and the definition of lead poisoning. As a result of public health activities, municipalities restricted the use of lead as a pigment in paint and in the 1960s new attention was directed to the potential long-term damage caused by this mineral. Finally, in the

1970s and 1980s, the federal government banned lead in paint and in gasoline, signaling a major victory for public health.

The establishment of OSHA and other government regulatory agencies, combined with a growing movement among environmental activists and labor unionists, signaled a serious challenge to business. After World War II the production of new petrochemical synthetic materials gave rise to a new set of concerns. Unlike lead, many of these chemicals and products were of unknown toxicity. Because they were so new, there was little history by which to judge the potential problems they posed for the broad community. When the chemical industry's own research indicated the possible carcinogenicity of vinyl chloride, the industry embarked on a serious effort to mislead the public and avoid federal regulation. But in 1974 the deaths of four workers in one plant from an extremely rare cancer forced the chemical industry to inform state and federal officials of these deaths. In the case of lead, no federal agencies existed to oversee the regulation of environmental and work-related diseases until the 1970s. By the time the dangers of vinyl were suspected, the EPA and OSHA had been established, a much stronger environmental movement was evolving, and a portion of the labor movement was focused on occupational disease. After sustained battle over the regulation of vinyl chloride, the new federal agencies initiated strict controls over the industry. But this was a pyrrhic victory. In the years following the vinyl crisis, the business community mounted a sustained public relations and political offensive that caused OSHA to be more wary of confrontations with industry.

During the 1980s, when the Reagan administration constrained OSHA, NIOSH, and EPA, many struggles to confront environmental dangers shifted to communities. Citizens of Louisiana, driven by a growing sense of the danger posed by a chemical industry that seemed out of control, asserted their right to defend their communities and forced the chemical industry, which dominated Louisiana politics, to deal with their demands. In the 1990s in Convent, Louisiana, hundreds of people organized and used the media, the law, and especially the threat of federal intervention to prevent a multinational corporation from placing one of the world's largest polyvinyl chloride plants in their rural, poor, and overwhelmingly African American Mississippi River town. One EPA official called Convent the "poster child for environmental justice." It was a defining moment in the century-long struggle to get industry to acknowledge and respect public health. Moreover, this was the first time the federal government acknowledged the importance of environmental justice on behalf of an economically depressed African American community in opposition to industry's preferences.

In the beginning of the century, Mrs. Emmers—poor, powerless, and frightened for her family—raised her voice to inform the company where her husband worked and the president of the United States that her daughter had been poisoned by lead from the plant. She asked for help, but received none. In Convent, people like Mrs. Emmers—also poor and powerless—raised their voices against industry. Their success was the result of more than a half century of struggle in which the public became less willing to trust their well-being to industry and decided instead to take control of their fate. Of course, the victory in Convent was small: the company had the resources to build elsewhere and pollute another community. It is for this reason that the movement to control industry is moving to a larger arena.

The struggle over environmental exposures continues with uneven results. Certainly there have been successes. Lead, identified as a major danger to children in the 1920s, was largely controlled as an environmental threat in the 1980s and 1990s. Standards regulating exposure of workers and community residents to vinyl are considered models of effective government regulation. Chief executive officers (CEOs) of major corporations must reconcile their fiduciary responsibilities to their stockholders with their environmental responsibilities to the public. They must, for example, reduce toxic air and water emissions from their plants in order to satisfy government regulations. In order to protect its interests, industry has escalated its efforts to oppose the work of environmental groups. Organizations such as the Business Roundtable, made up of the CEOs of two hundred of the largest corporations in the country, have intensified their lobbying efforts among government officials and established well-funded and large offices in Washington. Through political contributions, "message ads," support for pro-industry legislators, and direct contact with members of the executive branch—at the very highest levels—industry attempts to protect its interests.

The effect of environmental toxins does not end simply because regulators have done their job. The effects of lead and vinyl will be felt for generations. Recent studies show that all Americans carry in their bodies materials not normally found in human tissue and whose health effects may not be understood for many years. Because of their developing physiology, children especially are at risk. The walls of millions of homes are still coated with lead paint, which poses a serious threat to children. The landfills of our country are absorbing millions upon millions of pounds of polyvinyl chloride that will deteriorate, releasing vinyl chloride monomer, a known carcinogen, into the air and groundwater. The casings and components of computers, a commonplace of contemporary American life, are among these causes of pollution. Computer monitors, on average, contain four pounds of lead, and millions of them are crowding landfills and leaching into drinking water. Even new methods of waste disposal pose new problems—for example, the burning of plastics, particularly vinyl, produces dioxins in all but the most efficient incinerators.

Policy makers are faced with what to do about suspected toxins when there is uncertainty or ambiguity in the science used to judge risk. Industry members continue to argue that it is irresponsible to sacrifice new products and undermine fiscal prosperity by halting product development before the data conclusively indicate danger. But many public health advocates argue that the precautionary principle should prevail: when society is faced with devastating health problems as a result of using potentially toxic chemicals, those chemicals should be held in abeyance until they are proven safe.

In the 2000 presidential election debates between Al Gore and George W. Bush, the political value of scientific ambiguity was apparent in discussions about global warming. When Gore asserted the seemingly self-evident fact that American society had an obligation to reduce emissions that were harming the environment, Bush countered that all the facts were not in and that more research was needed before policy makers should act. The call for more scientific evidence is often a stalling tactic. The inability of science in the 1920s to prove that lead in gasoline, for example, was dangerous resulted in severe damage to children a half century later. The inability of scientists to agree about whether or not there is a problem with the use and disposal of plastics and the willingness of industries to use new chemicals before they are proved safe may also have terrible consequences for society. The possibility of hormone disruptions and mutagenic (causing genetic change) and teratogenic (causing abnormal embryonic development) effects from exposure to chlorinated hydrocarbons require new paradigms of science. Public health professionals argue that placing untested, potentially harmful chemicals on the market is not worth the risk. In December 2000, delegates from 122 nations (including the United States) agreed to ban dioxin and eleven other highly toxic chemicals that are "persistent organic pollutants that dissolve slowly, travel easily and are absorbed by living organisms, including humans."[6]

The activities of the lead and vinyl industries with regard to the known dangers of their products are not exceptional. Lying and obfuscation were rampant in the tobacco, automobile, asbestos, and nuclear power industries as well. In this era of privatization, deregulation, and globalization, the threat from unregulated industry is even greater. In fact, a deeper schism than ever separates the broader population's concerns about industrial pollution and the current political establishment's infatuation with market mechanisms and voluntary compliance. For this reason it is imperative for future policy decisions that all citizens and those with responsibility for the public's health be aware of industry's response to environmental danger.

THE HOUSE OF
THE BUTTERFLIES

Lead Poisoning among Workers
and Consumers

Throughout world history, industry managers and laborers alike understood that work was dangerous. But it was not until the beginning of the twentieth century that reformers began a concerted effort to ameliorate the worst aspects of industrial civilization. The growing concern over safety and health issues for American workers developed during the first decade of the twentieth century in the wake of revolutionary social and economic changes.[1] In little more than three decades Americans had witnessed an unprecedented population explosion in its cities and manufacturing centers. Work for most laborers had become so dangerous that some newspapers and magazines published exposés of "the Death Roll of Industry," which sent "to the hospital or the graveyard one worker every minute of the year."[2]

Accidents took the lives of thousands of workers who built the skyscrapers and railroads, who worked in mines and tunneled through the rock underneath and around America's cities to build subways and water tunnels. Indeed, in the late nineteenth and early twentieth centuries, America's industrial accident rates were among the worst in the world. Less apparent were the diseases that afflicted those working with new toxins. In the early twentieth century, practices within the steel, rubber, textile, and chemical industries ultimately forced Americans to confront the huge costs in health that we traded for industrial dominance.

While much attention was paid to industrial accidents that took an immediate toll, a few industrial toxins like lead, mercury, and phosphorus, which caused acute symptoms as well as chronic disability, also became the focus of intense reform efforts. In 1908, the occupational physician Alice Hamilton noted that lead had endangered workers as far back as "the first half century after Christ." She pointed out that "lead is a most potent producer of abortion, and it is very rare that a woman lead worker bears a healthy child at term."[3] Throughout her distinguished career, Hamilton was deeply involved in uncovering the relationship between lead and disease in the American workforce. She first worked among poor families as a member of the famous Hull House Settlement in Chicago and did most of her pioneering work on lead poisoning while living there. By investigating systematically, she and others found that workers in the battery, painting, plumbing, ceramics, pottery, and other industries were at high risk for death and disease. Because of her continuing involvement in protecting the dispossessed—the poor, the immigrants, the factory workers—she was able to observe the special dangers lead posed to the unborn. For many decades she advocated protectionist regulations for women at work, particularly in lead-using industries.[4]

Such efforts in the United States to protect workers were part of a broader effort to "preserve the race" in the face of the massive dislocations of urbanization and mass production. In England in 1911, Thomas Oliver wrote an article titled "Lead Poisoning and the Race" in which he focused on the corrupting effect of lead: "Lead poisoning develops insidiously; the metal acts upon the cells of particular organs of the body, deranging their function and structure, so that life is gradually brought to a close by the intervention of disease of organs, such as the kidney or nervous system, years after it may be the person has been near lead."[5] Not only were women and men workers at risk, but also children were seen as especially susceptible to lead's deleterious effects. In a 1912 monograph, Thomas Legge, another English authority on occupational hazards, observed that "young persons are regarded as more liable to lead poisoning than adults."[6] At the First National Conference on Industrial Diseases, held in Chicago in 1910, Alice Hamilton presented results from her landmark studies of lead poisoning in Illinois industries. She noted that lead was a hazard in lead smelting and the making of white lead and that the "painting trades yield the largest number of victims, especially if we add to ordinary painters the so called mechanical artists who use white lead for retouching advertisements." She noted that painters "have not so far been helped by improvements in their trade."[7] Her studies appeared in popular as well as medical journals such as the *Journal of the American Medical Association*.[8] Also in 1910 she went directly to the largest lead company in the country, National Lead, and delivered a speech on the need for protection against lead poisoning in Europe and America. She made the important point that "the study of the past thirty years has shown that lead enters the body through inhalation and swallowing, not through the skin."[9] In a summary

belief that for interior painting which is not exposed to the weather, zinc paints are as good, if not better, than white lead paints, not only from the hygienic point of view, which was known, but from the commercial."[25] The vitality of the European labor movements, not to mention their greater willingness to become involved in political struggles (by contrast with the American Federation of Labor), helped push the issue of interior paints onto the public-policy agenda outside the United States.

A number of countries banned or restricted the use of white lead for interior painting. These included France,[26] Belgium, and Austria in 1909; Tunisia and Greece in 1922; Czechoslovakia in 1924; Great Britain, Sweden, and Belgium in 1926; Poland in 1927; Spain and Yugoslavia in 1931; and Cuba in 1934.[27] In 1922 the Third International Labor Conference of the League of Nations recommended the banning of white lead for interior use,[28] ultimately deciding "that white lead be prohibited entirely for paints for interiors; that women and children under 16 years of age be not employed where white lead was used in the manufacture of paint, and that countries now using white lead have six years . . . to comply with these regulations." The conference also decided that in outdoor paint, "white lead be limited to 2%."[29]

Even in the United States, which refused to sign the International Labour Office (ILO) ban, growing awareness about the lead threat to painters was prompting calls to limit its use in indoor painting. Much as in 2001, when those outside the government demanded attention to global warming despite the refusal of the Bush administration to sign the Kyoto Protocol, those outside the administration of Warren G. Harding pushed for controls over painters' exposure to lead. The Painters District Council in Chicago suggested that among the measures useful in preventing lead poisoning would be the "prohibition of white lead in interior painting."[30] The Brotherhood of Painters, Decorators, and Paperhangers of America, an organization representing 125,000 members, predominantly house painters, stated that "the use of white lead is a grave menace to the health and lives of painters and should be forbidden."[31] The Workers Health Bureau, a labor advocacy group, proposed a labeling law in New York state for poisonous paint materials.[32] One such bill was introduced in February 1924.[33] In Massachusetts, the Legislature considered and ultimately rejected a code that would have limited the exposure of painters to "dangerous poisons such as lead" and would have prohibited the use of lead "in all interior painting of public buildings."[34]

By 1929, the Committee on Lead Poisoning of the Industrial Hygiene Section of the American Public Health Association remarked on "the improvement in substitute paint bases, such as lithopone," noting that they were now "essentially as acceptable as white lead or other lead compounds" with the added benefit of potentially lowering the incidence "of severe or fatal lead poisoning."[35] By the early thirties, lithopone, titanium and zinc oxides were capturing an increasing percentage of the market and were being marketed as "nonpoisonous," in contrast to "poisonous" lead pigments.[36]

But just as industrial hygienists, managers, and physicians were beginning to take meaningful steps to protect the workforce from lead in the paint industry in the 1920s, a more devastating threat was arising: tetraethyl lead was being added to gasoline to increase engine power in automobiles.

In the early 1920s General Motors found itself on the verge of bankruptcy. Ford's Models A and T had simply proven so durable—nearly indestructible—that people were not buying cars from GM. The company decided to try to save itself with a new marketing strategy. To compete with the unchanging Tin Lizzie, GM offered increasingly powerful cars whose styling and features were changed yearly in the hope that consumers would be seduced by a desire for newer cars. Owners of a four-year-old car would be faced with a spiffier and more powerful automobile. By building obsolescence into the vehicles, GM guaranteed itself a steady market. GM's fortunes turned around, and by 1927 Ford abandoned the Model T and joined in the automotive "arms race" of ever-changing exteriors and ever-increasing power.

Historian William Kovarik points out that in the early twentieth century a number of automobile fuels—gasoline, ethanol, alcohol, and various blends of these and other fuels—were competing in a wide-open market. Most early automobiles, like Ford's Model T, had low compression engines, and central to the creation of powerful, large automobiles was the development of a more efficient fuel that could drive cars at greater speed. Kovarik argues that alcohol and ethanol blends were the first fuels capable of providing power to the new engines, which demanded high octane, a measure of gasoline's power. The advantage of these fuels was that they were renewable and nonpolluting.[37]

But these very advantages worked against their adaptation as a motor fuel, since General Motors, with its interlocking directorate relationship with the DuPont Company and the petrochemical industry, sought to develop a fuel it could patent and profit from.[38] Tetraethyl lead, developed in 1922 by Thomas Midgley Jr. ("the Father of Ethyl Gas") at the General

Motors Research Laboratory in Dayton, Ohio, promised to raise the compression at which gasoline burned, thus eliminating the "engine knock" that decreased power. General Motors quickly contracted with DuPont and Standard Oil of New Jersey to produce tetraethyl lead. Ethyl, the brand name for "leaded gas" (that is, gasoline containing the additive tetraethyl lead), was placed on sale in test markets on February 1, 1923. In 1924, DuPont and GM created the Ethyl Gasoline Corporation to produce and market it.[39]

In the very year that Midgley and his co-workers at General Motors Research Corporation heralded the discovery of this anti-knock compound, scientists in and outside of government warned that tetraethyl lead might be a potent threat to public health. William Mansfield Clark, a professor of chemistry, wrote to A. M. Stimson, assistant surgeon general at the Public Health Service, in October 1922 warning of "a serious menace to the public health." He noted that in the early production of tetraethyl lead "several very serious cases of lead poisoning have resulted." He worried that its use in gasoline would result in atmospheric pollution, for "on busy thoroughfares it is highly probable that the lead oxide dust will remain in the lower stratum."[40]

Stimson advised that the Service "be provided with some experimental evidence tending to support this opinion" and suggested that it was in the province of the Division of Chemistry and Pharmacology to investigate the dangers.[41] The director of that division felt that such an investigation would take "a considerable period of time, perhaps a year," and that the results would be of little "practical use since the trial of the material under ordinary conditions [of use] should show whether there is a risk to man." He recommended instead that the Public Health Service depend upon industry itself to provide relevant data.[42]

A month later, H. S. Cumming, the surgeon general, respectfully asked Pierre S. DuPont, chairman of the board of General Motors, whether the public health effects of tetraethyl lead manufacturing and use had been taken into account. Thomas Midgley himself responded that the question "has been given very serious consideration . . . although no actual experimental data has been taken." Even without experimental data, GM and DuPont were confident that "the average street will probably be so free from lead that it will be impossible to detect it or its absorption."[43]

DuPont and GM recognized that, given the general apprehension about the potential hazards of tetraethyl lead, a private, in-house study of its safety would be met with skepticism. Rather than conduct their own investigations, therefore, they arranged for the General Motors Research

Corporation to pay for an investigation by the U.S. Bureau of Mines at government facilities. The bureau was trusted by industry and often performed testing as a service to the mining and metal industries. GM, through prime negotiator Charles Kettering, requested one other proviso: that "the Bureau refrain from giving out the usual press and progress reports during the course of the work, as [Kettering] feels that the newspapers are apt to give scare headlines and false impressions before we definitely know what the influence of the material will be."[44] The concern about adverse publicity and leaks to newspapers was so great that the bureau insisted on using "Ethyl" instead of "lead," even in internal correspondence. Since the bureau had agreed to a blackout of information, one official asserted, "if it should happen to get some publicity accidentally, it would not be so bad if the word 'lead' were omitted as this term is apt to prejudice somewhat against its use."[45]

The willingness of the Bureau of Mines to impose a gag on its own scientists and even to avoid accurate scientific terminology in favor of a trade name reflected the tentativeness with which the bureau (and the administration of President Calvin Coolidge) approached the giant corporations. This can be seen clearly in the subsequent agreements between this government agency and GM, DuPont, and the newly created Ethyl Gasoline Corporation while the critical research into the health effects of tetraethyl lead progressed. The first agreement, in September 1923 between the General Motors Research Corporation and the Bureau of Mines, allowed relative freedom for the bureau to report its final conclusions.[46] By June 1924, General Motors sought much greater control over the final product, demanding, in addition to the ban on all publicity in the popular press, that "all manuscripts, before publication, will be submitted to the Company for comment and criticism."[47] The bureau acquiesced, but in two months the Ethyl Corporation asked for still more modifications: that there be a dollar limit on the maximum expenses the company would incur and "that before publication of any papers or articles by your Bureau, they should be submitted to them [Ethyl] for comment, criticism, and *approval*" (emphasis added). These changes were incorporated into the new contract, which gave the Ethyl Gasoline Corporation, in effect, veto power over the research of the United States government.[48]

Ironically, when it appeared that the preliminary research results pointed toward the safety of tetraethyl lead, GM, DuPont, and the government violated their own agreement to release no information until the study was complete. In July 1924, five months before the preliminary report was released, GM's director of research, Graham Edgar, wrote to

Dr. Paul Leech of the American Medical Association that the results of the Bureau of Mines' research would show "that there is no danger of acquiring lead poisoning through even prolonged exposure to exhaust gases of cars using Ethyl Gas." He further erroneously assured the AMA that "poisoning from carbon monoxide would arise long before the concentration of lead would reach a point where even cumulative [lead] poisoning is to be feared."[49]

Many public health leaders and scientists saw the federal government as colluding with GM, DuPont, Standard Oil, and Ethyl to certify the safety of tetraethyl lead. Yandell Henderson of Yale University, a leading public health physiologist, wrote an angry letter to Royd R. Sayers, the coordinator of the government's activities as the bureau's chief surgeon and also as a surgeon in the U.S. Public Health Service, pointedly rejecting an offer to take part in the government's research. "As regards your suggestion that you might assign us [at Yale's Laboratory of Applied Physiology] a part in the investigation which you are carrying out for the General Motors on tetra-ethyl lead, I feel that I should want a greater degree of freedom of investigation and finding—in view of the immense public, sanitary, and industrial questions involved—than the subordinate relation which you suggest would allow. It seems to me extremely unfortunate that the experts of the United States government should be carrying out this investigation on a grant from the General Motors."[50] C. W. Deppe, the owner of a small car company, Deppe Motors, was much blunter: "May I be pardoned if I ask you frankly now, does the Bureau of Mines exist for the benefit of Ford and the G.M. Corporation and the Standard Oil Co. of New Jersey, and other oil companies parties to the distribution of the Ethyl Lead Dopes, or is the Bureau supposed to be for the public benefit and in protection of life and health?"[51]

The dangers posed by the widespread introduction of leaded gasoline were finally brought to the public's attention by newspaper reports of some odd goings-on at Standard Oil's Bayway labs in Elizabeth, New Jersey. Over the course of five days, five workers died and thirty-five others showed severe neurological symptoms of organic lead poisoning. In total, forty of forty-nine workers in the tetraethyl lead processing plant were severely poisoned.

Ernest Oelgert of Elizabeth, a laboratory worker, died strangely on Sunday, October 26, 1924. Witnesses declared that he had been hallucinating on Thursday, had become severely paranoid, and on Friday was running around the plant "in terror, shouting that there were 'three coming at me at once.'" By Saturday, he had been forcibly restrained and taken to Reconstruction Hospital in New York City, where he died the next day. Although the company officials denied any responsibility, none of the other workers were surprised. They all knew that Oelgert worked in what they all called "the looney gas building," an experimental station secretly established the previous year. Only forty-five workers were employed in the laboratory, and their fellow laborers had already made them the object of "undertaker jokes and farewell greetings." Standard Oil officials suggested that "nothing ought to be said about this matter in the public interest."

The headlines of a front-page story in the *New York Times* the next day reported "Odd Gas Kills One, Makes Four Insane." The *Times* quoted one of the supervisors at the Bayway facility who said "these men probably went insane because they worked too hard." The father of the dead man, Ernest Oelgert, however, "was bitter in denunciation of conditions at this plant" and told reporters that "Ernest was told by the doctors at the plant that working in the laboratory wouldn't hurt him. Otherwise he would have quit. They said he'd have to get used to it."[52]

By Monday, another worker had died and twelve others were hospitalized from what everyone at the plant called "insanity gas." Terror-stricken workers were being carted away to New York City in straitjackets, hallucinating, convulsing, and screaming about the visions appearing before their eyes. It soon became clear that the victims had been poisoned by a gasoline additive called tetraethyl lead. As the workers continued to be hospitalized and as the New York newspapers began to pick up the story, it became more and more difficult to deny its significance. By Friday, as the fifth victim of "looney gas" died—and as three quarters of the laboratory's workers lay in hospitals—the New York City Department of Health, the city of Philadelphia, and various municipalities in New Jersey had banned the sale of leaded gasoline. The *New York Times,* the *New York World,* and all the regional newspapers were blaring out front-page headlines such as "'Mad Gas' Claims Third Victim," "Bar Ethyl Gasoline as Fifth Victim Dies," and "Gas Madness Stalks Plant." These deaths stimulated renewed concern about the potential public health dangers from the exhaust produced by leaded gasoline, despite Standard Oil's assurance that no "perils existed in the use of this gas in automobiles."[53]

In some ways this was an extreme example of a typical scenario overtaking workers all across America. In industry after industry—rubber, steel, petrochemical, and automobile—workers were coming in contact with new chemicals that were making them sick and even killing them. In the first two decades of the century, muckraking magazines had produced dramatic headlines about phossy jaw among match makers, many of whom were children working with phosphorous, radium poisonings among the young women who painted watch dials in New Jersey, silicosis among granite cutters in Vermont, and lead poisoning among painters. *Everybody's, Charities and the Commons, World's Work*, and *The Outlook*, all widely circulated magazines, had exposés of "the work that kills" and "the lead menace."

But the crisis at Standard Oil's plant in Bayway, New Jersey, was different. Very quickly it became clear that more was at stake than the lives of a few workers. Public health officials and the public who read the daily accounts of dying workers understood that the gas that was killing the workers also could kill or harm ordinary citizens breathing air polluted by automobiles or who were pumping gas at the rapidly growing network of filling stations across the country. The horrendous experiences with poison gas in World War I less than a decade earlier had heightened public concern over the new substance, also called a "gas," that was making headlines in many major cities. With little distinction between the organic lead that was poisoning workers in the Standard Oil plant and the inorganic lead that would be spewing from the exhaust pipes of cars, newspapers fanned the fears that a toxic gas would soon be inhaled by millions of Americans. Industry leaders understood that if they could not contain the developing crisis, millions upon millions of dollars would be at risk. The questions: how to contain it, and what would containment mean?

On the one hand, the gasoline and lead industry had to develop a program to prevent dramatic outbreaks of "loony gas poisoning" within the plant if it were to quell public outrage generated by lurid headlines above photographs of sickened workers being taken to hospitals in straitjackets. On the other hand, industry had to convince the public that, far from being a generalized threat to their health, poisonings by industrial products could be solved, or at least confined behind the walls of a factory. Occupational health issues were exactly that: problems borne by the workforce but no threat to the public at large. This was part of a broader effort on the part of major corporations to improve their public image and undercut the popular suspicion that they were "soulless" entities that were "greedy and ruthless in their pursuit of profits."[54]

Amid daily newspaper reports on health conditions at the plant,[55] the company continually denied management's responsibility for the tragedy. Thomas Midgley, Ethyl's second vice president and general manager, appeared at a press conference and said that true responsibility for the crisis rested with the workers, who, "regardless of warnings and provision for their protection, had failed to appreciate the dangers of constant absorption of the fluid by their hands and arms." Midgley and other company representatives argued that the workers should have known from the precautions taken by the company that lead could be dangerous: "The rejection of many men as physically unfit to engage in the work at the Bayway plant, daily physical examinations, constant admonitions as to wearing rubber gloves and using gas masks and not wearing away from the plant clothing worn during work hours should have been sufficient indication to every man in the plant that he was engaged 'in a man's undertaking.'"[56]

Many people outside the industry reached different conclusions. The prosecutor in Union County, New Jersey, asserted that he was "satisfied many of the workers did not know the danger they were running. I also believe some of the workers were not masked nor told to wear rubber gloves and rubber boots."[57] The New Jersey commissioner of labor said he had never been informed that the workers in the Bayway plant were potentially in danger. "Secrecy surrounding the experiments was responsible for the Labor Department's lack of knowledge of them," an official said.[58] Under the relentless pressure of daily revelations and investigations, Standard Oil acknowledged, after the fifth victim died, "that it was known that this gas had collected a previous toll of death and insanity before the forty-nine employees were exposed to it at the Elizabeth plant."[59]

The day after the fifth victim died, and in the midst of growing public fear of this new chemical, the Bureau of Mines released its preliminary findings on the possible dangers of leaded gasoline to the general public. The *New York Times*'s headline summed up the report: "NO PERIL TO PUBLIC SEEN IN ETHYL GAS/BUREAU OF MINES REPORTS AFTER LONG EXPERIMENTS WITH MOTOR EXHAUSTS/MORE DEATHS UNLIKELY." They also reported "the investigation carried out indicates the danger of sufficient lead accumulation in the streets through the discharging of scale from automobile motors to be seemingly remote." The report exonerated tetraethyl lead.[60]

Yet, the circumstances of the workers' deaths put in doubt the credibility of the Bureau of Mines's findings. Scientists and labor activists found fault with the report. E. E. Free, editor of the prestigious journal *Scientific American*, was skeptical of R. R. Sayers's assurances that the Bureau of Mines could find no evidence of lead poisoning in the study animal subjects.[61] Cecil K. Drinker, editor of the *Journal of Industrial Hygiene* and professor of public health at Harvard University, and Dr. David Edsall, dean of the Harvard Medical School, were also critical. In early January 1925, Drinker wrote Sayers a pointed critique that concluded: "As an investigation of an important problem in public health ... [the report] is inadequate."[62] Occupational physician Alice Hamilton concurred with Drinker's position and noted the "desirability of having an investigation made by a public body which will be beyond suspicion."[63]

This attack by scientists, public health experts, and labor activists on the quality and integrity of the report prompted those who championed the introduction of lead into gasoline to begin a counteroffensive. Dr. Emery Hayhurst, of the Ohio Department of Health, emerged as one of the key figures in the attempt to "sell" tetraethyl lead to the American public. Hayhurst is of special interest in this period because of his established reputation as a respected and independent industrial hygienist. But what was not known about Hayhurst was that at the same time when he was advising labor organizations such as the Workers' Health Bureau on industrial hygiene matters, he was also working for the Ethyl Corporation as a consultant.[64] Correspondence between Hayhurst and the Public Health Service indicates that Hayhurst was supplying advocates of tetraethyl lead with information regarding the tactics to be used by their opponents. Indeed, even before the Bureau of Mines issued its report, Hayhurst had decided that tetraethyl lead was not an environmental toxin and advised the Bureau of Mines to include a statement that "the finished product, Ethyl Gasoline, as marketed and used both pure or diluted in gasoline retains none of the poisonous characteristics of the ingredients concerned in its manufacture and blending."[65]

Even more damning was that in another letter to R. R. Sayers of the Public Health Service, sent as the attacks on the report were mounting, Hayhurst secretly provided criticisms that the Workers' Health Bureau had developed so that the government could be prepared to reply. The Workers' Health Bureau had specifically refrained from sending these comments to the government; Hayhurst violated their trust.[66]

Hayhurst and Sayers also worked together to build public and professional support for the position of the Bureau of Mines and the Ethyl Corporation that tetraethyl lead was not a public health danger. Sayers urged that Hayhurst counter the criticisms of Drinker and Edsall with a review or editorial of his own in support of the report. Hayhurst replied that he had prepared an editorial for the *American Journal of Public Health* and that the unsigned editorial proclaimed, "Observational evidence and reports to various health officials over the country ... so far as we have been able to find out, corroborated the statement of 'complete safety' so far as the public health has been concerned."[67]

Nonetheless, this back-channel effort was incapable of quelling the doubts about the safety of leaded gasoline or the integrity of the Bureau of

Mines report. The press kept the public's attention focused on collusion of the Bureau of Mines and private industry. It was soon reported that other workers had died handling tetraethyl lead at the DuPont chemical plant at Deepwater, New Jersey, and at the General Motors Research Corporation site in Dayton, Ohio. As the Workers' Health Bureau researchers catalogued the deaths and illnesses of workers, they found that since September 1923 at least two men had died at Dayton and four others at Deepwater.[68]

The *New York Times*, in fact, published an article specifically about the difficulties that editors and reporters had in following the story; the article also noted that there was nothing in the *Record*, the local New Jersey paper, about the death of Frank W. "Happy" Durr, who had worked for DuPont for twenty-five years. Durr had literally given his life to the company. He began working at DuPont as a child of twelve and died, from exposure to tetraethyl lead, twenty-five years later. The editor of the *Record* told the *Times:* "I guess the reason we didn't print anything about Durr's death was because we couldn't get it. They [DuPont] suppress things about the lead plant at Deepwater. Whatever we print we pick up from the workers." The *Times* further described how it was almost impossible to get information from the local hospital about the source of the workers' problems, indicating the sway that DuPont held over medical staff. Nonetheless, the *Times* uncovered more than three hundred cases of lead poisoning among workers at the Deepwater plant during the previous two years. The workers knew that something was amiss there and had dubbed the plant "the House of the Butterflies" because so many of their colleagues had hallucinations of insects during their bouts of lead poisoning: "The victim pauses, perhaps while at work or in a rational conversation, gazes intently at space and snatches at something not there." The *Times* reported that "about 80% of all who worked in 'the House of the Butterflies,' or who went into it to make repairs were poisoned, some repeatedly."[69]

As a result of the continuing public disquiet over the Bureau of Mines report, scientists and public health leaders expressed their concerns to Hugh Cumming, the surgeon general of the Public Health Service, who was contemplating calling a national conference to assess the tetraethyl lead situation. Haven Emerson, the eminent public health leader and professor of public health at Columbia University, spelled out in a frank letter to Cumming the concerns of public health officers. He suggested that the report was having "a widespread, and to my mind harmful, influence on public opinion and the action of public agencies." He believed that it would be "well worthwhile to call those whom you intend to a conference promptly. ... The impression is gaining way that the interests of those who may expect profit from the public sale of tetraethyl lead compounds have been influential in postponing such a meeting."[70]

Despite some indication that R. R. Sayers opposed such a conference and may have delayed it,[71] the surgeon general announced at the end of April 1925 that he was calling together experts from business, labor, and public health to assess the tetraethyl lead situation. Cumming stated that leaded gasoline "is a public health question of extreme seriousness ... if this product is actually causing slow poisoning and serious effects of a cumulative character."[72]

On May 20, 1925, the conference convened in Washington with every major party represented. In the words of one participant, the conference gathered together in one room "two diametrically opposed conceptions. The men engaged in industry, chemists, and engineers, take it as a matter of course that a little thing like industrial poisoning should not be allowed to stand in the way of a great industrial advance. On the other hand, the sanitary experts take it as a matter of course that the first consideration is the health of the people."[73]

The conference opened with statements from General Motors, DuPont, Standard Oil, and the Ethyl Corporation outlining the history of the development of leaded gasoline and the reasons why they believed its continued production was essential. The companies made three points: that leaded gasoline was essential to the industrial progress of America; that any innovation entails certain risks; and that deaths and illnesses occurred at their plants because the men who worked with the materials were careless and failed to follow instructions.

While others stressed the importance of tetraethyl lead as a means of conserving motor fuel, Frank Howard, first vice president of Ethyl, provided the most complete rationale for the continued use of tetraethyl lead in gasoline. "You have but one problem," he remarked, attempting to characterize the position of his opponents. "Is this a public health hazard?" He countered by observing that "unfortunately, our problem is not that simple." Rather, he argued, automobiles and oil were central to the industrial progress of the nation, if not the world. "Our continued development of motor fuels is essential in our civilization," he proclaimed, and the development of tetraethyl lead, after a decade of research, was an "apparent gift of God." Howard, by casting the issue in this way, put his opponents on the defensive, making them appear to be reactionaries whose limited vision could permanently retard human progress and stunt the nation's economic growth. "What is our duty under the circumstances?" he asked. "Should we say, 'No, we will not use a material [that is] a certain means of saving petroleum? Because some animals die and some do not die in some experiments, shall we give this thing up entirely?'"[74]

Since tetraethyl lead was a key to the industrial future of the nation, the companies argued, some sacrifice would be required. Dr. H. C. Parmelee, editor of the trade journal *Chemical and Metallurgical Engineering,* stated, "The research and development that produced tetraethyl lead were conceived in a fine spirit of industrial progress looking toward the conservation of gasoline and increased efficiency of internal combustion motors." In the end, he said, "its casualties were negligible compared to human sacrifice in the development of many other industrial enterprises."[75]

The final part of the industry's position was that it was workers, and not the companies, who were at fault for the tragedies at Bayway, Deepwater, and Dayton. Acknowledging that there were "certain dangers" inherent in the production of this essential industrial product, the Standard Oil Company asserted that "every precaution was taken" by the company to protect its workers. According to Thomas Midgley Jr., "the essential thing necessary to safely handle [tetraethyl lead] was careful discipline of our men. ... [Tetraethyl lead] becomes dangerous due to carelessness of the men in handling it." In an earlier statement to the *New York World,* Midgley explained what this discipline consisted of: "The minute a man shows signs of exhilaration [a euphemism for acute lead poisoning] he is laid off. If he spills the stuff on himself he is fired. Because he doesn't want to lose his job, he doesn't spill it."

Midgley's own recklessness and inconsistency were revealed at a news conference in which he sought to downplay the toxicity of tetraethyl lead. When asked by a reporter if it was dangerous to spill the chemical on one's hands, Midgley dramatically requested that "an attendant bring in a quantity of pure tetraethyl." He "washed his hands thoroughly in the fluid and dried them on his handkerchief. 'I'm not taking any chance whatever,' he said. 'Nor would I take any chance doing that every day.'" He washed his hands with tetraethyl lead despite the fact that he had only a year before taken a prolonged vacation in Florida on account of his own symptoms of lead poisoning.[76]

Those who opposed the introduction of leaded gasoline disagreed with every fundamental position of the industry representatives. First, they believed that it was wrong to accept that progress entails inevitable risks; rather, they believed, the federal government had to assume responsibility for protecting the health of the nation. Second, opponents pointed out that what we would now call inorganic lead compounds were already known to be a slow, cumulative poison that should not be introduced into the general environment. Third, they rejected the notion that workers were responsible for their own poisoning. Fourth, and most important, because they believed that the public health should take precedence over the needs of industry, they argued that the burden of proof should be on the companies to prove tetraethyl lead was *safe* rather than on opponents to prove that tetraethyl lead was dangerous.

Dr. Yandell Henderson, a Yale physiologist, emerged as one of the strongest critics of the industry. He told the conference that lead was a public menace, as serious as the infectious diseases then affecting the nation's health. He was horrified at the thought that hundreds of thousands of pounds of lead would be deposited every year in the streets of every major city of America and that "the conditions will grow worse so gradually and the development of lead poisoning will come on so insidiously . . . that leaded gasoline will be in nearly universal use and large numbers of cars will have been sold . . . before the public and the government awaken to the situation."[77]

Unlike industry spokespeople, who defined the problem narrowly—as an occupational hazard—and maintained that individual vigilance on the part of workers could solve the problem, Henderson believed that leaded gasoline was a public and environmental health issue that required federal action. Harriet Silverman of the Workers' Health Bureau underlined the absurdity of the industry's position: "I ask you gentlemen to consider the fact that you are asked to allow a man to be subjected to contact with a poison which is considered hazardous by the leading scientists of the country. And when you expose them to that poison out of which the manufacturers are making profits, the manufacturers penalize those men by making them forfeit a day's wage."[78]

Opponents were extremely concerned that the industry equated the use of lead with industrial progress. Reacting to the Ethyl Gasoline Corporation representative's statement that tetraethyl lead was a "gift of God," Grace Burnham of the Workers' Health Bureau said it "was not a gift of God when those 11 men were killed or those 149 were poisoned." She angrily questioned the priorities of "this age of speed and rush and efficiency and mechanics" and said that "the thing we are interested in in the long run is not mechanics or machinery, but men." A. L. Berres, secretary of the Metal Trades Department of the American Federation of Labor (AFL), also rejected the prevalent notion that "the business of America was business." He told the conference that the AFL opposed the use of tetraethyl lead. "We feel that where the health and general welfare of humanity is concerned, we ought to step slowly."[79]

The country's foremost authority on lead, Dr. Alice Hamilton, agreed with those who believed there was no way to know how to regulate leaded gasoline so that it would be safe. Only a ban would suffice. "You may control conditions within a factory," she said, "but how are you going to control the whole country?"[80] In a more extended commentary on the conference and the issues that it raised, Hamilton stated, "I am not one of those who believe that the use of this leaded gasoline can ever be made safe. No lead industry has ever, even under the strictest control, lost all its dangers. Where there is lead some case of lead poisoning sooner or later develops, even under the strictest supervision."[81]

Most public health professionals did not agree with Henderson and Hamilton. For the vast majority of public health experts at the conference, the problem was how to reconcile the opposed views of advocates of industrial progress and those frightened by the potential for disaster. Although everyone hoped that science itself would provide an answer to this imponderable dilemma, the reality was that all evidence to this point was ambiguous. No one in the 1920s had a model for explaining the apparently idiosyncratic occurrence of lead poisoning.

Convinced by industry that oil supplies were limited and there was an extraordinary need to conserve fuel by making combustion more efficient, most public health workers believed that there must be overwhelming evidence that leaded gasoline actually harmed people before it should be banned. Industry advertisements compared tetraethyl lead to vitamins, suggesting that automobiles would run inefficiently without the additive.

Dr. Henry F. Vaughan, president of the American Public Health Association, said: "Certainly in a study of the statistics in our large cities there is nothing which would warrant a health commissioner in saying that you could not sell ethyl gasoline." He agreed that there should be further tests and studies of the problem but that "so far as the present situation is concerned, as a health administrator I feel that it is entirely negative." Dr. Emery Hayhurst of the Ohio Department of Health argued that the widespread use of leaded gasoline for twenty-seven months "should have sufficed to bring out some mishaps and poisonings suspected to have been caused by tetraethyl lead."[82] Given that it didn't, he was prepared to declare leaded gas safe.

In private, however, Hayhurst and others admitted their private doubts. One investigator from Columbia University, Frederick Flinn, who had not spoken at the conference, expressed his fears in a personal communication

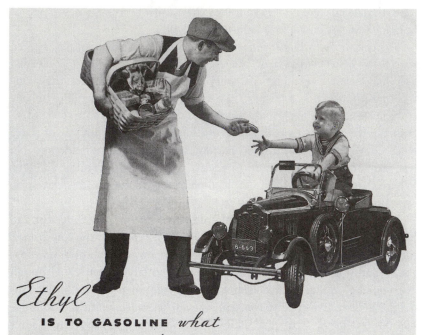

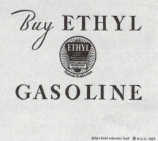

Ethyl

IS TO GASOLINE *what* VITAMINS *are to* FOOD

DOCTORS SAY, "Give your children fruit. It adds needed vitamins to the nourishment they get from other foods."

Oil companies say, "Give your car Ethyl. It evens the explosions of gasoline inside the engine; delivers more of gasoline's energy to your motor as *power*, leaves less of it as *waste* heat."

But oil companies go one step farther. They add Ethyl to *good* gasoline —and sell you Ethyl Gasoline already mixed in the right proportion.

And this month, oil companies are announcing an even higher standard of quality for Ethyl Gasoline—offering you still greater value for your gasoline money.

The new high compression cars, built by automobile companies to take advantage of Ethyl's universal distribution, *require* this better motor fuel. Older cars find Ethyl a real economy because it prevents harmful knock, overheating and power-loss.

Stop at the Ethyl pump tomorrow. You'll notice the difference immediately. Ethyl Gasoline gives you more power on hills, faster pick-up and less gear-shifting in traffic, a smoother, more responsive motor. It is the correct motor fuel for your car. Ethyl Gasoline Corporation, New York City.

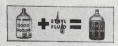

Buy ETHYL

ETHYL

GASOLINE

Ethyl fluid contains lead. © E.G.C. 1932.

1. Ethyl is to gasoline what vitamins are to food. In this advertisement, the Ethyl Corporation equates leaded gasoline to vitamins and links children, food, lead, and automobiles. Source: *Ladies' Home Journal* (June 1932), 55.

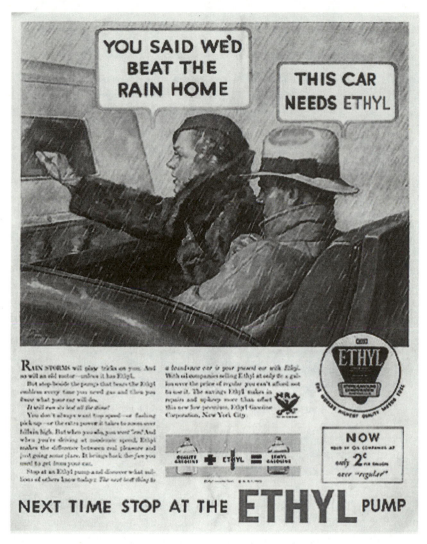

2. This car needs ethyl. The Ethyl Corporation promotes its lead gas additive, comparing it favorably to nonlead fuels. Source: *Saturday Evening Post* (1933).

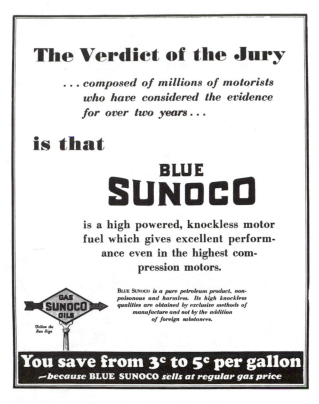

The Verdict of the Jury

. . . composed of millions of motorists who have considered the evidence for over two years . . .

is that

BLUE
SUNOCO

is a high powered, knockless motor fuel which gives excellent perform-ance even in the highest com-pression motors.

GAS SUNOCO OILS

Follow the Sun Sign

BLUE SUNOCO is a pure petroleum product, non-poisonous and harmless. Its high knockless qualities are obtained by exclusive methods of manufacture and not by the addition of foreign substances.

You save from 3ᶜ to 5ᶜ per gallon
—because BLUE SUNOCO sells at regular gas price

3. The verdict of the jury. After the controversy over tetraethyl lead, other gas companies promoted their nonleaded products as nonpoisonous and the choice of the people. (March 1929). Source: Hagley Museum. Acc. 84.247.5 po 90-251, 8-3.

to R. R. Sayers of the Public Health Service and the Bureau of Mines: "The more I work with the material [tetraethyl lead] the more I am confused as to whether it is a real public health hazard," he began. He felt that much depended upon the special conditions of exposure in industry and on the street, but in the end stated he was "convinced that there is some hazard—the extent of which must be studied around garages and filling stations over a period of time and by unprejudiced persons." As Flinn had per-formed studies for the Ethyl Corporation, it is not surprising that he ended his letter by saying that "of course you must understand that my remarks are confidential."[83]

Emery Hayhurst was even more candid in his private correspondence to Sayers. He told Sayers that he had just received a letter from Dr. L. R.

Thompson of the Public Health Service saying that "lead has no business in the human body. . . . That everyone agrees lead is an undesirable hazard and the only way to control it is to stop its use by the general public." Hayhurst, however, acknowledged to Sayers that political and economic considerations influenced his scientific judgment. "Personally I can quite agree with Dr. Thompson's wholesome point of view, but still I am afraid human progress cannot go on under such restrictions and that where things can be handled safely by proper supervision and regulation they must be allowed to proceed if we are to survive among the nations. Dr. Thompson's arguments might also be applied to gasoline and to the thousand and one other poisons and hazards which characterize our modern civilization."[84] Despite the widespread ambivalence on the part of public health professionals and the opposition to any curbs on production on the part of industry spokespeople, the public suspicion aroused by the preceding year's events led to a significant victory for those who opposed the sale of leaded gasoline. At the end of the conference, the Ethyl Gasoline Corporation announced that it was suspending the production and distribution of leaded gasoline until the scientific and public health issues involved in its manufacture could be resolved. The conference called upon the surgeon general to organize a blue ribbon committee of the nation's foremost public health scientists to study leaded gasoline. Among those asked to participate were David Edsall, professor of clinical medicine at Harvard University; Julius Stieglitz, professor of chemistry at the University of Chicago; and C.-E. A. Winslow, professor of public health at Yale University.

For Alice Hamilton and other opponents of leaded gasoline, the conference appeared to have yielded a positive result, placing the power to decide the future of an important industrial poison in the hands of university scientists. "To anyone who has followed the course of industrial medicine for as much as ten years," Hamilton remarked one month after its conclusion, "this conference marks a great progress from the days when we used to meet the underlings of the great munitions makers [during World War I] and coax and plead with them to put in the precautionary measures. . . . This time it was possible to bring together in the office of the Surgeon General the foremost men in industrial medicine and public health and the men who are in real authority in industry and to have a blaze of publicity turned on their deliberations."[85]

The initial euphoria over the apparent victory of "objective" science over political and economic self-interest was short-lived. The blue ribbon committee, under pressure to deliver an early decision, designed a short-term, and thus very limited, study of garage and filling station attendants and chauffeurs. Researchers studied four groups of workers in Dayton and Cincinnati, totaling only 252 people. Of these, 36 were controls employed by the city of Dayton as chauffeurs of cars using gasoline without lead, while 77 were chauffeurs using leaded gasoline over a period of two years. Also, 21 others were controls employed as garage workers or filling station attendants where unleaded gasoline was used and 57 were engaged in similar work where tetraethyl gas was used. As another means of comparison, 61 men were tested in two industrial plants in which there was known to be persistent exposure to lead dust. In just seven months, the committee concluded their study, finding that "in its opinion there are at present no good grounds for prohibiting the use of ethyl gasoline . . . provided that its distribution and use are controlled by proper regulations." They suggested that the surgeon general formulate specific regulations to be enforced by the states.[86]

Although it appears that the committee rushed to judgment, it must be pointed out that this group viewed their study as only interim, to be followed by longer follow-up studies in the coming years. In their final report to the surgeon general, the committee warned:

> It remains possible that if the use of leaded gasoline becomes widespread conditions may arise very different from those studied by us which would render its use more of a hazard than would appear to be the case from this investigation. Longer experience may show that even such slight storage of lead as was observed in these studies may lead eventually in susceptible individuals to recognizable lead poisoning or to chronic degenerative diseases of a less obvious character.

Recognizing that their short-term retrospective investigation did not address the issue of long-term effects, the committee concluded that further study by the government was essential:

> In view of such possibilities the committee feels that the investigation begun under their direction must not be allowed to lapse. . . . It should be possible to follow closely the outcome of a more extended use of this fuel and to determine whether or not it may constitute a menace to the health of the general public after prolonged use or other conditions not now foreseen. . . . The vast increase in the number of automobiles throughout the country makes the study of all such questions a matter of real importance from the standpoint of public health and the committee urges strongly that a suitable appropriation be requested from Congress for the continuance of these investigations under the supervision of the Surgeon General of the Public Health Service.[87]

These suggestions were never carried out. For the next four decades, all studies of the use of tetraethyl lead were conducted by laboratories and scientists funded by the Ethyl Corporation and General Motors. In direct contradiction to the recommendations of the committee, Robert Kehoe, a physiologist who had originally helped formulate the industry's position, supervised the studies for Ethyl. He explained that since "it appeared from their investigation that there was no evidence of immediate danger to the public health, it was thought that these necessarily extensive studies should not be repeated at present, at public expense, but that they should be continued at the expense of the industry most concerned, subject, however, to the supervision of the Public Health Service." It should not be surprising that Kehoe concluded that his study "fails to show any evidence for the existence of such hazards," nor did the Public Health Service supervise his work.[88]

Since there was no immediate danger that could justify the removal of this toxin, industry used this rationale to justify another sixty years of leaded gasoline. This is an unfortunate testament to the power of industry's conception that a valuable (profitable) product should continue to be used until it was proven to be hazardous to consumers. For most of the twentieth century, this need to prove danger prevailed over the public health community's traditional precautionary model that toxic materials should not be used unless they could be demonstrated not to present a health risk.

The industry was successful in defining the issue as an occupational problem that remained largely undetected outside of the industrial setting. And Kehoe, a professor of physiology at the University of Cincinnati College of Medicine, continued to have his industry-supported laboratories and emerged in the following decades as a virtual commissar of lead toxicology. He, more than anyone, was responsible for promulgating the view that it was "normal" for certain amounts of lead to be in all human beings and that people had natural mechanisms for eliminating it and controlling it as a threat. Until the 1960s, there was no challenge to this position.

Kehoe fought the environmental model of lead poisoning. Yet, he saw that children were being lead poisoned as a result of ingesting lead-based paint. Ironically, while he was a staunch defender of the Ethyl Corporation and its use of lead in gasoline, he became part of a reconceptualization of risk and responsibility of industry as it related to childhood lead poisoning from paint, a movement that ultimately opened the door to a critique of environmental lead poisoning in general. This, in turn, resulted in the end of tetraethyl lead as the premier additive in gasoline.

A Child Lives
in a Lead World

In the first half of the nineteenth century paint manufacturing was a distinctly local affair, often controlled by druggists, whose access to a variety of mineral compounds and dyes led them to develop paints as a sideline.[1] Paints were composed of two primary materials—the liquid medium (usually linseed oil, turpentine, or flatting oils) and pigments (usually lead, but also zinc, titanium, or other metals). Transporting large amounts of heavy metals like lead from one part of the country to another was an enormous and quite complex task. Manufacturers increasingly found it most expedient to haul their supplies across the prairies from the mines to Lake Michigan, and from there to Buffalo by ship. Hundreds of tons of ore from mines in Missouri, Kansas, Oklahoma, and southern Illinois were refined in local smelters. The "custom of the smelters [in Illinois and Missouri] to offer the product of their furnaces daily, at public auction" made it necessary for buyers of lead to assign agents to the mines year-round in order to guarantee that they could bid against others and maintain a reliable source. The lead was then loaded onto "a caravan of ox-teams" that lumbered across the great plains northward pulling heavy wagons with tons of lead ingots.[2]

By the late nineteenth century, the trunk lines of the transcontinental railroad, the development of an extensive communications network, and the evolution of the modern corporation allowed for an enormous burst of technological and entrepreneurial activity. This, combined with an exploding domestic market, catapulted the United States into its position as the largest lead-producing nation in the world. Entrepreneurs in major industrialized cities centralized production. Towns like Pittsburgh and St. Louis, Milwaukee, Buffalo, and Chicago grew into manufacturing centers and transportation hubs, drawing their produce and meats from the rich midwestern farm and grazing lands and their iron, lead, and zinc from the mines of Minnesota, Missouri, Kansas, Oklahoma, and Montana. Train cars more reliably transported metal than oxen or even steamboats had. Once in the city, the metal was loaded on barges and transported across the Great Lakes or down the Mississippi River to huge manufacturing plants where it would be refined into a host of consumer goods from paint and face powders to pipes and toy lead soldiers.

TO MAKE OUR HOMES BEAUTIFUL

In the late nineteenth century, millions of working-class Americans moved into single-family homes throughout the United States. Historian Oliver Zunz documents that in the period between 1880 and 1920 in Detroit "owning a home . . . was not a middle class phenomenon . . . [but] was more an emblem of immigrant working-class culture."[3] Historian Margaret Garb notes a similar pattern in Chicago where urban and suburban communities developed as the city spread from along Lake Michigan into the Illinois countryside.[4] While the 1920 census showed that only 46 percent of all Americans were homeowners (and the percentage was much lower in most major cities), by the end of the 1940s home ownership had become the norm.[5] The single-family house was defined "as the healthiest, most moral, and most secure place to shelter the American family."[6]

These new homes boasted amenities not available to any but the wealthy earlier in the nineteenth century. Even for working-class families, indoor plumbing (the pipes and fixtures of which used huge quantities of lead[7]) replaced the overflowing outdoor privy, except in the tenements of large cities. Immigrant workers turned to private builders and savings and loan associations for the $900 needed to finance the construction of small houses in the growing industrial communities of the Midwest. Workers could afford a small two-bedroom house that comfortably slept a family of four. For $1,900 a bathroom with running water and flush toilets connected to the new sewer and water systems would be included.[8] In addition, iceboxes, telephones, and electric lights (all of which used lead) became common among more upscale families and were even within reach for the most marginal of middle-class families. Lead was needed for pipes, for solder for plumbing, and for sealing the cans that became increasingly common in the homes of urban workers far from the farm.

Higher standards of cleanliness called for the use of washing machines, irons, vacuums, and plumbing, all of which used lead.[9] And perhaps most significantly, the growing American middle class also developed a taste for brightly colored, clean walls dependent on paint, which usually contained lead. The lead industry quickly capitalized on this new style and standard of cleanliness. It sought to "make colorists of us all," emphasizing lead paint's "durable, hygienic, clean and washable" qualities that served "to make our homes beautiful."[10]

In the late nineteenth century the means of producing lead-based pigments, which remained the predominant basis for paints until the 1930s, was substantially improved as methods for producing lead carbonate, or "pure white lead," were perfected. Although the method for producing lead carbonate had been known for many centuries, it was complicated and expensive to produce until the "Dutch process" was developed in the seventeenth century. For much of the eighteenth and nineteenth centuries, the Netherlands and England were the centers of the white lead industry, slowly perfecting the Dutch process, making lead carbonate cheaper and cheaper to produce.[11]

It had long been known that lead corroded when exposed to certain acids, creating a pure white powder. The Dutch process used pots and platforms designed to maximize the efficiency of the chemical process. One pound of refined lead was placed in a cone-shaped pot to which a small amount of vinegar had been added. These pots were placed on beds of horse manure (or tannin), approximately four feet thick; another layer of horse manure was stacked on boards that rested on the pots. Over time the manure decomposed, producing heat that warmed the acid and created acid vapors, which ate away at the lead to create lead acetate. In all, "a completed stack contained five to ten tiers and as many as two thousands pots." Carbon dioxide emanating from the "manure decomposed the basic lead acetate and produced basic carbonate white lead, a whitish, scaly and brittle product." The entire process took three to four months. Because the white lead was too uneven to use in paint, it had to be ground, rolled, and dried over and over again to produce a very fine powder. Painters mixed the powder with linseed oil or flatting oil to produce the paint that would be spread on the nation's walls.[12]

By the turn of the century the druggist who produced paint as a sideline and the local foundry that poured lead into casts for toy soldiers for local merchants were replaced by corporations like National Lead and Eagle-Picher.[13] National Lead was founded in 1891 as a holding company after the breakup of what was called the Lead Trust. (The Sherman Antitrust Act of 1890, passed largely to prevent collusion among manufacturers, also broke up the Lead Trust.) The Lead Trust was a merging of thirty-one lead firms organized by a group of financiers to secure "intelligent cooperation in the business of smelting, refining, corroding, manufacturing, vending, and dealing in lead and all its products."[14] By 1890 the trust "controlled the manufacture of 80 per cent of white lead, 70 per cent of red lead, 15 per cent of linseed oil [used to mix paint], and 9 per cent of lead pipe produced in the United States."[15] It brought together all but three of the largest lead producers.[16]

By 1893, the newly formed National Lead Company was the most powerful of the lead companies, and lead pigment was its signature product. It manufactured 65,000 tons of white lead annually, compared to a total production of 25,000 tons by the other nine American producers combined.[17] National Lead, like other pigment manufacturers, such as Eagle-Picher and Anaconda, was a vertically integrated company, owning everything necessary for the production of lead products, including smelters, factories, and paint companies. Thus it had a tremendous stake in encouraging the use of lead pigment in paints. But even though National Lead controlled the market for lead pigments by 1900, it could not control the amount of its product that any of the hundreds of individual paint producers used. Most of these companies produced "mixed paints," which contained not only lead carbonate and lead sulfate, but also other pigments such as titanium and zinc.[18] Hence National Lead embarked on a fifty-year campaign to promulgate the view that "pure white lead" was the pigment of choice. Beginning in 1906, with the introduction of the Dutch Boy Painter, the young boy in a workman's cap, clogs, and overalls with a paintbrush in his hand, as its advertising symbol, National Lead linked lead, whiteness, healthfulness, prosperity, and purity with its "pure white lead" product.

THE EMERGENCE OF CONSCIOUSNESS ABOUT THE HEALTH OF CHILDREN

As lead became an integral part of new middle-class life in the cities and the suburbs in the late nineteenth century, changes were happening in medicine and public health that would eventually lead to the discovery of lead's effect on children. Pediatrics was developing as a specialty. New technologies and skills dramatically improved the care of young patients. The nineteenth century saw the growth of children's hospitals, where pediatric surgeons could reset the deformed bones of children afflicted with rickets. In the twentieth century there arose a growing network of infant and child welfare clinics. These hospitals and clinics became teaching centers for doctors who focused on the special problems of childhood.[19]

For much of American history, children had worked alongside their parents in the fields and eventually in factories. During the early twentieth century, reformers began to view children's victimization in the factory and on the farms as a symbol of retrograde exploitation and primitive ideas about children's use value. The public health community began to focus on the broad array of childhood diseases. By World War I, when draft boards rejected 25 percent of draftees for physical and psychological problems, it was clear that America had been neglecting its children.

Better nutrition, housing reforms, the introduction of pure water supplies and sewerage systems, and better street cleaning led to a generally cleaner, more sanitary urban environment for children. The horse, which deposited up to twenty-five pounds of manure and two quarts of urine on city streets every day, was replaced by the electric streetcar and trolley in the 1890s and by the automobile in the early 1900s. The numerous granaries needed for the maintenance of nearly 200,000 horses in New York City began to disappear, making it easier to control the huge rat and rodent problem linked to the spread of lice and tick-borne diseases.[20] Similarly, the creation of public health stations that provided pasteurized milk[21] and settlement houses that provided emergency shelter, visiting nurses, and educational programs for mothers and their children also improved the chances of childhood survival. The development of maternity hospitals as well as pediatric and foundling hospitals further improved the conditions for children.[22]

The vast majority of public health and medical workers gauged their professional success by how much they improved the care of the mother and child and eradicated infectious disease. They worked to improve sanitation and living conditions, to improve prenatal care for the mother, and to intervene medically to prevent deaths at birth and immediately afterward. As a result there was an extraordinary decline in the rate of infant and early childhood deaths during this time. Virtually every cause of death could be fitted into the bacteriological, social reform, and sanitary models that dominated the thinking of political progressives, settlement house social reformers, and public health and medical professionals. Even convulsions and the symptoms that accompanied brain injuries could be explained as a result of physical trauma during birth or of bacterial infections of the brain or central nervous system.

Until the 1920s, except for a few extraordinary observations, few health professionals ever broke free from the prevailing paradigms to envision other causes for convulsions, mental retardation, or other diseases of infancy and childhood. In some ways this improvement in children's health set the stage for the identification of childhood lead poisoning. As more families settled in the booming cities, more and more children were exposed to lead. Children were brought into hospitals and clinics suffering from severe convulsions, tremors, and listlessness. A few physicians noted that some children had the blue line above the gums that was characteristic of occupational lead poisoning and were thus alerted to the possibility that children were ingesting lead. Still, lead poisoning went grossly underdiagnosed for much of the first half of the twentieth century, as periodic epidemics of infectious diseases like diphtheria, measles, and influenza continued to focus attention on bacterial agents.[23]

THE IDENTIFICATION OF LEAD POISONING IN CHILDREN

Physicians, first in Australia and then in the United States, began diagnosing cases of lead poisoning among children from lead chromate used as a dye for cakes, from lead in foil candy wrappings, and from lead in paint on verandas, porches, toys, cribs, and woodwork. Public health officials, preoccupied by infectious childhood diseases and the demands for better medical and prenatal services, were slow to pick up on the cases of lead poisoning that were being reported. Ironically, the lead industry itself was most attuned to the incidence of lead poisoning because it feared that attention in the media could devastate the expanding consumer lead market. By the 1920s, that market included not simply lead paint, but also lead pipes, lead car batteries, and lead in gasoline. Over the next thirty years, the industry embarked on a program to obscure the relationship between lead, paint, and children's deaths and illnesses.

The medical literature on lead poisoning and children can be traced back to the treatise of Louis Tanquerel des Planches in 1848. He remarked on children placing lead-painted toys in their mouths and developing lead colic.[24] As early as 1887 medical authorities in the United States noted cases of children coming down with lead poisoning. David Stewart, for example, reported in *Medical News* that nine members of a single family developed lead poisoning from lead chromate used to dye bread yellow.[25] In the nineteenth century lead chromate was often added to lead sulfate to form what was called "chrome yellow," a coloring agent used by bakers and candymakers. In 1889, an article in *Science* reported on the deaths of two children from the ingestion of baked confections that contained chrome yellow.[26] In 1892, Australians J. Lockhart Gibson and A. Jefferis Turner reported that one of Brisbane's lead-poisoned children was "remarkably fond of sweets and chewing things." One boy chewed the foil covering chocolates "to make pellets to pelt other boys." Others were so delighted by the taste of the foils that covered sweetmeats that they chewed them with the foil still on them.[27] In the United States, a physician, noting that toys were often made of lead and painted with lead paint, wondered how important it might be to guard against its use if "infants and older children, [and] especially young babes, refer all objects to the mouth."[28]

In the late nineteenth and early twentieth centuries, the literature on lead poisoning among children continued to accumulate in Australia, England, and the United States. In 1896 the *American Medico-Surgical Bulletin*, for example, reported on a nine-month-old baby poisoned by painted lead soldiers. It hypothesized that the paint was a possible source of poisoning.[29] In Australia in 1897, A. Jefferis Turner documented "lead poisoning among Queensland children." He listed a series of cases and noted that lead poisoning was widespread among children between the ages of three and twelve.[30] J. Lockhart Gibson's 1904 article in the *Australasian Medical Gazette*, "A Plea for Painted Railings and Painted Walls of Rooms as the Source of Lead Poisoning amongst Queensland Children," which was based on evidence he gathered as a clinician in Queensland, was among the first in an English-language publication to directly link lead-based paint to disease in children.[31]

A few years later, Gibson reported on cases of ocular neuritis in children and held that poisoning was due to paint powder that came off of verandas and the walls of rooms. He urged that "the use of lead paint within the reach of children should be prohibited by law."[32] In 1907 American physicians learned of the Queensland studies from David Edsall of Harvard University, who noted their significance in a chapter he contributed to the textbook *Modern Medicine*.[33] The Australians continued to document the role of lead paint in the poisoning of children, publishing in medical journals in their own country and also in the prestigious *British Medical Journal*.[34]

The first American documentation of cases of childhood lead poisoning from paint came in 1914 when Henry Thomas and Kenneth Blackfan, physicians at the Harriet Lane Home, a children's facility affiliated with Johns Hopkins Hospital, detailed a case of a boy from Baltimore who died of lead poisoning from white lead paint bitten from the railing of his crib. Five days before admission, the child began to complain about "pain in his face and head, to be restless at night, and to look ill." He began vomiting and rapidly deteriorated. He then began to convulse and went into a coma, and when he entered the hospital he was comatose with his head thrust forward "and his arms and legs . . . extended and spastic."[35] In 1917, Blackfan published an article that reviewed the extensive English-language literature on lead poisoning in children. In his case histories he noted that children were poisoned by gnawing on lead and concluded his review with the recommendation that children should be prevented from eating or mouthing painted items. He described children who first became "fretful, peevish and often very restless at night." Their appetite was poor and their gums began to bleed, and soon pain shot up and down their legs. Their stomachs began to ache, and they became constipated. Their muscles became "so painful as not to permit of the weight of the bed-clothing." They developed a waddling gait, walking only on the "outside of the feet." They dragged their toes, and their legs swung out sideways as they walked. Soon, seizures occurred and some died.[36]

In the 1920s, clinicians produced a drumbeat of articles linking lead-based paint to lead poisoning among children.[37] These early casualties were signs of a much deeper problem that was not being addressed. Isaac Abt argued in his standard text on pediatrics that childhood lead poisoning was "more common in children than generally supposed,"[38] a point that was echoed over and over in the coming years. In 1924 the *Journal of the American Medical Association* published an article by John Ruddock showing that the true extent of lead poisoning in children was understated because there were "many mild cases . . . manifested by spasms or colic, the true nature of which are never suspected."[39] In 1926, Charles F. McKhann, a Harvard physician, detailed seventeen case studies, concluding that lead poisoning was "of relatively frequent occurrence in children" and was usually associated with the ingestion of lead paint.[40]

At the time (and even in some cases to the present), the lead industry and its defenders argued that the real "culprit" was the child.[41] They were able to do so because in the 1920s many viewed a child's lead poisoning as the result of pathological behavior on the part of the child. Some of the physicians reporting cases of lead poisoning in children described the poisoning as a consequence of another condition, pica, which was often considered an abnormal craving for nonedible substances; to make such a diagnosis put the child's own behavior in question, for pica was often associated with mental retardation. Others, however, argued that the problem was not the child's behavior but the fact that there were too many opportunities for children to put lead in their mouths. For these physicians, pica, if the term was used, was a normal habit, not a pathology. This distinction had enormous social and political implications for the lead industry: if the ingestion of lead was defined as due to the pathology of a small number of individual children, then the lead industry could justify the continued use of lead. But if this gnawing and mouthing were a habit normal in children, then the number of potential victims of poisoning would be increased astronomically and the industry's responsibility less easily skirted.

Today, defenders of the lead industry argue that the medical literature was long dominated by the view that only certain children engaged in the "perverse" behavior of sucking on objects and were thus at risk. However, even a cursory review of the articles that reported on childhood lead poisoning reveals no such clear-cut understanding of the term "pica." In many articles it was described as part of children's normal behavior or a mild habit. *Holt's Diseases of Childhood,* a standard pediatrics text, noted that pica was a habit that was not confined to mentally deficient children; the 1940 edition noted, "Most of the children who acquire [lead poisoning] do so during the first few years of life when it is natural for them to put things in the mouth. The abnormal persistence of this trait, pica, in older children may be followed by lead poisoning."[42]

Others echoed the view of pica as a habit, rather than a pathological condition. Charles McKhann and Edward Vogt, in a 1933 article in the *Journal of the American Medical Association* argued that there were different forms of pica and that "in the majority of cases of lead poisoning due to ingestion of paint, the pica has apparently been merely a pernicious habit, unrelated to any underlying abnormal condition."[43] McKhann and Vogt noted that "the incidence of lead poisoning is highest in infants and small children in whom teeth are erupting and in whom there is a great tendency to put things into the mouth."[44]

For the most part, sucking on fingers covered with lead dust, placing toys and other objects in one's mouth, biting fingernails, and chewing cool, sweet objects like painted windowsills or lead soldiers were understood as normal behavior for young children. In the evolving field of psychology, developmental theorists and psychoanalysts identified a variety of stages of child development; the early years were viewed as a stage when children tended to put any object they could grasp into their mouths. For Freudians, this was deemed the "oral" stage. Many who observed children simply noted that, in the normal act of teething, children would chew and gnaw on objects.

Childhood lead poisoning was a condition arising both from a set of behaviors typical of young children and the opportunity to ingest a poison. From the very beginning of the literature on lead poisoning, it was clear that this was an unusual condition, one that could not simply be attributed to abnormal behavior, but an environmental disease in that it was related to the widespread availability of the poison itself. Unlike arsenic or other toxic substances, which had limited availability and were distributed with warning or skull-and-crossbones labels to let people know their danger, lead was everywhere and there was no warning as to its hazards. As John Ruddock put it, "a child lives in a lead world."[45]

PIGMENT MAKERS KNEW OF
LEAD PAINT'S DANGER TO CHILDREN

Whatever the cause of children's ingesting lead, the fact that such ingestion caused poisoning was well established by the time the lead industry organized the Lead Industries Association (LIA) in 1928. The LIA was organized at a moment when American industries were establishing trade associations in part in response to the urgings of Secretary of Commerce Herbert Hoover, who during the 1920s promoted the "associative state," which emphasized cooperation between government and industry. More than one thousand such trade associations were organized in that decade. Coming after a period of intense public scrutiny in the Progressive era, when many Americans became deeply suspicious of the developing power of giant corporations, such associations provided a universally rosy image of the companies they represented. Through mass marketing and public relations campaigns, the corporation was promoted as a less formidable, more humane, and generally progressive force in American life.[46]

The LIA's organizational meeting at New York's Roosevelt Hotel was attended by representatives from the National Lead Company, St. Joseph Lead Company, and several smaller lead companies. This was a traditional trade association that sought, in its own view, "to combat the substitution of other metals and products for lead," to expand the market for lead so that "old uses of lead might be increased and new uses found," and to gather "better statistical information regarding lead than is now available."[47] The LIA was a vertical trade association, representing "the various links in the chain from mine to finished product as represented by mining companies[,] smelting and refining companies, and corporations fabricating the multitudinous lead products." They banded together because "what affects one link in the chain is apt to influence others."[48]

While some industry groups, like the National Safety Council, primarily concerned themselves with specific occupational safety and health problems (as well as nonindustrial issues such as highway safety), the LIA devoted much of its energy and resources to creating a safe and healthful image for its deadly product.[49] Unlike the National Safety Council, which promoted "Safety First" with billboards, posters, and educational campaigns within and outside the factory, the LIA did everything in its power to obscure the health dangers associated with lead.

Although one of the stated purposes of the trade association was "to decrease the prevalence of occupational diseases due to lead in industry,"[50] promoting a positive image soon became one of its leading objectives. As the LIA's president, Edward Cornish (the past president of National Lead),[51] put it in 1933, it was "important to remember that the lead industries must have the good-will of the public for it is more often subjected to unfavorable comment than other metal industries. Publicity which shows the important work our metal is discharging in the world helps to build up good-will and respect for lead."[52] The industry knew that further evidence of the dangers from lead in paint could undermine public confidence in lead and ultimately destroy the industry's market. It was necessary for the industry to mount a counteroffensive.

Felix Wormser, the LIA's secretary, led the industry's battle against negative publicity from 1928 through 1947. Wormser, a graduate of Columbia University with a degree in mining engineering, had begun his career as a gold miner and surveyor in Oregon's Blue Mountains along the Snake River. After a short stint with the Department of the Interior and with publisher McGraw Hill, he became a consultant for the St. Joseph Lead Company before joining the LIA when he was 34 years old.[53] With the LIA's founding, Wormser made combating lead's growing negative image a prime focus of his career, calling for an "impartial investigation which would show once and for all whether or not lead is detrimental to health under certain conditions of use."[54]

The LIA contracted with Harvard University's young lead researcher, Dr. Joseph Aub, who had already worked with the National Lead Company, to continue his "medical research on lead poisoning" and lead metabolism in adults,[55] never addressing questions about lead's effect on children. In 1921 National Lead's president, Edward Cornish, gave Harvard Medical School a check for almost $14,000—equal to about $140,000 today—as part of a coordinated contribution of the lead industry to fund "a thorough study of lead poisoning." Cornish wrote to David Edsall, then the dean of Harvard's Medical School, stating that lead manufacturers, as a result of "fifty to sixty years" of experience, agreed that "lead is a poison when it enters the stomach of man—whether it comes directly from the ores and mines and smelting works . . . as well as the ordinary forms of carbonate of lead, lead oxides and sulfate and sulfide of lead."[56] Two years later Cornish again wrote Edsall, noting the dangers of both ingested and inhaled lead: "We have long realized the necessity of enforcing the rule of wearing respirators in dusty places as well as washing the hands and face carefully before eating."[57]

Researchers supported by the industry served the same purpose for the lead pigment industry that the Kettering Institute at the University of Cincinnati, headed by Robert Kehoe, served for the leaded gasoline industry. If the lead industry sponsored research on lead, it would be seen as a responsible and progressive force.[58] For the next three decades, Kehoe's research at Kettering and Aub's research at Harvard would determine the nation's agenda for all toxicological research on lead.[59]

Aub and Kehoe, while not always in agreement about the implications of the research, continued to express industry's preferred view—that lead was a normal part of the human environment and that certain amounts of lead could be safely absorbed without pathological consequences. Aub's work centered on lead metabolism among adults subject to occupational exposures, never on childhood lead poisoning. Aub also questioned the legitimacy of individual allegations of workers' deaths or illnesses from lead poisoning; thus Aub earned the trust of the lead industry.[60] Aub's research was never fraudulent nor secret, but it focused on such a narrow range of questions that, while important for uncovering the physiology of lead poisoning, it never touched on the pressing issues of the dangers of lead paint to children.

Even in the midst of the Great Depression, when a steep decline in lead prices reduced the industry's revenues, the LIA continued to provide financial support for Aub's efforts. In Wormser's mind, the unrelenting attacks on lead as a toxic substance made it crucial for the industry to "emphasize the question of the general health hazard of lead." Speaking for the lead industry, "we should always be in the forefront so far as medical knowledge of lead is concerned."[61] As late as 1942, when the LIA gave Aub $3,500,[62] Wormser described Aub's work as "our medical research at Harvard Medical School."[63]

But in the early years of the depression, the lead industry faced another problem besides sagging revenues. Information about the dangers of lead that had appeared in professional journals was beginning to find its way into the popular press. In 1930, the *United States Daily* (a newspaper "Presenting the Official News of the Legislative, Executive and Judicial Branches of the Federal Government and of Each of the Governments of the Forty-Eight States") ran a front-page story stating that "lead poisoning as a result of chewing paint from toys, cradles and woodwork is now regarded as a more frequent occurrence among children than formerly, and all children's hospitals, realizing the extent of the dangers from this source, are coming to use a lead-free paint on their beds, toys, furnishings and interior decorations." The story quoted a U.S. Public Health Service official who said that "small amounts of lead which may cause only chronic lead poisoning in an older person may be of sufficient quantity to cause acute poisoning, leading to death, in an infant."[64]

This information did not lead Wormser and his association to consider addressing the very real problems of lead poisoning in children. Instead, at an LIA board of directors meeting three weeks later, Wormser, in response to the article and another in the New York *Daily News*, complained that "of late we have received much undeserved publicity in newspapers damaging to lead products." Renewed energy would be needed to counteract what Wormser called "such unfair and unfavorable publicity." The LIA would take "any remedial steps if necessary," along with its ongoing medical research, but would in the meantime initiate "a program of vigorously investigating each alleged case that arises." This meant that when a case of lead poisoning was mentioned, the industry would question the accuracy of the diagnosis and its link to lead ingestion. Further, the LIA would publish "literature showing the useful role of lead in industry." Together, these acts "may help to improve the situation"[65]—that is, improve lead's image in the public mind.

Also in 1930, the Metropolitan Life Insurance Company issued a report stating that "chronic lead poisoning occurs much more frequently among infants and young children than has been generally supposed. It would be a more prominent item in both morbidity and mortality records but for the fact that the condition is often unrecognized by physicians." Among the seventy-five pediatricians interviewed for the study, one Boston physician, Charles F. McKhann, "stated that fifty cases of lead poisoning in children had been seen in a single Boston hospital during the last six years . . . as the result of chewing paint from cribs, woodwork or toys."[66] The company's *Statistical Bulletin* concluded that "education of parents concerning this hazard would be a definite, forward step in public health education."[67]

Responding to Metropolitan Life's survey, Dr. Isaac Abt, author of *Abt's Pediatrics*, wrote to Louis Dublin, the author of Metropolitan's report and a vice president of the company, to concur that "lead poisoning in children is not uncommon." Dr. Harold K. Faber, professor of pediatrics at the Stanford University School of Medicine, wrote that he was "surprised that the subject had not come to the attention of your Company long ago" and that "every pediatrician of experience keeps it in mind when he is dealing with cases of convulsions without fever, severe secondary anemias with constipation and abdominal pain, and the like."[68]

Prompted by the revelations in the *United States Daily* and the Metropolitan Life report, the Lead Industries Association took actions that, while giving the appearance of addressing the danger of lead in consumer products, were intended only to (falsely) allay pediatricians' fears and mislead doctors about the extent of the danger that children were exposed to. In November 1930 the LIA sent manufacturers a short note, which it later portrayed as a "survey": "We are conducting an investigation to ascertain if any lead paint is being used to paint or decorate cribs, children's beds or furniture. Will you therefore, kindly let us know if it is your practice to use any white lead in painting this type of furniture. A return envelope is enclosed and a simple notation at the bottom of this letter will suffice. Thanking you for your cooperation."[69] They received replies from only 12 companies, all but one of which said they did not use lead paint on their products.[70] Although the LIA had no sense of whether these companies were representative—or whether their replies were truthful—they proceeded to use this "survey" in the most self-serving way, assuring medical researchers that although children had been poisoned by lead paint on toys and cribs in the past, "the lead industry and the manufacturers of cribs and toys . . . have cooperated by substituting other types of pigments for the lead pigments formerly used."[71]

It soon became clear, however, that the reality was quite different. In 1935 the U.S. Children's Bureau, founded two decades earlier in the Department of Labor to improve children's health, surveyed various toy companies about their use of lead and the presence of lead in their products. The A. Schoenhut Company described how it received a large order from Macy's in 1932, and how Macy's returned one quarter of the order saying it contained lead. Schoenhut had these toys tested and found that this was true. Subsequently they "took this question up with quite a number of paint manufacturers and everyone was willing to sign an agreement that the paint furnished would be non-poisonous, but only a few agreed that they would furnish materials that were entirely free of lead."[72] Similarly, the Newark Varnish Works "found that lead in the form of Lead Chromate was being used extensively in colored finishes."[73]

The LIA also failed to ensure that parents would not use lead paint on children's toys and furniture. During the depression new toys were often too expensive, so many parents repainted used toys and cribs. Because paint cans did not carry warnings about the dangers of lead paint, and would not for another quarter of a century, most parents were unaware of the serious health hazard this paint posed to their children. Unknowing parents let children repaint their own bikes, toy trucks, and scooters with paint that could poison them. One of the few warnings about the dangers of lead in paint came in a *Consumers Union Report* in 1936: "Repainted toys should be avoided unless there is some way of being assured that lead-free paints were used. In some cities, old toys are collected and repaired and repainted for distribution to children in poor families at Christmas time. There is always the danger that persons unaware of the hazard will use ordinary lead paints. In one city, children were employed to do the repainting, and many of them were poisoned by the lead paints provided for the work."[74]

Even painters in the industry appear to have been unaware of the potential hazard to children. In a 1933 issue of *Painter and Decorator*, an article about painting wooden toys ignored any mention of a lead paint hazard: "A priming coat of linseed oil and red lead . . . works well on most of the toy woods. If a light colored finish is to go on, enough white lead can be used, in lieu of red lead, to lighten this first coat. The paint on toys in these times has to be regarded for exterior as well as for interior use, because of the extensive use of the toy in yards and on the sidewalks."[75]

Given that parents were often not aware of the dangers from lead paint, it is not surprising that children continued to be diagnosed with lead poisoning. In 1931, Charles F. McKhann delivered a paper before the American Neurological Association in Boston, in which he asserted that "the most common cause of ingestion of lead appears to be the habit of small children of chewing paint from toys, cribs or woodwork of the house."[76] Also in 1931, Edward Vogt, from the Infants' and Children's Hospital in Boston, delivered a paper, later published in the *Journal of the American Medical Association*, in which he noted that "the most frequent source of lead . . . is from paint off the furniture, woodwork and toys. As everyone knows, infants have a common tendency during the teething period to chew at anything they can get into their mouths."[77]

Evidently the work of McKhann and Vogt was worrisome to the Lead Industries Association. In the spring of 1931 Wormser "visited Boston for the purpose of discussing the subject of lead poisoning in infants with some of the medical profession there who have caused us to receive some unfavorable publicity about lead." He later reported to his board of directors that "the visit was worthwhile."[78] We do not know what transpired in these meetings, but their tenor can be gleaned from a 1933 correspondence between Ella Oppenheimer of the United States Children's Bureau and Louis Dublin of Metropolitan Life. When Oppenheimer asked for information from the Metropolitan Life survey cited above, Dublin wrote back: "Please be advised that our *Bulletin* article received a great deal of publicity against which there was strong remonstrance by the Lead Industries Association. You will readily understand that we wish to avoid any controversy with the lead people. Please, therefore, do not mention the Metropolitan in connection with whatever releases you may make. We have the entire case in our files and if you wish to see all the correspondence . . . it will be placed at your service."[79] Given that one of the most respected and established insurance companies in the United States was intimidated by the LIA, it is no wonder that lead poisoning among children received so little publicity in the years between World War I and World War II.

DISPOSING OF EACH SITUATION AS IT ARISES

Throughout the 1920s and 1930s, physicians continued to identify as hazardous the lead paint on woodwork, windowsills, door frames, toys, and cribs. But the lead industry maintained that the sole concern about lead poisoning in children during the inter-war years related to the problem of lead-painted toys and cribs that children would gnaw or suck on. Once industry had "resolved" that problem by sending out the "survey" to reassure public health officials that there were no leaded paints on children's toys and cribs, they regarded the problem as so much history. The industry failed to warn parents of the dangers or to make sure that their paint with lead was not promoted for interior use.

(To this day, the industry claims that it has always been a responsible corporate citizen. When Gale Norton, the secretary of the interior under President George W. Bush, was questioned at her confirmation hearing in January 2001 about her role as a lobbyist for NL Industries, formerly known as National Lead, she maintained that the lead industry, unlike the tobacco industry, had "a record of responsible corporate behavior . . . [and] as scientific evidence became available as to problems, they responded to those problems." She maintained that it was not until the 1940s that knowledge about paint on interior surfaces was recognized as a problem and that then the industry removed lead from paint products intended for interior surfaces.[80])

While the industry maintained publicly that the toy manufacturers themselves had solved the problem, the industry worried privately that its attempt to control the issue was failing.[81] More and more information about lead's harmful effects was appearing in the medical literature. "Hardly a day goes by but what [sic] this subject receives some attention at the headquarters of the Association," Wormser told the LIA's annual meeting in 1935. "We are constantly investigating alleged cases of lead poisoning and endeavoring to correct misstatements about lead poisoning, to calm misapprehension about the toxic properties of the metal." So serious was the threat of negative publicity, Wormser told the members, that "if all other reasons for the establishment of a cooperative organization in the lead industries were to disappear, the health problem alone would be sufficient warrant for its establishment."[82]

By the 1930s and 1940s, even defenders of the lead industry began to question the LIA's position. Robert Kehoe, who had been the primary defender of the safety of lead in gasoline, declined to defend lead paint when presented with evidence of its dangers to children. He acknowledged to physicians that "the preventive aspect of this problem should...be greatly stressed" since poisonings occurred "at the period when children are most likely to eat abnormal things and to chew various objects in their environment." Kehoe argued that "strenuous efforts must be devoted to eliminating lead from their environment."[83]

It is difficult for us to understand what small amounts of lead were capable of killing children. The proceedings of the American College of Physicians, published in the *Canadian Journal of Public Health,* included the report of a study done in a Toronto hospital from 1919 to 1933. The authors, John Ross and Allan Brown, were adamant that the prevention of lead poisoning in children required "the elimination of these paints from the immediate environment of the child during the second and third years of life." This idea had been percolating throughout the medical community for at least fifteen years. But Ross and Brown added a new dimension to the problem by attempting to quantify the startlingly small amounts of lead a child needed to ingest to develop symptoms or even die. "The amount of lead per unit of painted surface has recently been estimated. On one square foot of a surface painted with ordinary house paint of the lead-zinc oxide type there would be 5.8 grams of metallic lead, while on a similar area painted with yellow toy enamel (lead chromate) there would be 1.86 grams Pb. A fatal case of lead poisoning in our series was found to have ingested not more than two-thirds of a gram of metallic lead," or approximately a two-inch-by-two-inch chip of one coat of paint. Given this, "it would seem advisable to prohibit the use of lead containing paints for toys, children's furniture, and for interior work."[84]

A gallon of ready-to-apply paint contained a great deal of lead. Mixing directions required a half-and-half mixture of white lead and oil, with the result that each gallon of paint contained about 16 pounds of white lead.

In the early 1930s lead poisoning remained primarily a concern to the lead industry and a few physicians and public health professionals. To the extent that the general public was aware of the danger represented by lead paint, a huge advertising and promotion campaign assuaged their fears, leading them to believe that lead was safe and that paint, even containing lead,

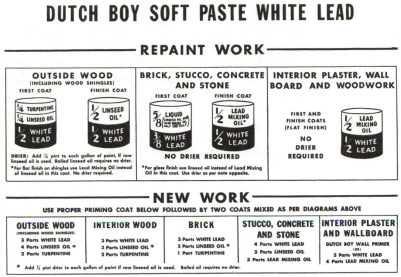

4. Volume mixing directions. From the 1920s through the 1940s, National Lead published *The Handbook on Painting*, which included formularies telling painters and consumers how to mix lead paint for interior and exterior uses. This illustration, reproduced throughout most of the 1940s, shows the proportions of white lead needed for interior plaster, including wallboard and woodwork, long identified as sources of lead paint affecting children. Source: *The Handbook on Painting* (1950).

was benign and wonderful for decorating their homes (see chapter 3). But the industry still had reason to worry. Nontoxic zinc- and titanium-based pigments became more readily available during the 1930s. If it became public knowledge that lead was killing children to the extent that physicians were documenting, the competing pigments, some of which were already displacing lead as the leading pigment, could devastate the industry. A prohibition of lead in paint became more feasible as alternatives were developed.

In 1931 the *American Journal of Public Health* published a short item stating that substituting zinc for lead in paint would protect children. Since children were being poisoned because of eating "paint on cribs, woodwork and toys," the writer believed, "it seems obvious that the simple precaution of using zinc paints in these cases should be resorted to."[85] Titanium-based pigments could also replace lead, and in fact an increasing share of the market was being taken over by companies selling paint with nonlead pigments. National Lead itself, despite continuing to produce and market lead carbonate, its signature product, had acquired the Titanium Pigment Company and a significant interest in the Titan Company, a Norwegian pigment manufacturer during the 1920s, thereby broadening its product line and protecting itself against the erosion of the lead pigment market.[86]

Even the National Safety Council noted that "the most obvious method of preventing lead poisoning is to substitute for lead and its compounds other materials that are non-toxic."[87] Feeling extremely threatened, the industry was vigilant about challenging those who dared to propose substitutes, particularly when their proposal was offered as a means of preventing lead poisoning. President Edward Cornish bragged to LIA members: "Wherever we have detected competitors of lead materials using the argument of lead poisoning as a means of furthering their sales, we have protested this practice."[88] The association continued to use its tried and true approach. "We have continued privately to investigate any attacks on lead that have appeared in the press and which have the semblance of being merely wishful thinking. Our vigilance pays dividends in enabling us to correct many inaccurate statements about lead that would ordinarily go unchallenged."[89]

Meanwhile, the LIA fought any proposed regulation, legislation, or action by the states that would restrict the use of its paint on walls. In 1934, when the Massachusetts Department of Labor sought to regulate the "use of white lead in painting buildings," Wormser went to state officials and reached what he called "a satisfactory adjustment." He told the LIA, "It was particularly important to obtain a hearing and settlement in Massachusetts[,] otherwise we might have been plagued with an extension of similar restrictive painting legislation in other States, affecting the use of white lead." By then it was "the most important outlet for pig lead metal."[90] This was in keeping with the LIA's broader attempts to derail government regulation. "The Association has continued to act for its members in legislation affecting the lead industries, such as, . . . miscellaneous contacts with numerous Government Departments on health legislation, standards and other matters," the LIA reported to its members.[91]

The intensity of the battle to maintain lead pigments was heightened by competition the industry was facing from lithopone and titanium during the 1920s and the 1930s and beyond. By 1929 lithopone, a zinc-based pigment, had outstripped white lead as the primary pigment for paint, and titanium pigments "were moving in carload lots." The lead industry was saved from disaster by dramatically increased sales of lead for storage batteries, power cable sheathing in the electrical industry, and increasingly, from the sale of Ethyl leaded gasoline.[92]

BALTIMORE LEAD CASES

The campaign by the LIA to shape public consciousness and to defeat isolated voices of opposition was successful in keeping clinicians' worries out of the public eye and even out of the public health community's line of vision until the 1940s. The one exception to this was Baltimore, which was the first and only American municipality before the 1950s to develop, according to historian Elizabeth Fee, "an extensive public health program on childhood lead paint poisoning."[93] The city organized health education campaigns, housing inspections, lead abatement campaigns, and passed some of the early labeling laws. Baltimore's role in uncovering childhood lead poisoning began in 1917 when Kenneth Blackfan of Johns Hopkins Hospital in Baltimore reported on cases of lead poisoning in children from the Harriet Lane Children's Home in Baltimore. But it was Huntington Williams, appointed Baltimore's commissioner of health in 1931, who brought Baltimore to the forefront of public health knowledge. Baltimore's sensitivity to this issue may have been due to Williams's unique vision and also to the early identification of fifty-nine cases of lead poisoning, many among children, caused by the burning of battery casings that poor African-Americans had used for heat in the early years of the Great Depression.[94] When two additional cases of lead poisoning in children were found to be caused by "chewing paint from windowsills, beds, tables, chairs and other pieces of furniture in their homes," the Baltimore city health department was already aware of lead's effect on children and thus warned parents that "paints often contain large quantities of lead compounds."[95] In 1935, the health department began "the unprecedented step of offering free laboratory diagnostic tests to assess the blood lead levels of any person with suspected lead poisoning."[96] During the first three years of the program, fifty-seven cases of lead paint poisoning in children were confirmed. Throughout the 1930s, the department continued to document that paint was a major cause of childhood lead poisoning and used the radio to warn residents: "Every year there are admitted to the hospitals of Baltimore a number of children with lead poisoning caused by eating paint. Most of these children die, but those who live are almost equally unfortunate because lead poisoning leaves behind it a trail of eyes dimmed by blindness, legs and arms made useless by paralysis, and minds destroyed even to complete idiocy."[97]

The dedication of Williams and the Baltimore city health department to uncovering lead-poisoned children was remarkable, given the enormous effort that such an undertaking required. It was nearly impossible to get children tested for suspected lead poisoning because of the difficulty of the tests themselves, the limited number of laboratories capable of performing them, and legal restrictions that limited testing to occupational, not environmental, exposures. In the decades before World War II, the "estimation of lead in [one] 24-hr urine specimen occupied a technician for two full days." In Massachusetts, which boasted one of the most sophisticated academic infrastructures, "only one laboratory maintained by the State Division of Industrial Hygiene was equipped and acknowledged to be competent to attempt it." Even there, it was impossible to test children's blood or urine because "by law, this laboratory was forbidden to do such examinations in any but industrially oriented cases."[98]

Diagnosis was all the more difficult because the symptoms among the children were not generally the most obvious or severe, encephalopathy being observed only "from time to time." But the children had symptoms such as anorexia, vomiting, cramps, constipation, irritability, headaches, peripheral neuritis, and "anemia with stippling of the red blood cells." X rays of the children's abdomens "usually showed the shadows of paint chips in the gastrointestinal tract," and X rays "of the long bones demonstrated condensation of the zones of provisional calcification."[99]

These difficulties led some to abandon the laboratory as a method for diagnosis and to depend upon clinical diagnosis instead. One physician particularly believed "that a well-founded clinical diagnosis of lead poisoning would be as reliable as one based on chemical recognition of lead in the blood or urine of the patient."[100] But even though it was difficult to establish proof of lead poisoning through blood tests, some insisted that only those tests could provide biological and physiological "proof."[101]

By 1942, "Baltimore City health officials concluded that fatal lead poisoning was in fact far more prevalent among children than adults; 86 per cent of the recorded deaths were those of children, with an average age of death of two and one half years."[102] Recognizing that the problem was related to lead paint in the dilapidated slum housing of the city, "Huntington Williams persuaded Mayor Howard Jackson that a new city ordinance was needed to deal with the problem." Titled the "Hygiene of Housing Ordinance," the 1941 law authorized the commissioner of health to order the removal or abatement of anything in a building or structure found to be "dangerous or detrimental to life or health."[103]

Baltimore's efforts illustrated that if you looked for lead poisoning among America's urban children, you generally found it. As the Baltimore public health department systematically screened children, more and more cases of lead poisoning were uncovered. "Of the 202 deaths from lead poisoning in persons under 15 years of age which were reported in the entire United States registration area (1936 population about 128,052,000), 49 deaths or 24.3 percent of the total were from the city of Baltimore." Between 1931 and 1940 there were 135 reported cases of childhood lead poisoning in Baltimore, 37 of which were associated with the use of storage battery casings. Of the other 99 children diagnosed with lead poisoning, the average age was two and a half years and "practically all had a history of pica associated with the chewing of objects painted with lead-containing paints."[104] The LIA understood better than any other entity, whether it be the federal Children's Bureau, Public Health Service, or Commerce Department or state and local health departments, that lead was a severe danger when it was ingested.

But the LIA still failed to warn people of the dangers. One Baltimore physician, Dr. Edward Park, long remembered the terrible role that the LIA played in trying to undermine reports of lead poisoning. Park worked at Johns Hopkins' Harriet Lane Home, where the first American cases of childhood lead poisoning were uncovered in 1914. He remembered the "secretary to some organization of paint companies," undoubtedly Felix Wormser, would "come often to the Harriet Lane and insisted that we were all wrong in our diagnoses of lead poisoning."[105] Far from seeking to uncover cases of lead poisoning, throughout his long career at the LIA, Wormser spent long hours finding ways of undermining documentation of cases.

UNPLEASANT READING FOR THE LEAD PRODUCER

By late in the Great Depression, the lead industry's success in controlling information through sponsorship of research, challenges to the accuracy of reports of lead poisonings, and even intimidation had begun to diminish. The popular press began picking up on the medical reports about lead poisoning that had been reported in professional journals. In 1939 and 1940 Wormser regularly reported to the LIA's members that "the large amount of space given to lead by medical columnists in the daily press, by the medical profession, by consumer organizations and by authors of scientific subjects has increased the amount of attention that we have had to give to the subject of lead toxicology."[106] In January 1941, "Lead poisoning matters continue to absorb a large amount of time of the Association." Yet, the association continued to make it a policy "to protect our interests from unwarranted attacks and undeserved publicity on lead poisoning. . . . The

greatest attacks on lead now occur among so-called 'consumer organizations' who make statements about lead that are decidedly unsupportable
from a scientific standpoint."[107]

By June 1943, Wormser was complaining that meeting "attacks on lead
due to its toxic qualities . . . is apparently endless."[108] The LIA felt bom-
barded from all sides by articles and opinions that cited lead paint as a
deadly poison for children. Yet, America's leading pediatricians were shocked
to note that despite the accumulating body of scientific knowledge, no regulations were in place to protect children from lead. L. Emmett Holt's textbook, *Diseases of Infancy and Childhood,* concluded that "lead poisoning
is one of the common and most serious forms of intoxication recognized in
childhood." Holt lamented, "In spite of the rather high incidence of cases
of lead poisoning there are no laws in this country to prevent the use of
lead paint in children's toys and furniture." He urged that paint be labeled
"so that one may ascertain that lead is an ingredient."[109]

In December 1943, *Time* magazine discovered the issue of children poisoned by lead from paint and made it national news, the first time that lead
paint became a broad public issue. The basis for *Time*'s report was an article published by Drs. Randolph Byers and Elizabeth Lord of Boston's Children's Hospital in the *American Journal of Diseases of Children* that noted
that parents' lack of awareness of the dangers of lead-based paint led many
to use it on toys, cribs, "windowsills and other places." Children, it was
pointed out, then chewed the objects, leading to a variety of physical and
nervous disorders. "All but one child, Dr. Lord discovered, were school fail-
ures. Only five had normal I.Q.s, and four of the five were so erratic that
they could not learn easily."[110]

In a preliminary report on the *Time* piece, the LIA maintained that the
assumption regarding the relationship between lead poisoning in babies
and later mental retardation was not proven and that "many of the alleged
cases of lead poisoning were probably nothing of the kind."[111] Wormser
believed that the paper was "open to serious criticism on many important
points, both from the economics of the situation and the medical aspects"
and that the case was "far from proven." He took solace in a conversation
he had with Harvard's Joseph Aub, who told him that "he felt that children
that have sub-normal appetites, or the disease known as 'pica' which
caused them to chew on inedible articles, were sub-normal to start
with!"[112] The *Time* article, which Wormser conceded was "unpleasant reading for the lead producer," was simply another example of where "lead has
been unfairly attacked in the public press."[113]

Wormser visited Dr. Byers in Boston and had a discussion with him that Wormser characterized as "frank and friendly."[114] Byers would remember the meeting differently. In 1980 he recalled that following the publication of his article, "Dr. Lord's and my results were challenged at once by the Lead Industries and their lawyers."[115] Christian Warren, author of the authoritative study of lead poisoning, *Brush with Death,* writes: "According to Byers the Lead Industries Association threatened to sue him for a million dollars, but this threat could have been nothing more than the stick to complement the carrot they planned to extend," which was money to support Byers's research for up to ten years. Warren concludes that "Felix Wormser had to come up to Boston to do damage control in the time-honored way he had dealt with Harvard's researchers since the 1920s: by buying their cooperation with research funds."[116]

The *Time* article was a turning point for the industry. Not only did it bring lead paint poisoning to national attention, but it also shifted the terms of the lead-poisoning discussion. Before Byers and Lord, the medical community had focused on the dramatic effects of acute lead poisoning—convulsions, coma, and death. But Byers and Lord documented subtler, long-term effects of lead poisoning upon children who appeared to be recovered from a first acute episode. The study, then, was the first that documented that lead's effects were not due only to the death of brain tissue, but also to the interference of children's neurological development.[117] As Warren puts it, "the simple epidemiological and statistical tools employed by Byers and Lord would never cut muster today," but few could not "acknowledge the fundamental impact of [their] study."[118]

Wormser, to be sure, was one of those few; but by the mid-1940s even his natural allies in the leaded gasoline industry were privately urging the LIA to abandon its long-held policy of protecting lead paint at all costs. The tetraethyl lead defenders came to believe that the unyielding defense of lead in paint could harm portions of the industry that produced lead for other uses than lead paint. J. H. Schaefer, a senior official at the Ethyl Corporation, which manufactured tetraethyl lead for gasoline, worried that the LIA's attempt to deny lead paint's toxicity to children could ultimately backfire. In a June 1944 letter to Wormser, Schaefer urged him to quit stonewalling the public, "because certainly there are a sufficient number of legitimate cases of lead poisoning of children."[119] Robert Kehoe, director of the Kettering Laboratories of the University of Cincinnati and a firm defender of the innocuousness of leaded gasoline, also argued that the paint industry's position was indefensible. Shortly after the publication of the

Byers and Lord article in the *American Journal of Diseases of Children* and the *Time* piece, Wormser wrote to Kehoe critiquing Byers and Lord's work. He worried that "other doctors will accept as authoritative this paper of Byers and Lord and probably build upon it still more fantastic assertions." But, Wormser acknowledged, "if what this article describes is correct, then we have indeed a most serious public health hazard."[120] Kehoe wrote back that "I fear that you will be disappointed by my answer, for I am disposed to agree with the conclusions arrived at by the authors, and to believe that their evidence, if not entirely adequate, is worthy of very serious consideration." He wrote that in his own work he had seen "serious mental retardation in children that have recovered from lead poisoning."[121]

Throughout the 1930s and 1940s, Kehoe argued strenuously, in private, for the avoidance of lead on any surface a child could come in contact with. In 1945 he advised the Colorado health department that people should

> be careful to avoid the use of lead compounds in any large extent on surfaces within the environment of small children. Small children crawl about on the floor and contaminate themselves pretty generally with any kind of dust or dirt that is within their environment. Eventually everything they get on their hands goes into their mouths, and therefore considerably greater opportunities exist for the dangerous exposure of small children of a variety of materials that have no important influence on the adult with more circumspect personal habits. . . . It is well known that children are more susceptible to the effects of lead absorption than are adults and also that clinical lead poisoning as seen in the child is a more serious disease than it is in the adult, generally speaking.[122]

The LIA continued during the World War II years to portray this growing body of scientific literature as "prejudice against lead" rather than the documentation of a serious public health concern.[123] The LIA still sought to cast doubt on virtually every report of lead poisoning, focusing on the reports' methodological problems rather than the underlying reality.[124] In December 1945 the LIA became more deeply alarmed by the detrimental effect that antilead reports could have on their market and stepped up its efforts to depict these reports merely as propaganda. The LIA called for a concerted effort to undercut the existing literature by shifting the debate from the consumer to the worker. "If it can be demonstrated . . . that the production of various lead articles can be attended with no detriment to health of the worker even though, as is well known, exposure may be of a high order, then public alarm over public exposure to lead, which is of a much lower order, should subside." Further, the LIA sought to continue to proselytize the public: "The dissemination of accurate publicity about lead to newspapers, magazines and radio should be organized specifically through a professional agency such as our own advertising agency."[125]

When the New York *Daily News* "printed on its front page a photograph of some women lying prone in a factory loft and carrying the caption 'lead fumes victims,'" Wormser visited the editorial staff of the newspaper and "protested the printing of this photograph."[126]

Wormser's relentless denials in the face of a barrage of information about the dangers of lead in paint began to make him look foolish. Robert Kehoe, meanwhile, let it be known to his Ethyl Corporation contacts that Wormser was dead wrong about the benign impact of lead on children. "I cannot fail to be somewhat critical of the comments of Mr. Wormser on various phases of the subject of lead poisoning in children. Whatever he may wish to think about this matter, lead poisoning in children is all too frequent. When it occurs, it is usually a very serious disease, and for this reason the warnings given to the public through various avenues are likely to be useful, and therefore should not be unduly criticized, even if they do contain some misinformation."[127] When Wormser claimed that toy and crib manufacturers had ceased using lead-based paint on these items,[128] Kehoe responded that he could "show him records of a number of cases that are fully authenticated even to his satisfaction." "Mr. Wormser takes the position that since reliable manufacturers do not supply playpens and the like that have been painted with lead paint, that all this [concern] is a tempest in a teapot."[129]

By the mid-1940s physicians began to directly challenge Wormser in a way they never would have done before. In 1946 in Boston, after Wormser gave the opening address at an American Medical Association conference on lead poisoning, one doctor brushed aside Wormser's assurances that children were no longer getting lead poisoning from nibbling on cribs: "The next time Mr. Wormser comes to Baltimore, I will show him a repainted crib which caused at least three cases of lead poisoning."[130] A representative of Consumers Research wrote to Wormser objecting that "no one could possibly know that" lead paint is not used for interiors because that "would imply a knowledge of the behavior of builders and just ordinary people all over the country, which no human being could possibly have."[131] In fact, in the following years National Lead itself continued to market leaded paint to painters, trumpeting its use on "interior plaster and wallboard [and] enamel undercoats."[132]

At the 1946 conference, Kehoe indirectly challenged Wormser: "More lead poisoning in children has occurred than we would like to think about.

The number that are actually reported in medical literature have very little relationship to the number that actually occur. Lead poisoning in a child
is a serious disease."[133]

In 1948 Manfred Bowditch, former director of the Division of Occupational Hygiene of Massachusetts, became the director of health and safety
of the LIA, succeeding Felix Wormser as chief spokesperson on health-
related issues.[134] (Wormser had rejoined St. Joseph Lead Company, becoming vice president in 1948. In 1953 Wormser would become assistant secretary of the interior for mineral resources under President Dwight
Eisenhower and served until 1957, when he returned once more to St.
Joseph.[135]) Kehoe wrote to congratulate Bowditch and encourage him to
break with the denials of the past and confront forthrightly the problems
lead was causing. Bowditch should pay attention to "more effective control
of lead exposure, both in the community at large, but more particularly in
the lead trades. My impression is that these industries, by and large, have
not taken full advantage of the available information that now enables satisfactory control to be achieved."[136]

In the late 1940s, sensing that professional opinion seemed to be turning against the industry's position and that pressure for regulatory activity was increasing, the LIA, as many corporations had since the 1920s,
sought to reshape its image.[137] For the first time it acknowledged that it
could play a role in educating the public about the dangers of lead. The
LIA collaborated with the Metropolitan Life Insurance Company to educate parents about "the soundest approach to the problem of preventing
childhood lead cases."[138] But at the same time, it was still seeking to protect its declining market by assailing charges of lead's deleterious impact
on health; agreeing in April 1948 to join with the American Zinc Institute to cease attacks on each other's products arising because of issues
of "toxicity."[139] But the damage had already been done. Over the next
several years the popular press highlighted the havoc that lead paint
wreaked on children's lives. Not until 1971 would action finally be taken
by the federal government to prevent the use of lead paint on interior
surfaces.

The ability to mass-produce lead carbonate for use as a pigment in paint
helped create an industry that for a century depended upon a poison and
its distribution throughout the environment. The industry's success could
be measured by the tons of the toxin it could mine, process, and distribute.
Happily for the industry, the reorganization of American society during
the twentieth century increased the demand for lead. But at the same time
the dangers from lead were becoming more apparent. The lead industry

had to find ways to neutralize the popular idea that lead killed people and had to create a positive image that would encourage consumers to use this deadly material on the walls of its homes where its children would come into contact with it. The tension between creating a healthful image for the toxin and addressing the public health concerns of the professional community would ultimately prove too intense for the long-term solvency of the lead pigment industry. The industry eventually phased out lead for use in interior paint. In the meantime, for half a century, the industry deflected attention from the dangers of its product and perpetuated, in Christian Warren's words, a "silenced epidemic."[140]

CATER TO THE CHILDREN

The Promotion of White Lead

The girl and boy felt very blue
Their toys were old and shabby too,
They couldn't play in such a place,

The room was really a disgrace.
But all at once they chanced to spy
The Dutch Boy Painter passing by.
"Oh Mother!" each one cried with joy,
"Please let us play with that nice boy!"...

"This famous Dutch Boy Lead of mine
Can make this playroom fairly shine
Let's start our painting right away
You'll find the work is only play."
      (National Lead Company, *The Dutch
      Boy Conquers Old Man Gloom,* 1929)

The response by the lead industry to reports on the dangers of lead was a cynical thirty-five-year advertising campaign to convince people that lead was safe, and the most insidious part of this campaign was the industry's marketing to children. Beginning in 1918, just as the studies of the Harriet Lane Home in Baltimore confirmed that lead paint was a danger to children, the industry undertook a sustained advertising and promotion campaign designed, in the words of National Lead's trade magazine, *Dutch Boy Painter,* to "cater to the children"[1] while convincing their parents and the public health community that lead "helps to guard your health." This elaborate and decades-long public relations campaign was intended to shape the public image of lead, emphasizing its "healthful" qualities and suggesting that it was essential for the social and economic progress of the nation.

In ads throughout much of the first half of the century, National Lead continually marketed not only its individual products, but also lead in general. A series of advertisements in *National Geographic* in the early 1920s extolled lead's critical place in modern American life. Lead, used in the production of fertilizers and insecticides, would protect customers "from

Cater
To The Children

Do you make it a point in your store to show courtesy to your youthful customers? Do you give them the same consideration and attention that you do the older folks, or do you brush them aside as of less importance?

Have you stopped to think that the children of today are the grown-ups of tomorrow and that a child is particularly quick to remember a kindness and slow to forget a slight or an injustice?

A busy parent sends a child —perhaps a shy little girl— to make a purchase. If there is a choice of stores, the child naturally makes a practice of going where she is made to feel welcome and where she is waited on promptly. She wins approval for doing her errand quickly and it takes less time from her own interests.

This is one of the seemingly small matters which many successful merchants consider worth attention.

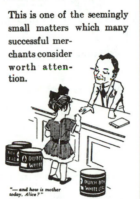

"— and how is mother today, Alice?"

5. Cater to the children: From 1906, when the National Lead Company adopted the Dutch Boy logo, children were a central element in the company's advertising campaigns. Source: *Dutch Boy Painter* (January/February 1918), advertising section.

famine" and keep "the wolf from the door."[2] In another ad directed at the new automobile-buying public, National Lead explained how important lead was in the production of every part of the car—in its batteries, radiators, lightbulbs, gas tanks, gasoline, even tires.[3]

Lead was presented as integral to the scientific revolution that was transforming the very way Americans saw the world. It was used in optics— ordinary cameras and eyeglasses as well as in "lens-making [which] has made the planets in the universe objects as familiar to astronomers as are the chickens in a barnyard to a farmer's wife." Likewise it contributed to our ability to see the smallest microorganisms. "With the help of magnifying lenses man has developed the serums that protect humanity against diphtheria, typhoid, and other diseases."[4] In all of these ads, the objective was to extol the benefits of lead in general and to convince the public that they would really feel the loss if lead in paint were eliminated: "It is in paint that lead would be missed the most. No matter where you go you can see and touch this important product."[5] No mention was made of the dangers of lead—that workers were poisoned, children died, women miscarried, people were affected by convulsions or palsies.

National Lead's ad campaign was also designed to promote its own line of Dutch Boy white lead paint. National Lead's logo of the little Dutch Boy, sitting on scaffolding with a paintbrush in one hand and a bucket of paint beside him, became a part of American consumer culture, appearing in thousands of issues of popular and trade magazines from *Good Housekeeping* and *Better Homes and Gardens* to *Lead* and *Painter and Decorator* throughout the early decades of the century. (Also appearing frequently was Sherwin-Williams's "cover-the-earth" logo: a can of paint pouring over the entire world.)

The early twentieth-century demographic movement to single-family homes, often on the fringes of growing cities, was accompanied by uncertainty about the way one was to function in these new environments. Most of America's new suburbanites, previously apartment dwellers, had little experience with maintaining a lawn, garden, and home. The lead paint industry wasted no time in seizing this enormous marketing opportunity.[6] In brochures, booklets, and advertisements, the industry dispensed tips on the fine points of middle-class living. In a booklet titled "Decorating the Home," the National Lead Company illustrated "up to the minute effects obtainable with white lead paint." The booklet sought to portray the role of paint in both the traditional and the modern home. The cover showed a grand house surrounded by huge trees and a well-manicured garden. In the first few pages, illustrations of Tudor, colonial, and southern colonial exteriors and interiors suggested stability and tradition: the handsomely painted cornices and trim, the fireplace, with a model schooner sitting on the mantelpiece, a picture of a bearded patriarch hung over a crammed bookcase, a room filled with Victorian furniture.[7]

Modern homes, the captions informed readers, were equally in need of lead paint, particularly the Dutch Boy brand. National Lead informed the new homeowner that even the "bungalow type of home depends largely on its surroundings." "To make it stand out, the color scheme selected for its decoration should usually offer a striking contrast to the surrounding houses." The booklet sought to answer questions for new homeowners: "What color scheme should I select to bring the interior walls of my home into harmony with the furnishing and hangings of the

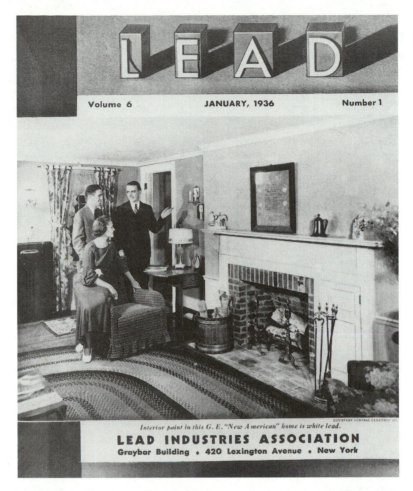

6. *Lead* magazine cover. This idealized scene of a family in their living room
tells the reader that the "New American" home can be covered in white lead.
Source: *Lead* 6 (January 1936).

various rooms? Can I obtain . . . washableness, sanitary qualities, and rich
texture? What paint is the most economical, offers the most in looks and
surface protection?"[8]

Most of the book focused on interior design and the use of color. On
walls, floors, and ceilings one should use "delicate, neutral tones, with ceilings lightest, walls darker, floors darkest, and trim either a deeper or lighter
shade than the side wall color." The color illustrations in the book told how
to finish one's home in order to "create a happy state of mind." Paint

became intimately linked with middle-class status, success, and stability. "For the decoration of the living room walls, tans, medium brown, warm gray, old blue, gray-green, and other soft colors are excellent," National Lead advised. Other examples of a bedroom, living rooms, and hallways completed the illustrations.[9]

National Lead cleverly appealed to the new middle class's aspirations to imitate the lifestyle of the wealthy. "Interior finishes once found only in the houses of the rich" were "now made available for every home by white-lead and flatting oil."[10] Ads by National Lead in the *Saturday Evening Post* and *National Geographic* stated: "Up to a short time ago such handsome finishes were a luxury that only the wealthy could afford. Today, however, a new flat paint puts similar interior finishes within the reach of all, not only for woodwork but for walls."[11]

Similarly, the industry recognized another potential market in the rising class of apartment builders, owners, and renters who would be replacing old-fashioned wallpaper with paint. Ads for Dutch Boy showed interiors of the Bryn Carlton Apartments in Los Angeles, all "decorated with Dutch Boy Lead Mixing Oil and Dutch Boy White-Lead." The lead industry positioned ads in *Modern Hospital, Buildings and Building Management, Hotel Management, National Real Estate Journal, Building Modernization, Architectural Record,* and *Architectural Forum*—publications that would reach builders, decorators, and managers in hospitals, hotels, and apartments.[12] The *Dutch Boy Painter,* National Lead Company's trade magazine, which regularly reached 95,000 dealers and housepainters, became an extremely valuable place to advertise white lead paints and colored pigments for interiors.[13]

Even in the 1930s, when the industry felt under siege from continuing reports of childhood poisonings from woodwork and interiors covered with lead paint, the industry continued its advertising campaign. In a National Lead promotional booklet titled "The House We Live In," the company called upon its readers to consider that white paint was not the only choice one had. In the section "What Color for the Woodwork?" the booklet suggested that woodwork could have "deeper tone" or a variety of decorative options of the consumer's or the interior decorator's own choosing.[14] By promoting lead paint for interiors, through pictures of entrance halls, living rooms, woodwork, dens, dining rooms, and kitchens, the industry reminded the reader of paint's versatility. Lead paint was recommended even in children's rooms and nurseries.[15] Paint was a flexible, versatile, durable, economical, and all-purpose wall covering that provided the consumer with the ultimate in hygiene, choice, protection, and modern convenience, the promotions asserted, never hinting that their product caused deaths, convulsions, and brain damage in children in Baltimore, Boston, and elsewhere.[16]

The company continually linked its product to purity and whiteness, reminding customers that no other paint could possibly match "pure white lead" for hygienic qualities. White surfaces were thought to be more hygienic than darker surfaces. White tile in the bathroom and white walls in kitchens and other areas of the house were stressed, those areas being especially prone to lurking germs that carried diseases.[17] Americans developed an "obsession with whiteness," equating it with cleanliness and perhaps with national purity, leading immigrants and second-generation Americans to embrace white. "In those days, them people believed in white wood," Nancy Tomes quotes one working-class daughter of immigrants as saying. "If it wasn't white, Grandma would hollar [*sic*]."[18]

Purity, whiteness, and paint were linked with efficiency and professionalism as well. The *Carter Times,* the trade publication for the Carter White Lead Company, which later merged with National Lead, suggested that the use of "pure white" would enhance business and reassure customers. Offering the example of a plumbing firm in a western city that had sought the advice of an efficiency expert, the magazine advised readers to "paint your shop pure white, outside and inside; dress your employees in white with white shoes and white caps, give them white canvas bags, in which to carry their tools and let them wear these white clothes while at work, not merely going to and from a job. Advertise yourself as 'The White Plumber.'"[19]

The image of purity was particularly appealing to some readers' nativist feelings. Many of the companies' products were used with tints and coloring, as we noted above. But, by emphasizing the underlying whiteness of lead paint, the companies were playing with cultural biases, namely the prevailing culture of racism in America. "White is associated with the Aryan race, and its members, vain as they are, naturally assume that no other hue is quite as honorable," explained one commercial art booklet in the 1930s just as Adolf Hitler was consolidating power in Germany. In the United States, becoming "white" was a critical component in immigrants' assimilation. "To say that a man is white," the booklet asserted, "is an Americanism."[20]

Middle-class consumers who could not afford an army of servants to clean walls or maintain the house would, advertisers hoped, be swayed by the notion that "cleanliness depends upon washability and consequent freedom from dirt and other impurities. Economy has to do with cost and years of wear." These "results are best reached by the use of paint made with pure white-lead."[21] Throughout the Great Depression and World War II, advertisements promoted the virtually unlimited uses of lead paint. "White-Lead Lasts!" screamed one such ad. "'The more lead the better the paint' is an axiom that the paint trade and public accept without question."[22] When you "step up the white-lead in your formula ... you automatically step up the quality and durability of your paint," the industry boasted.[23]

Although one consumer advocate, as early as 1915, was quite clear about lead's toxicity, the truth couldn't compete with the public relations campaign waged by National Lead and the Lead Industries Association (LIA). Harvey W. Wiley, the former head of the Bureau of Chemistry of the Department of Agriculture and later with *Good Housekeeping* magazine, where he established the Good Housekeeping Seal of Approval, discussed the differences between wallpaper and paint. He pointed out that "paint containing lead at once sounds its warning. As a matter of fact, lead is a subtle poison and, above all others, a cumulative one.... Thus, a zinc paint, from a sanitary point of view is better for indoor use."[24]

SOWING THE SEEDS OF MORE BUSINESS

Despite the accumulating evidence that lead-based paint put children at risk for seizures and death in their very homes, the industry still saw no reason to warn parents. In fact, in the late 1910s and early 1920s, the industry commenced a more troubling advertising campaign aimed at capitalizing on the popularity of National Lead's little Dutch Boy. The campaign stressed that lead was a benign product that adults could use in creating a happy environment for their children. The campaign was also targeted at the children themselves. Through the clever marketing of an assortment of giveaways, rhymes, and games, lead found its way into the hearts and minds of children and therefore the next generation of customers—that is, if they survived their childhood exposures to lead-based paints. By being associated with the cheerful Dutch Boy, dressed in workman's garb, lead could be seen as useful, efficient, and benign. The Dutch Boy's varied activities alerted children and parents alike to the endless possibilities of lead paint. The activities of National Lead were part of a much broader trend within American industry in general and the paint industry in particular to increase sales by marketing to children.[25]

National Lead was the most aggressive of the pigment manufacturers in promoting the use of lead in children's toys and games, reminding

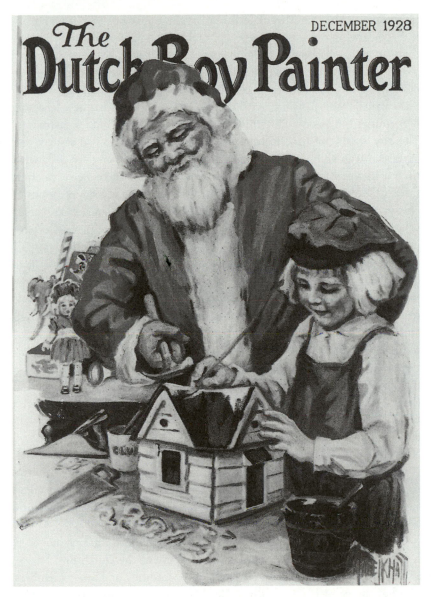

DECEMBER 1928

The Dutch Boy Painter

7. Santa Claus. This cover of the National Lead Company's trade magazine conveys the message that children can be encouraged to use lead paint on toys. Source: *Dutch Boy Painter* (December 1928).

customers of the qualities of lead that made it most useful. It was malleable, heavy, and resistant to rust and mold, giving substance and shape to toys. In one ad, the company bragged that "lead takes part in many games," detailing the ways that lead was used in baseballs, footballs, rubber balls, golf clubs, and fishing sinkers. Lead was also an essential part of toys: "The little boy's eyes shine with excitement as he takes his new lead soldiers out of the box on Christmas Day," National Lead told its customers. The boy would not have to worry about rust or mold, the ad assured the parents. Meanwhile "his sister peacefully plays with her new dolls with their lead-weighted eyes and her miniature furniture and other toys often made of lead."[26] Another ad celebrated the advantages of lead in shooting, always a fascination for young boys and older sportsmen. Lead's "great weight in minimum bulk" made bullets "pierce the air with unswerving velocity."[27]

National Lead's marketing of toys and sporting goods was not incidental, but part of an intentional campaign to make palatable the buying of lead products for children and to influence the next generation of consumers. In a promotion to paint distributors, the company advised store owners "Do Not Forget the Children—Some Day They May Be Customers."[28] It urged dealers to hand out a "children's paint book," which carried a "message to the grown-ups, while its jingles and pictures amuse the little ones." The paint books, a series of "Paint Book[s] for Boys and Girls," were to be handed out "to the little ones in store, [or] mailed out to them, or used in prize contest[s]."[29] ("Paint books" were booklets devoted to pictures—mostly featuring the little Dutch Boy—that could be colored in with water paints that were included in the books.) Filled with rhymes and poems and accompanying drawings, they promoted just the sort of parent-child read-aloud experience that is so much in vogue today—except for the fact that the subject matter valorized an insidious poison.[30]

One paint book, *The Dutch Boy's Lead Party*, extolled the advantages of white lead over nonleaded paints. Its cover showed the Dutch Boy, bucket and brush in hand, looking at lead soldiers, lightbulbs, and other members of what the paint book called the "lead family." Throughout the booklet the Dutch Boy carries a bucket inscribed "Dutch Boy White Lead."[31] The National Lead Company explained to parents that "the drawings afford [the child] pleasure," for the "story of lead, told in rollicking jingles," was meant to "capture his interest." But, again, the book was intended to do more than merely entertain the child; inside its pages there was a booklet for parents "so that a decisive paint message is placed in the hands of both

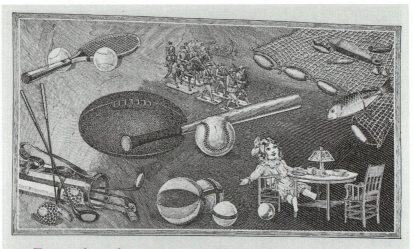

Lead takes part in many games

LEAD whistles back and forth in every play on the baseball diamond. It is at the bottom of every football scrimmage. It leaps back and forth across the tennis net. Lead influences every stroke the golfer takes, and is the fisherman's helper in making his catch.

How lead gets into these sports

Wherever toughness is required in rubber, lead is added to it. Thus lead in the form of litharge—or red-lead, that other lead oxide—is in the rubber core which is in every high-grade baseball. It helps to make the rubber bladders of footballs and basketballs, and is in tennis and other rubber balls.

Lead is also in many baseball bats and in the heads of wooden golf clubs, because it adds weight and helps to balance them. Pulverized lead is used in some golf balls to give them the necessary weight.

Lead helps the fisherman

Lead sinkers are used in fishing to carry the hook down to the desired depth. The heavy weight of lead for its bulk makes it the proper metal to use. And it will not rust.

This metal often covers the shanks of fish-hooks and weights down large fishing nets.

Lead in the nursery

The little boy's eyes shine with excitement as he takes his new lead soldiers out of the box on Christmas Day. Made of lead, they will not rust or mold as did the toy soldier of Field's "Little Boy Blue."

His sister peacefully plays with her new dolls with their lead-weighted eyes and her miniature furniture and other toys often made of lead. Toy-makers use lead extensively because it can be easily shaped and moulded into many forms.

Save the surface and you save all—Dutch Boy

Lead for preservation

Despite the widespread use of lead in the sport and play of the world, perhaps it is in preserving and beautifying buildings, inside and out, that lead performs its most useful service. Dryness and decay deface and destroy. But white-lead paint protects from the ravages of weather.

It is false economy to put off painting houses until deterioration makes expensive repairs necessary. Hence, property owners are heeding the warning, "Save the surface and you save all."

The professional painter, careful of his reputation, uses what he calls "lead-in-oil," a mixture of pure white-lead and pure linseed oil, for outside work. He uses white-lead and flatting oil, with coloring matter added, to make a smooth, beautiful paint of any color, for interior work.

Look for the Dutch Boy

NATIONAL LEAD COMPANY makes white-lead of the highest quality and sells it, mixed with pure linseed oil, under the name and trademark of *Dutch Boy white-lead.* The figure of the Dutch Boy is reproduced on every keg of white-lead and is a guarantee of exceptional purity.

Dutch Boy products also include red-lead, linseed oil, flatting oil, babbitt metals, and solder.

More about lead

If you use lead, or think you might use it in any form, write to us for specific information.

8. Lead takes part in many games. National Lead suggests that lead is a mainstay of toys and games for children and adults alike. Source: *National Geographic* (ca. 1923).

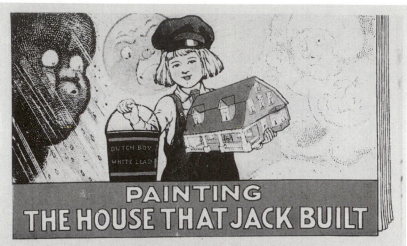

Do Not Forget the Children—
Some Day They May Be Customers

We are not even overlooking the children in our campaign for a record paint business this fall. The children's paint book, which is reproduced in only two colors above, carries a paint message to the grown-ups, while its jingles and "pictures" amuse the little ones. Moreover, in the back of the book there is a special paint message to the parents.

By all means do not hand out these children's paint books at random. One way is to hand a copy to each youngster who comes into your store *with a parent*. Parents appreciate little attentions of this sort paid their children. They like to trade at stores where the youngster is not overlooked. Another effective method is to mail the paint books to the children of prospective customers. Accompany the book with a pleasant little personal letter, working in subtly a few references to your store and the "Save the Surface" idea. There are other ways to distribute these clever little books, which you no doubt will work out to your advantage. Order a supply of these children's paint books today.

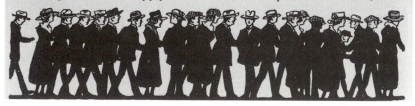

9. Do not forget the children. The Dutch Boy, carrying a bucket of white lead, reminds readers of this trade journal to court customers by offering children's "paint books." Note the stereotypical black cloud threatening the house protected by white lead paint and the Dutch Boy. Source: *Dutch Boy Painter* (August 1920), 126.

parent and child." Through the marketing campaign to children "business is built for the present and insured for the years ahead."[32]

Some booklets shamelessly capitalized on universally adored stories and fairy tales by placing the Dutch Boy in them. "The Dutch Boy in Story Land" partnered the Dutch Boy with Little Red Riding Hood in defeating the evil wolf, with Alice in her Adventures in Wonderland, with Cinderella in her pursuit of a prince, and so on.[33] The Dutch Boy and his lead paint were written into even the most common events in a child's life.

> Rover's house was painted white
> By "NO-Lead" paint, quite clean and bright.
> It was the best "No-Lead" could do—
> It surely made the house look new.

But the forces of nature soon attacked the house, making it look decrepit. The Dutch Boy came to the rescue, riding a bar of lead, and saved Rover's house:

> "That horse you ride is quite a steed!"
> "He is," the Dutch Boy said, "indeed,
> He is my Hobby—thoroughbred,
> Which means my mount is thoro lead."[34]

By the Great Depression, so much information about lead paint's danger to children had accumulated that even the LIA would acknowledge the inappropriateness of using lead paint on children's toys and furniture. Still, the National Lead Company continued in its Dutch Boy campaign to promote lead's use in children's rooms. In another "Paint Book for Boys and Girls," published in 1929, National Lead suggested that its paint "conquers Old Man Gloom":

> The girl and boy felt very blue
> Their toys were old and shabby too,
> They couldn't play in such a place,
> The room was really a disgrace.

But, just then, the Dutch Boy appears:

> But all at once they chanced to spy
> The Dutch Boy Painter passing by.
> "Oh Mother!" each one cried with joy,
> "Please let us play with that nice boy!"...

The little Dutch Boy tells the family that lead paint could remedy this terrible state of affairs:

This famous Dutch Boy Lead of mine
Can make this playroom fairly shine
Let's start our painting right away
You'll find the work is only play.

The Dutch Boy paints the children's walls and furniture, as Old Man Gloom watches.

Then Old Man Gloom cried: "It's a fact
That I will have to change my act.
My work is all undone!" He said,
"By Dutch Boy art and Dutch Boy Lead!"[35]

The booklet shows the Dutch Boy mixing white lead with colors and painting the walls and the dresser. Finally as the children play in their bright room with a freshly painted dollhouse and rocking chair, Old Man Gloom slinks off in defeat.[36]

Ads in professional and popular journals were also used to reinforce the image of lead as a boon to children. At every opportunity, even as the evidence of its danger to children grew, the ads sought to link lead paint to cleanliness, durability, and safety. In one of its most insidious promotions, National Lead depicted a crawling infant reaching out to touch a painted wall. "There is no cause for worry when fingerprint smudges or dirt spots appear on a wall painted with Dutch Boy white-lead."[37] The explicit message is that lead paint could be easily cleaned, but the equally important *implicit* message was that toddlers were safe touching, crawling, and playing near lead-painted walls and woodwork. This assurance was being offered despite the fact that the pigment manufacturers knew that toddlers were dying from chewing, sucking on, and ingesting paint from cribs, woodwork, and toys.

Even in the 1930s, the focus on children continued. To emphasize lead paint's benign qualities, National Lead depicted a child in a bathtub scrubbing himself with a brush. His Dutch Boy cap, clothes, and shoes were slung on a chair along with a paintbrush and a can of Dutch Boy All-Purpose Soft Paste. The caption read "Takes a Scrubbing with a Smile."[38] Other Dutch Boy ads depicted children painting houses and carrying paint. In 1930 the company bragged that its children's paint books were "good, sound advertising" and that "kids just 'eat it up.'"[39] The *Dutch Boy Painter,* in a 1933 article titled "Stencils—Types of Stencils . . . How to Use Them," noted that "humorous designs such as cartoons, caricatures, and pictorials . . . are for use in recreation rooms, game rooms, bars, etc. Juvenile designs . . . are, of course, for use in nurseries, kindergartens, play rooms or

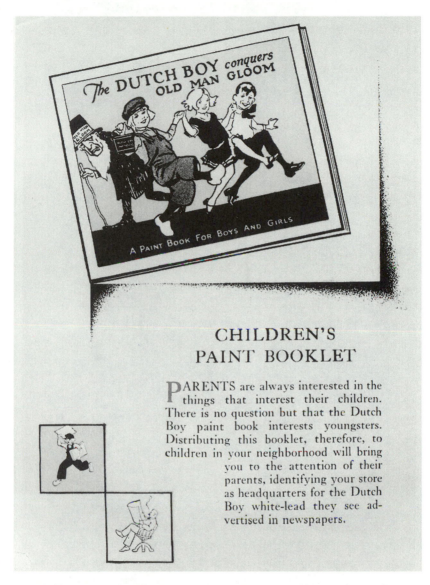

CHILDREN'S PAINT BOOKLET

PARENTS are always interested in the things that interest their children. There is no question but that the Dutch Boy paint book interests youngsters. Distributing this booklet, therefore, to children in your neighborhood will bring you to the attention of their parents, identifying your store as headquarters for the Dutch Boy white-lead they see advertised in newspapers.

10. Children's paint booklet: The Dutch Boy Conquers Old Man Gloom. This advertising booklet shows how paint can be used on toys and in children's rooms to lift the youngsters' moods. Source: *Dutch Boy Painter* (January/February 1929), 20.

Give Coupon to Father or Mother

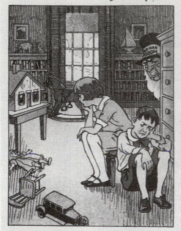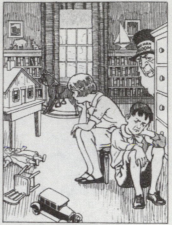

The girl and boy felt very blue
Their toys were old and shabby too,
They couldn't play in such a place,
The room was really a disgrace.

All gray and old with nothing bright,
It surely was a sorry sight,
And yet'that poor neglected room
Was the delight of Old Man Gloom.

Give Coupon to Father or Mother

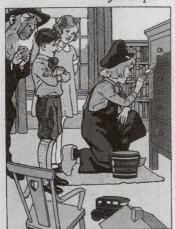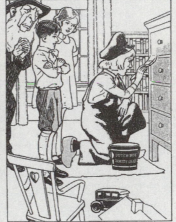

And as the work went on and on
The old and shabby room was gone
And sunny colors, soft and gay,
Made it a lovely place to play.

Then Old Man Gloom cried: "It's a fact
That I will have to change my act.
My work is all undone!" he said,
"By Dutch Boy art and Dutch Boy Lead!"

11a & 11b. Dutch Boy conquers Old Man Gloom, panels. These two pages promote lead paint for use in children's rooms. The first, composed of a color panel to be used as a template for the duplicate black and white panel to be colored in by the child, shows children in a gloomy room of dull colored toys and furniture. The second shows the same room after the Dutch Boy brightened it up with leaded paint. Note the Dutch Boy painting the furniture and the bright toy truck and dollhouse. Source: *National Lead booklet* (1929).

Finger Prints

THERE is no cause for worry when finger-print smudges or dirt spots appear on a wall painted with Dutch Boy white-lead. A little soap and water will remove them easily without harming the paint or marring the beauty of the finish. Painted walls are sanitary, cheerful and bright.

We carry a complete line of painting supplies including Dutch Boy white-lead, linseed oil, flatting oil, brushes and all other accessories.

Visit our store and let us help you plan your home decoration.

Dealer's Name and Address Here

No. DF-25

12. Fingerprints. This ad, one of several suggested to paint dealers, conveys to parents that white lead on interior walls is not only easy to clean but also sanitary for young children. Source: *Dutch Boy Painter* (August 1927), 117.

other places where children gather."[40] In one article in its trade magazine, *Lead,* an illustration of a model interior shows a child's nursery.[41] National Lead also promoted the use of lead paint in schoolrooms, showing a teacher with a classroom of children. The text of the promotion suggested that summer was the best time to "get after the school trustees to have each room repainted" with "flat paint made of Dutch Boy white-lead and flatting oil." Who could benefit more from a fresh coat of lead paint than "a band of husky young ones"?[42] Many of these ads appeared in the 1920s, but some ads and promotions directed at children appeared in the 1930s when the industry claimed it was exhorting manufacturers of toys and children's furniture to stop using lead paint on their products. But it is clear that the industry continued its campaign to promote the very uses of lead that it claimed to be combating.

National Lead Company was particularly pleased with its Dutch Boy logo as a marketing device.[43] The broader marketing community as well admired National Lead for such effective advertising. In 1949, *Modern Packaging* noted:

> The appeal [of its advertising] was particularly strong to children and the company has never overlooked the opportunity to plant the trademark image in young and receptive minds. One of the most successful promotions for many years was a children's paint book containing paper chips of paint from which the pictures (including, of course, several Dutch Boys) could be colored. A coupon in the book invited parents to write in for a booklet on house painting. The company will still loan a Dutch Boy costume—cap, wig, shirt, overalls and wooden shoes—to any person who writes in and asks for it for any reasonable purpose, and the little painter has graced thousands of parades and masquerades.

The magazine nominated Dutch Boy Paint for its "packaging Hall of Fame" in its cover story.[44]

This marketing of the Dutch Boy image was seen as an essential element of National Lead Company's profitability.[45] Throughout his long and inglorious existence, the Dutch Boy sought to appeal to children at least as much as to their parents. Dutch Boy costumes, puppets, dolls, potholders, rings, and other paraphernalia were sold, lent, and given free as souvenirs to entire generations of children.

A SANITARY SURFACE WHICH BEAUTIFIES

In addition to appealing to children, National Lead aligned itself with the growing public health movement that viewed the old clutter of Victorian homes as a haven for germs and disease. The themes of order, cleanliness, and purity that were hallmarks of the efforts to reform and sanitize American life were quickly incorporated into the industry's promotional materials. Such publications as "How Paint Promotes Public Health" and the

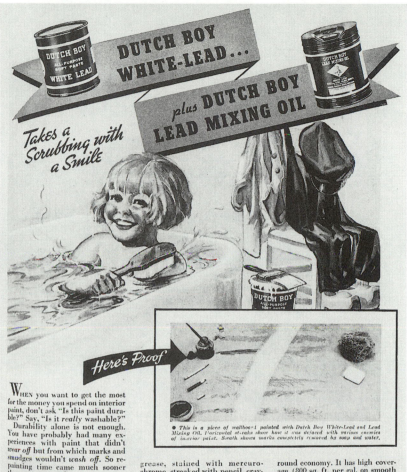

DUTCH BOY
WHITE-LEAD...

plus DUTCH BOY
LEAD MIXING OIL

Takes a Scrubbing with a Smile

Here's Proof

● *This is a piece of wallboard painted with Dutch Boy White-Lead and Lead Mixing Oil. Horizontal streaks show how it was defaced with various enemies of interior paint. Swath shows marks completely removed by soap and water.*

When you want to get the most for the money you spend on interior paint, don't ask "Is this paint durable?" Say, "Is it *really* washable?"

Durability alone is not enough. You have probably had many experiences with paint that didn't *wear off* but from which marks and smudges wouldn't *wash off*. So repainting time came much sooner than was expected.

Flat paint made with Dutch Boy White-Lead and Dutch Boy Lead Mixing Oil has all the durability for which white-lead is famous. In addition, this paint is washable in the full sense of the word. Its beauty is not impaired by hard scrubbings. Those scrubbings really get you somewhere. Stubborn stains and dirt actually do "come out in the wash".

For proof, take a look at the test panel above. It was walked on for a week. Then it was smeared with grease, stained with mercurochrome, streaked with pencil, crayon and lipstick, daubed with shoe blacking. *But despite this hard treatment, washing with soap and water left the panel looking as clean as when first painted.*

Now consider briefly this paint's many other advantages. It has all white-lead's characteristic richness, solidity and depth, a paint of unusual beauty. Because of its excellent sealing power, it stops suction and hides fire cracks.

Finally, this paint gives you all-round economy. It has high coverage (800 sq. ft. per gal. on smooth plaster), mixes quickly, spreads easily. Add up those three qualities, and you have *low first cost.* Then add long wear and *real cleanability*, and you have low cost per year.

NATIONAL LEAD COMPANY

111 Broadway, New York; 116 Oak St., Buffalo; 900 W. 18th St., Chicago; 659 Freeman Avenue, Cincinnati; 1213 West Third St., Cleveland; 722 Chestnut St., St. Louis; 2240 24th St., San Francisco; National-Boston Lead Co., 800 Albany St., Boston; National Lead & Oil Co. of Penna., 316 Fourth Ave., Pittsburgh; John T. Lewis & Bros. Co., Widener Bldg., Philadelphia.

13. Takes a scrubbing with a smile. This ad, depicting the Dutch Boy taking a bath, suggests that white lead paint can be scrubbed clean. An unstated message is that children can safely come in contact with lead paint. Source: *National Geographic* 48 (April 1937), 35.

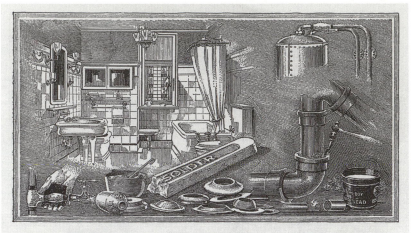

Lead helps to guard your health

YOU wouldn't live today in a house without an adequate plumbing system. For without modern plumbing, sickness might endanger your life.

Lead concealed in the walls and under the floors of many modern buildings helps to give the best sanitation.

Lead pipe centuries old

Lead, therefore, is contributing to the health, comfort, and convenience of people today as it did when Rome was a center of civilization. Lead water and drainage pipes more than 1800 years old have been found in exactly the condition they were in when laid.

In some cities today the law specifies that lead pipe alone may be used to bring water from street mains into the building.

In drainage systems are lead traps made of lead pipe bent into the shape of the letter S, so that a little water will stay in the bend and prevent gases which collect in the pipe from getting out through the house.

The malleability of lead also makes it easy to change the direction of any pipe through the use of lead bends.

Joining the pipes

A plumber easily "wipes" a joint or repairs a pipe leak with lead and tin solder. Because this alloy melts at the low temperature of 358 degrees it can be applied without melting the lead pipe, which melts at 620 degrees.

Lead is also poured into the flanges of pipe-joints to make them absolutely tight. Pipe threads are painted with white-lead or red-lead to make a tight connection. Where vibration or movement of pipes may loosen a poured joint, lead wool is used; lead shredded into threads is packed into the joint in a dense, compact mass.

Rubber gaskets and ball washers containing lead prevent leaking at joints and faucets.

Lead is used to beautify the modern bathroom. Red-lead and litharge, both lead oxides, are important ingredients in making the glossy white enamel covering the iron bodies of tub and basin and the glazed tile walls.

Lead in paint

While lead is invaluable in assuring comfort and proper sanitation, its best-known and most widespread use is as white-lead in paint. Such materials as wood would soon deteriorate unless protected with paint. And the paints that give the most thorough protection against the weather are based on white-lead.

The loss of invested capital through failure to protect the surface of property adequately has led property owners to paint frequently and well. As days and months go by, more and more of them are learning the wisdom of the phrase, "Save the surface and you save all." And they are using white-lead paint to prolong the lives of their houses.

Look for the Dutch Boy

NATIONAL LEAD COMPANY makes white-lead and sells it mixed with pure linseed oil, under the name and trade-mark of *Dutch Boy white-lead.* The figure of the Dutch Boy is reproduced on every keg and is a guarantee of exceptional purity.

Dutch Boy products also include red-lead, linseed oil, flatting oil, babbitt metals and solder.

More about lead

If you use lead, or think you might use it in any form, write to us for specific information.

NATIONAL LEAD COMPANY

New York, 111 Broadway; Boston, 131 State St.; Buffalo, 116 Oak St.; Chicago, 900 West 18th St.; Cincinnati, 659 Freeman Ave.; Cleveland, 820 West Superior Ave.; St. Louis, 722 Chestnut St.; San Francisco, 485 California St.; Pittsburgh, National Lead & Oil Co. of Pa., 316 Fourth Ave.; Philadelphia, John T. Lewis & Bros. Co., 437 Chestnut St.

14. Lead helps to guard your health. This ad shows the variety of uses to which lead is put in the modern home, and particularly its plumbing fixtures. It proudly points out that in "some cities today the law specifies that lead pipe alone may be used to bring water from street mains into the building." Source: *National Geographic* (ca. 1923).

Dutch Boy Painter advised readers that "the easiest way to get rid of germs that have nested in your house and around your premises is: Clean-up and Paint-up."[46] Promotions emphasized that unlike wallpaper, felt, and other common wall coverings of Victorian America, lead paint could be washed, making it both sanitary and attractive.[47]

Even as clinicians were documenting that lead was a potent poison, National Lead ran an ad in *National Geographic* magazine promoting the idea that "lead helps to guard your health." "Lead," the ad proclaimed, "concealed in the walls and under the floors of many modern buildings helps to give the best sanitation." "Lead pipe" was "centuries old" and was as important now as it was for making Rome "a center of civilization."[48]

Throughout the twenties and thirties, National Lead linked lead to the most modern and efficient symbols of medicine and public health. It promoted the use of lead-based paints for hospital interiors in *The Modern Hospital,* calling tinted paint "the doctor's assistant," because of its cheerful coloring and its ability to be washed with soap and water. The company assured customers that lead paint was "an ideal paint for hospital walls" because it did "not chip, peel or scale."[49] National Lead's Department of Color Research and Decoration had "already served more than 600 hospitals, recommending color treatments, supplying color samples, sketches and formulas."[50]

Paint would help patients feel better: "Walls finished in cheerful tints are sure to have a restful, beneficial influence on a patient who has not much else to look at during the long, weary days spent in bed," the ad proclaimed.[51] "Certain colors not only create pleasurable sensations but produce mental reactions which are reflected in more rapid physical recovery."[52] The modern hospital administrator was told over and over "that color today has an important place in reception rooms, wards, corridors, private rooms, and solariums." Further, each room, with its own special function, demanded special attention, "exactly the [right] tints or shades."[53]

Yet the use of lead paint in hospitals was not without its dissenters. Even some within the paint industry worried. George B. Heckel, a former publicist for the New Jersey Zinc Company[54] and the long-time editor of *Drugs, Oils and Paints,* a trade journal of the industry, wrote in 1921: "I stake my life and my reputation in hand by stating at the outset, that I think that lead, in any form, except for plumbing, has no place inside the doors of a hospital.... The proper white pigments for interior hospital painting are zinc oxide, lithopone ... and very probably newly introduced titanox.... All of these are white, permanent, and innocuous."[55]

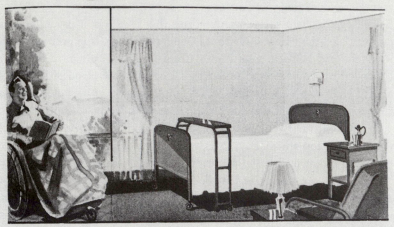

Sunshine stimulates...

GET SUNNY EFFECTS WITH COLOR

● Patients who show a tendency toward depression or morbidity during convalescence are frequently stimulated by the harmony and beauty found in the colors of nature.

The yellow sunlight...the cheering color combinations in flowers, in woodland scenes...when properly combined in hospital rooms, may play an important role in hastening recovery. Warm reds and yellows are recommended for patients of certain temperaments. Restful greens are frequently beneficial to nervous individuals.

Our Department of Color Research and Decoration has conducted exhaustive studies on the uses of color in hospitals and is equipped to apply this knowledge to the individual requirements of your hospital.

Superintendents and other hospital officials, as well as architects, are invited to consult this department regarding decorative problems. This service is offered without cost or obligation.

Address Department of Color Research and Decoration in care of our nearest branch.

NATIONAL LEAD COMPANY

New York, 111 Broadway   Buffalo, 116 Oak Street - Chicago, 900 West 18th Street — Cincinnati, 659 Freeman Avenue Cleveland, 820 West Superior Avenue   St.Louis, 722 Chestnut Street — San Francisco, 2240 24th Street — Boston, National-Boston Lead Co. 800 Albany Street — Pittsburgh, National Lead & Oil Co. of Pa., 316 Fourth Avenue — Philadelphia, John T. Lewis & Bros. Co., Widener Building.

15. Sunshine stimulates. This ad shows the cheering effects of a painted hospital interior. Source: *The Modern Hospital* 38 (February 1932), 15.

It is no surprise that the sole purpose of advertising is to promote a product and thereby increase revenues for a company. But the marketing of lead paint was particularly cynical in that it sought to turn the truth on its head. Lead was a toxin promoted as healthful. Though its reputation was soiled, it was touted for its white purity; though children were being poisoned, Dutch Boy was marketed to suggest that lead paint was benign for children, even fun.

In the years after World War I, National Lead employed military themes, depicting lead paint as a soldier vanquishing enemy germs. In one piece in National Lead's magazine, *Dutch Boy Painter,* titled "Why Paint Saves Lives," readers were told that "germs have killed a vastly greater number of people than have fallen in all the wars ever fought." Doctors and scientists had devoted their lives to the "wiping out of these enemies of man," the journal proclaimed, and "one of their most practical discoveries is that paint is a foe of germs." A hospital wall "need never afford a resting place for germs" when "every inch of surface in a hospital is painted." The lessons of the home could be learned by modern hospital administrators. But the opposite was also true: the hospital could train its patients in more modern ways of maintaining health. "The lesson learned by the modern hospital can well be put into practice in the home. In the kitchen where food is prepared, washable painted surfaces are unquestionably needed; sleeping and living rooms and particularly nurseries require the same protection. The ideal feature about paint in the home of course is the fact that the same operation produces a sanitary surface which beautifies."[56]

The theme of health continued to be used to promote leaded paint for the entire period between the wars. An article in *Dutch Boy Painter,* "How Paint Promotes Public Health," maintained that "a very real patriotic service can be performed by painters and dealers who get behind clean-up paint-up movements with their best efforts."[57] In 1943, Eagle-Picher advertised in *National Painters Magazine* that professional painters should use "four arguments with prospects—you'll find they really sell paint jobs." The fourth of these points was that "Eagle White Lead is just about the purest, safest, most fool-proof paint you or anybody else can use."[58] The industry appealed to government agencies to use lead paint. "Some means should be found for bringing steadily to the attention of various departments of the Government, . . . wherever competitively possible, the use of lead will be specified on Government projects."[59]

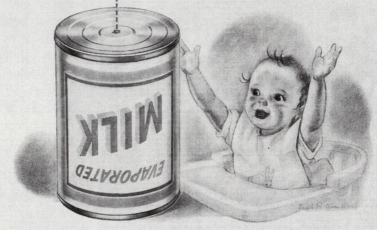

16. The drop of solder. Even after World War II, lead was promoted as a boon to children. Here, National Lead tells parents that lead solder is not a problem even in canning evaporated milk meant for babies. Source: *Saturday Evening Post* (February 23, 1946), 59.

THE LIA WHITE LEAD PROMOTION CAMPAIGN

During the 1930s and 1940s, as an increasing share of the pigment market was being taken over by lithopone- and titanium-based pigments, the lead industry realized that the stakes were getting higher and that a more coordinated approach was necessary. Even by the late 1920s the total consumption of lithopone was "eclipsing white lead,"[60] and by the 1930s and 1940s, mixed paints had slowly eroded the lead industry's share of the market because consumers had begun to respond to the convenience and ease of use of these paints. But to abandon lead as a pigment entailed more than a mere switch to a new product line. Because several of the leading companies, particularly National Lead and Eagle-Picher, were vertically integrated, it meant potentially giving up related interests in mines and smelters. The LIA made one last, gasping effort to reverse lead pigment's declining fortunes. It began the White Lead Promotion Campaign in 1938, on the eve of World War II.

The Lead Industries Association's White Lead Promotion Campaign was the largest activity ever undertaken by the LIA to increase sales of white lead in paint. According to the LIA, white lead in paint had always been a principal use of lead. Moreover, the amount of lead sold for other major products (storage batteries, cable coverings, buildings, etc.) was "dependent almost entirely upon economic and industrial factors which can be little affected by promotion and advertising."[61] Paint, on the other hand, could be promoted through direct appeals to consumers and painters and could therefore increase lead sales.

The problem for the lead industry was that mixed paints enjoyed several advantages over white lead: the mixed-paint industry outspent the white lead industry 10 to 1 in advertising and had many more salespeople in the field; mixed paint was more convenient and easy to use, as it required no complex measuring or mixing of white lead powder with linseed or flatting oil; and finally, mixed-paint manufacturers could boast that they used pigments other than white lead. Not only did the lead industry need to do something to increase sales, but it also had to address the "morale" problem in the industry resulting from the bad press lead was receiving. The LIA thus began a vigorous, coordinated advertising campaign to make the paint and lead industries realize that *"there was something to be said on behalf of white lead* after years of industry silence—and that *the people who produced white lead took pride in their product."*[62] Fearing that "white lead is also constantly subject to attack from the health standpoint,"[63] the LIA, taking a page out of other corporations' public-relations efforts in the 1920s and 1930s to recast public views of big business, focused much of its efforts on improving the image of white lead.[64] "It was the feeling of the lead industry . . . that unless something was done to at least arrest the rate of downward tendency as far as white lead was concerned, its whole future in the paint industry would become seriously, if not permanently, jeopardized."[65] The LIA argued, "White-lead will continue to lose its position in the paint industry unless some effort is devised to offset competitive attacks and to acquaint the public widely with the merits of the product."[66] The White Lead Promotion Campaign was "an important nation-wide effort to increase the consumption of white-lead in the United States and to combat the substitution of inferior pigments for white-lead."[67]

Part of the industry's task was to influence competing paint manufacturers (the zinc and titanium manufacturers) to stop attacking lead. Manufacturers who had abandoned or never used lead pigments, the LIA charged, were emphasizing the dangers of lead to the detriment of lead paint and pigment companies. The LIA claimed, "Prior to the initiation of this campaign white lead came in for specific attack in the advertising and literature of many paint manufacturers." It had, in its files, many examples of these attacks by "nationally known paint manufacturers." The campaign was judged a success by the LIA because it had "been able to induce several large paint manufacturers of national repute, to withdraw and cease all detrimental attacks of this kind."[68]

Contradictory pressures faced the lead industry as it pursued the increasingly untenable promotion of a dangerous product. On the one hand, it publicly proclaimed the value and safety of its product. On the other hand, industry privately worried about the legal ramifications of promoting a poison, especially the possibility of lawsuits from consumers made ill by paint and its ingredients. In July 1939 the Executive Committee of the National Paint, Varnish and Lacquer Association (NPVLA), a trade group representing pigment and paint manufacturers (some also in the LIA),[69] reported on a meeting of its Toxic Materials Committee at which a letter had been prepared for distribution to its Class A members about its "responsibility to the public . . . and the protection of the industry itself with respect to the use of toxic materials in the industry's products."[70] In a memo marked "CONFIDENTIAL—Not for Publication" and which the NPVLA said "should be given no other publicity," the association informed its members that "the vital factor concerning toxic materials is to intelligently safeguard the public. People may feel safer in buying materials whose danger they know rather than materials unknown to them." The committee's members believed that manufacturers should apply "every precautionary measure in manufacturing, in selling and in use where toxic materials are likely to or do enter a product." They noted that "children's toys, equipment, furniture, etc. are not the only consideration." They warned NPVLA members that toxic materials "may enter the body through the lungs ... through the skin, or through the mouth or stomach." They specifically noted that lead compounds, such as white lead, red lead, litharge, or lead chromates "may be considered as toxic if they find their way into the stomach." They reproduced for their members a set of legal principles established by the Manufacturing Chemists' Association (MCA), the trade association of the chemical industry, regarding the labeling of dangerous products. The first legal principle was, "A manufacturer who puts out a dangerous article or substance without accompanying it with a warning as to its dangerous properties is ordinarily liable for any damage which results from such failure to warn."[71]

The MCA suggested that warnings be included even when a product was widely understood to be dangerous. Further, it noted, "The manufacturer ... must know the qualities of his product and cannot escape liability on the ground that he did not know it to be dangerous." The NPVLA called on its members to make a "sincere effort in taking advantage of every possible precaution in the use of toxic materials in manufacturing, selling and in use."[72] The next year, another trade group, the Federation of Paint and Varnish Production Clubs, acknowledged the industry's responsibilities. "Now there is one obligation that I think we really have, not only to our worker in our plant, but to our customers. We ship out into the field various things that are intoxicant or dangerous if not properly used. Good sales service should see that our customer is educated along the lines of prevention of sickness and accident while consuming our products. The manufacturer must educate the public. He can't get out of it. It is just as important to do that as to make a good product."[73]

LIA members were actually part of this talk about responsibility to the public at the very moment that the LIA was promoting the use of white lead more vigorously than ever.[74] The LIA even promoted white lead among farmers and their children by starting a project in cooperation with 4-H Clubs. "A trial painting project had been started with Iowa's 4-H Clubs which are important key organizations for young farmers, and that this would probably spread to other states," campaign planners reported.[75] The LIA also sought to expand its markets in urban areas. In mid-October 1940 the LIA reported, "In the course of his work with government officials in the neighborhood of New York City, our representative also conducted a survey of painting practices of 36 real estate developments. A separate report of this survey has been sent to interested members."[76] Sales representative Seldon Brown reported to the LIA of his success with the Brooklyn Brewcourt Management Company: "Through a demonstration of the true costs of WL [white lead] as compared to MP [mixed paint] for interiors, Mr. Kilman plans to use WL on several jobs and probably all future work."[77]

In 1940 the campaign was expanded to encourage municipal, county, and state institutions to use white lead paint. Two representatives of the LIA, Seldon Brown and W. L. Frazee, traveled throughout the country for this purpose. Brown specifically marketed white lead paint for public schools, noting whether institutions he visited used mixed paint or white lead on both exterior and interior walls. The LIA claimed that Brown made a total of 427 calls in his first two years on the job, of which 380 were to state, county, and miscellaneous institutions. Brown would identify the person responsible for buying paint for the city or community, then the person in charge of buying paint for the school system. Brown was particularly insistent on pushing white lead for interior use. The superintendent for maintenance of Seattle's public school system was "completely sold on white lead for exteriors, but can't see [the] value of white lead for interiors and [I] was not able to convince him. It was suggested that a demonstration of white lead and flat wall paint be run for this department by a lead salesman."[78]

In Dearborn, Michigan, Brown visited John Whitehead, the Board of Education's maintenance supervisor, who informed Brown that "the Board of Education gave up using white lead some years ago." Brown informed the LIA that "they were considerably impressed by our WL data and agreed to try it on interiors on the strength of this information."[79] A day later, Brown contacted the business manager for the Highland Park, Michigan, Board of Education, John Smith, who "was very appreciative of the information we gave him last summer. [He] is completely sold on WL for exteriors and as a result of our data is now experimenting with WL on interiors."[80] In Lansing, Michigan, Brown reported that Harry Chamberlain, business manager for the Board of Education, told him that the school system was "using a MP which they claimed betters WL for interior work by their own tests." Brown informed the LIA that the board would "consider running further tests due to our data in favor of WL on interiors."[81]

It is difficult to understand how the LIA could send Brown and Frazee to promote the use of white lead in schools and other public buildings at a time when so much evidence existed that lead caused serious illness and sometimes death—particularly in children. The fact was that the LIA had been extremely successful in its efforts to keep the information about lead's potential dangers out of the public eye by challenging medical reports of lead poisoning and by portraying lead in its advertising campaign as a benign substance. Although other pigments were gaining in popularity because of their lower costs and greater ease of application, hard sells emphasizing lead paints' durability and long-term cost effectiveness, whether true or not, could still be successful.

Brown also reported on his ability to sell the virtues of white lead to those who knew little about it. In Flint, Michigan, the superintendent of maintenance for the Board of Education, William Barclay, was "very interested in our description of the qualities of interior WL. [He] said that he thought that WL was going out because he has heard so little about it. [He knew] nothing about WL for interiors. [But he] plans to run comparative tests between WL and present MP used on interiors."[82] In Kansas City, Missouri, Frazee was particularly proud of his work in convincing contractors and the school board superintendent to use white lead. "I called on a number of contractors as well as the superintendent...whom I have known for a great many years. I made some samples with white lead for him some three years ago and they have been using lead for the past two years and will use it again this year. They use it entirely on their interior wall work and are having wonderful luck." The Lead Industries Association also worked through the New Deal's National Youth Administration "in the preparation of a teacher's training manual covering exterior and interior painting on all types of construction." They expected this manual to "be used as text material by the 8,000 vocational agricultural instructors in high schools throughout the country."[83]

The LIA went directly to cities, hotels, and health departments. W. L. Frazee visited Little Rock, Arkansas, where he convinced a hotel manager to have "his entire hotel, inside and out, done with lead and lead reducing oil."[84] In Poplar Bluff, Missouri, he visited the manager of the "leading hotel," who "informed me that he had seen the white lead job in the Little Rock hotel and was now having the entire interior of his hotel painted with white lead, and had also started to redecorate his hotel at Sackston, Missouri."[85] In Pierce County, Washington, LIA representative Frazee visited the health department, where he "explained properties of interior white lead paint, stressing sanitary aspects of a highly durable and washable surface. This department is frequently asked for painting specifications, but have [*sic*] always felt that no brand name could be mentioned.... However, they say that they may be able to recommend Lead Industries Association white lead specifications as they mention no one company's product."[86]

In general, the White Lead Promotion Campaign consisted of an advertising campaign, the placement of articles promoting the use of white lead in trade and popular journals, and mailings to paint dealers around the country. National Lead extolled the cooperative nature of the campaign; it was "sponsored by the miner, smelter, refiner and white-lead manufacturer members of the Lead Industries Association.... A series of large-size advertisements in such widely read magazines as the *Saturday Evening Post, Colliers, American Home, Country Gentleman,* and *Better Homes and Gardens* will bring the white-lead story to the public in general and to home-owners in particular." The LIA was proud of the scope of the magazine campaign, for it would produce "67,570,526 separate messages that will be carried in the publications named."[87] The initial copy of the advertisement featured a miner as the industry spokesman, but a housepainter gradually replaced him. The ads originally promoted only white lead paste (or in dry form), but they later pushed ready-to-use and high-lead-content white paints as well.[88]

For the LIA the benefits of the campaign were not simply increased sales in the short run but "the good will it is building up for lead in general," association secretary Felix Wormser reported. "I have always felt that the cultivation of good will for our metal and publicity about the indispensable work it does for mankind is something that lead needs more than other common metals because lead in many forms is constantly under attack on account of its toxic qualities. Our campaign helps to meet this issue." Wormser added, "It is also noteworthy that attacks on white lead, which was one of the reasons for undertaking our campaign, have declined greatly and that more articles of national interest, specifically endorsing white lead, have appeared in the press during the last year than for any period to my recollection."[89]

Despite the best efforts of the members of the LIA, changes in paint technology were working against them. For many generations the industry had counted on the fact that consumers depended on the skills of painters trained in the exacting process of mixing, matching, and hand-painting delicate moldings, woodwork, and other exposed surfaces throughout the home. As fashions changed and large surfaces free of wood detailing, fabric, and wallpapers became popular, there was less need for skilled painters. Spray painting became feasible, and less-skilled workers could do the job. Homeowners who began fixing up their own houses became increasingly interested in ready-mixed paints (most of which contained little, if any, lead), that required few of the skills previously necessary.

For this reason the industry sought to capture more of the ready-mixed paint market by promoting ready-mixed lead paints in small quantities. It was "one of the fundamental objectives of the campaign . . . to make white lead available in convenience or ready-mixed form to the consuming public everywhere." The LIA applauded the "recent decision of the National Lead company to join an increasing list of paint manufacturers, (stimulated by our campaign) in producing a ready-mixed white lead paint for nationwide distribution."[90]

White lead was made available in more and more colors in prepared paint form. In addition, homeowner magazines ran white lead articles and in some instances asked the LIA for ready-written articles. One overall result of the campaign was improved relations with professional painters and contractors. The LIA asserted, perhaps wishfully, "A ground swell of white lead interest had been set in motion in important places affecting the consuming habits of the next generation. Vocational school instructors, 4-H club leaders and the like have eagerly received white lead promotional material and expressed a genuine desire for more."[91]

In 1941 Wormser reported to the LIA's annual meeting that "anxiety about [lead's] use . . . remains serious for our industry [for] hardly a day passes but what this office has to devote some attention to lead poisoning." He added, "The problem is how to obtain a better press for our products is indeed a troublesome one. Our promotional work and especially our national advertising helps to build up good-will for our metal." The LIA also acknowledged, "We have continued to keep our members posted on the most significant literature currently published about lead poisoning."[92] Even during World War II, when restrictions were placed on linseed oil and containers used to produce and distribute lead paint, the LIA continued to extol lead's virtues in paint.[93]

As late as 1952 the LIA promoted the usefulness of white lead as both an exterior and an interior covering. The new edition of the LIA book *Lead in Modern Industry* asserted that "white lead adds more desirable qualities to paint than any other white pigment and has practically no undesirable qualities to nullify its advantages." The book continued by saying that "the profitable application of white lead . . . is not confined to exterior use. Pure white lead paints can be utilized to advantage for interior decoration, particularly in public and traditional buildings where elaborate decoration is used and it is very expensive and inconvenient to repaint often."[94] For the first time it included a section on the "Safe Handling of Lead and

Its Products," noting that lead poisoning could occur when lead gained "entrance into the human system in measurable quantity" either through inhalation of vapors, fumes or dust or ingestion of lead compounds introduced into the mouth on the fingers." It maintained that "ingestion is by far the less important [danger] and is most often associated with children chewing on objects coated with paints containing lead." The chapter allayed readers' fears by maintaining that "since most inside paints and paints used by manufacturers on children's furniture and toys contain no lead, a hazard usually exists only if children are allowed to chew outside painted surfaces, like porch railings, or if parents inadvertently repaint furniture with outside house paint." But it failed to mention that older coats of paint were likely to contain lead and thus present a hazard. It commented on the condition of pica (which it defined as "abnormal appetite in children") and teething as possible causes for injury.[95]

Even Manfred Bowditch, who became the LIA's director of health and safety in 1948 after a long and distinguished career at the Massachusetts Division of Industrial Hygiene, appeared embarrassed by the level of misinformation emanating from his association. Writing to the Ethyl Corporation's consultant, Robert Kehoe, about the new edition of the industry's flagship publication, *Lead in Modern Industry*, he apologized for the virtual absence in the book of information about the health hazards of lead and implied that this was because of the resistance of various members of the lead industry to acknowledge lead's hazards. "Before yielding to the quite natural impulse to comment caustically on the meager section" on the toxicity of lead, he begged Kehoe, "please consider that the volume represents the thinking of our 70-odd member companies." His only defense was that "the book which it supersedes, published in 1931, made no mention of the toxicity of the metal which is our bread and butter."[96]

After the intense publicity generated by popular and professional articles, public health department studies, and internal correspondence objecting to the use of leaded paint for interiors, the LIA finally began to withdraw support for the promotion of lead in interior paints. In December 1952, the LIA decided to "discontinue all activities of the Association relating to the promotion of white lead in house paints." "It was apparently felt that the economic obstacles faced by white lead pigments nullify whatever technical advantages these pigments enjoy and thus further expenditures of money by the Association are not justified."[97]

The LIA's decision to cease direct promotion of leaded paint for interior surfaces was one step of the industry's broader acknowledgment, however halting, of lead paint's dangers to children and the consequential risk that the lead paint industry might not survive. Popular and scientific attention to the dangers of lead made it untenable to continue to promote lead paint. So did the move toward regulation by departments of public health and their officials, who began pushing more intensely for warning labels and outright bans of the use of lead in interior paints. Now the LIA, although no longer promoting lead paint for interior use, shifted its energy to fight any regulation that it perceived to be inimical to its interests.

Once again, it was the health studies from Baltimore that provided the most startling statistics on childhood lead poisoning and prompted other cities to conduct studies, which in turn led to regulatory activity. In 1949, Maryland's Toxic Finishes Law "made it unlawful to sell toys and playthings, including children's furniture, finished with any material containing 'lead or other substance of a poisonous nature from contact with which children may be injuriously affected,' unless such articles are so labeled as to show that the finish contains lead or other poisonous substance." The Baltimore Health Department in the May issue of "Health News" warned parents to "not buy paint for indoor use unless it is free from lead."[98] Immediately the LIA challenged the Maryland law by holding four "conferences with governmental authorities in Maryland." It claimed success for its efforts. "The campaign to remove this 1949 enactment from the statute books of the state was brought to a successful conclusion" when the governor signed the repeal, the association trumpeted to its members.[99] This was "among the most important activities" because the law was seen as "unworkable and a hardship on members and others," the LIA said.[100] The approach that the industry favored placed the burden for preventing lead poisoning directly on the family. "The only seemingly feasible means of coping with the childhood plumbism problem is that of parental education," it argued.[101]

In 1951, Baltimore's health commissioner adopted a regulation that stated: "No paint shall be used for interior painting of any dwelling or dwelling unit or any part thereof unless the paint is free of any lead pigment."[102] The next year the LIA, acknowledging that lead was viewed as a toxic substance, conducted a survey of "State and Territorial Warning Labeling Laws," which they sent to all state health and labor departments. The reply from Arkansas, which had no warning or label laws, was telling. The director of the Arkansas Division of Industrial Hygiene wrote that the office had received "information concerning apparent epidemics of lead poisoning among children which have occurred in the Baltimore City area. We intend to inform all our state and county health workers, and our physicians, to bring to the attention of the public the potential hazard of using lead based paints on children's furniture and toys, and on the interior of homes."[103] During this time the LIA was seeking to modify and repeal state regulations and other restrictions on the use of lead paint.[104]

The refrain from the lead industry—that childhood plumbism was not a serious problem—had grown old by the 1950s. J. Julian Chisolm Jr., a young physician associated with Johns Hopkins University Hospital, had much firsthand experience with the group of children who by the mid-1950s were unfortunately labeled "lead heads" by the young residents at the hospital. Chisolm, soon to emerge as a major figure in lead research, took issue with the industry's casual attitude toward what was obviously a serious medical problem affecting hundreds of children in the Baltimore area. "It is believed that at present the ingestion of lead-containing paint flakes is the most common source from which children obtain excessive quantities of lead," he noted in 1956. In his study of children at the Harriet Lane Home, he had inspected sources of lead contamination and found, like physican Kenneth Blackfan over thirty years before, that the "leading sources of lead were windowsills and frames, interior walls, including painted paper and painted plaster, door frames, furniture and cribs." Throughout the "dilapidated dwellings" where young children lived, Chisolm found that "flaking leaded paint is readily accessible." And he took umbrage that the industry blamed parents for the tragedy. "While the responsibility of parents to protect their children from environmental hazards is not denied, no mother can reasonably be expected to prevent the repetitive ingestion of a few paint chips when these are readily accessible."[105]

Also in Baltimore, Huntington Williams, the city's commissioner of health, had begun looking beyond the convulsions, seizures, and deaths of children. He noted, "Unrecognized plumbism, lead poisoning, in children may explain many obscure nervous conditions and convulsions of undetermined etiology." His conclusion: "Lead poisoning is cumulative."[106] New problems such as mental retardation, behavioral disorders, and learning difficulties were on the horizon and, as the LIA noted, "as our hygiene activities have expanded, the magnitude of our industry's health problems become more and more evident."[107] The daily press was playing a greater role in bringing lead to the attention of the general public. In one year the LIA collected "nearly 500 newspaper clippings featuring lead poisoning, often in sizable headlines." While it is unclear how many of these dealt with children, the LIA noted (internally) that "childhood lead poisoning continued to be a major problem."[108] Yet, despite its systematic attempt to collect this material, the industry still opposed warning consumers of the danger that the product posed to children.

Baltimore was particularly vexing because the local health department had been so assiduous in reporting and following cases. At one point in 1949, Manfred Bowditch complained in a letter that "these young Baltimore paint eaters are a real headache."[109] By the early 1950s, "the alarming number of cases of alleged lead poisoning, particularly in children, which are being reported" led the LIA to systematically attend "many meetings of organizations dealing with our own health problems." These included meetings of the American Medical Association, the American Public Health Association, the Greater New York Safety Council, and the National Safety Council.[110]

In a summary of his activities in 1952, Bowditch called childhood lead poisoning "a major 'headache' and a source of much adverse publicity." He counted 197 reports of lead poisoning in nine cities, of which 40 were fatal, although he noted that this was an "incomplete" estimate, especially for New York City. In New York, 44 cases were reported, of which 14 were fatal.[111] Between 1951 and 1953, according to George M. Wheatley of the American Academy of Pediatrics, as reported in the *New York Times,* "there were 94 deaths and 165 cases of childhood lead poisoning . . . in New York, Chicago, Cincinnati, St. Louis, and Baltimore."[112]

The LIA was caught in a bind. On the one hand it possessed numerous reports from health departments demonstrating the widespread nature of the lead paint hazard. On the other hand, the LIA was still fighting a rearguard action to show that the number of cases was exaggerated. To continue to do this, Bowditch confided to an industry colleague, would be "prohibitively expensive and time consuming."[113] Bowditch did not dispute that childhood lead poisoning existed as a result of children ingesting lead-based paint. But rather than concentrate on how to prevent lead poisoning—a first step toward which would be the warning of parents—Bowditch believed the LIA should focus on "securing more accurate diagnosis of lead poisoning or face the likelihood of widespread governmental prohibition of the use of lead paints on dwellings."[114] Robert Kehoe admitted in a personal letter that the problem was an issue not of diagnostics, but of the paint itself. If the elimination of lead paint "for all inside decoration in the household and in the environment of young children . . . is not done voluntarily by a wise industry concerned to handle its own business properly, it will be accomplished ineffectually and with irrelevant difficulties and disadvantages through legislation."[115]

By the mid-1950s the LIA was under siege.[116] There was an over-whelming amount of medical evidence concerning the dangers to children of lead-based paint. Reports of lead poisoning of children flowed from Baltimore and other cities. There was a plethora of articles in popular publications concerning the dangers of lead-based paint to children. Internal correspondence from leading lead authorities around the country declared that lead paint was a serious hazard. Even in the face of all this, the industry still refused to remove lead from paint or to warn consumers of the dangers of lead.

Many lead pigment manufacturers, however, had already developed new product lines of leadless or low-lead-content paints. National Lead promoted two lines of paint for interiors: one of them, known as the "black and yellow line" (for the design of the cans the paint was packaged in), contained the traditional white lead pigments and was earmarked for professional painters. The "blue and white line," containing mixed paints, was aimed at consumers. Its brand name, Wonsover, enticed homeowners with the ease of doing their own painting, implicitly promising it would cover in one coat. Many companies had produced mixed paints for decades, but for the National Lead Company to market them under the Dutch Boy brand was a dramatic concession, particularly because the company had long fought to maintain "pure white lead" as the industry standard. Even this concession was not total, however. Some of the new line also contained lead, though in far lower amounts than the traditional line,[117] despite Wormser's public assurance in 1946 that "so far as white inside paint is concerned there is no lead in it."[118] Likewise, in the early 1950s, Sherwin-Williams sold "House Paint" labeled "For Exterior or Interior Use" that contained from 14 percent to 23 percent lead carbonate and/or lead sulfate.[119]

The development of new mixed paints came amidst the growing recognition among lead producers that the market for lead was changing dramatically. A mere twenty years earlier, in 1929, white lead in paint accounted for 12 percent of lead's market while lead for gasoline, tetraethyl lead, was "a fraction of a percent." By the late 1940s the industry was much less dependent upon paint as an outlet for its product, relying after the mid-1920s on storage batteries instead. By 1949, white lead pigment accounted for less than 3 percent of the market, while tetraethyl lead consumed 11 percent and its use was increasing. Put differently, in 1929 the per capita consumption of lead in the United States was 15.9 pounds, with 2 pounds coming from lead paint and less than 0.1 pound from gasoline. By 1949, Americans were consuming about 11.6 pounds per person, and of that less than a third of a pound came from paint and 1.3 pounds from gasoline. Over the next generation, the emphasis of the lead industry in general and of the LIA specifically shifted to promoting the use of lead in gasoline and generally fighting a rear-guard, and ultimately doomed, action to maintain what remained of the lead paint industry.[120]

In 1953 the LIA began working with the American Standards Association (ASA), a group made up of representatives from the American Academy of Pediatrics, the American Medical Association, the American Hospital Association, the American Public Health Association as well as the LIA, the NPVLA, the Association of Casualty and Surety Companies, among others, to develop a voluntary standard to "Minimize Hazards to Children." A subcommittee made up of representatives of the LIA, National Lead Company, DeVoe and Raynolds Company, Sapolin Paints, DuPont, New York State Department of Health, the American Academy of Pediatrics, and the New York City Department of Health began to draft a standard that, "would not cause the paint industry any trouble."[121] A representative of Union Carbide chaired it, and its alternates were representatives of Sherwin-Williams, Glidden, and Benjamin Franklin Paint.[122] The ASA standard that was adopted reflected a growing consensus that paint used for interiors or any surface that children might chew on, should not contain more than 1% lead of its total weight. John H. Folger, who represented the NPVLA on the ASA Committee, told the NPVLA that the standard was "very innocuous."[123] The new standard would be used to combat local legislation, both in New York and elsewhere, that was seen by the industry as more stringent.

It was not until the early 1950s that the industry began to pay serious attention to another issue—the question of labeling lead paint as a hazardous material. In the spring of 1953, following reports of dozens of cases of lead poisoning in New York City, the city's Health Department began considering legislation to require warning labels that would identify lead as a "poison" or "dangerous."[124] Throughout 1954, a variety of city, state, professional, and industry groups addressed the issue of what type of warning New York City should require on lead paint sold in the city. In general, the city officials wanted warning labels on any paint containing more than 1 percent lead. In May 1954 the Department of Health of New York City "asked that a draft of a proposed sanitary code change be submitted to it in connection with paints and coatings containing excessive amounts of lead." It proposed the following wording: "No person shall have, keep or offer for sale in the City of New York any liquid coating material or paint which contains lead compounds of which the lead content

... is in excess of 1%." It also required a warning label: "Warning: This paint contains lead—unsafe—poisonous—and should not be used to paint children's toys or furniture, or interior surfaces in dwelling units which might be chewed by children."[125]

Some of the pigment manufacturers reacted negatively to the proposed warning. In 1953 and 1954 the LIA worked closely with the NPVLA to, in the LIA's words, "combat these moves" by the city.[126] Paul Whitford, a manager in the Eagle-Picher Company, wrote to the NPVLA that "the proposed section of the Sanitary Code, . . . demands the immediate and concerted effort of our committee to prevent the enactment of this legislation. The adoption of this proposal by the Department of Health by the city of New York, places an unprecedented stigma upon the Paint Industry by demanding the labeling of innumerable shelf goods and specialty products as unsuitable for use."[127] (Four years later, in 1958, when New York City was considering banning the use of lead paint on the interiors of buildings and apartments, Whitford would state that warning labels are "certainly in order and if properly enforced should remove much of the stigma and unfavorable publicity within the industry arising from the nutritional deficiencies of children."[128]) The NPVLA pushed for a very different warning that emphasized paint's flammability as well as its dangers from ingestion. While explicitly saying, "Do not apply on toys, furniture or interior surfaces which might be chewed by children," the word "poisonous" was conspicuously absent from its proposal.[129] The American Medical Association suggested in September of that year that the following warning be put on all paints with lead: "WARNING: this paint contains an amount of lead which may be POISONOUS and should not be used to paint children's toys or furniture or interior surfaces in dwelling units which might be chewed by children."[130]

On October 29, 1954, the New York City Department of Health adopted a warning label for paints with lead, but without the words "poison" or "poisonous." The NPVLA noted in a confidential internal document that although "originally the word 'poison' was proposed for the label of paints containing lead," it had been removed and the final wording was the "result of cooperation between the New York City Health Department officials and representatives of the New York [Paint Varnish and Lacquer Association] and National Paint, Varnish, and Lacquer Association."[131]

The LIA would also claim some credit: "The initial proposal of the New York City Health Department to require a poison label on all paints containing any lead whatsoever was ultimately modified through the establishment, at our instance, of a committee of the American Standards Association which evolved a standard permitting up to one per cent of lead in paints used on surfaces which 'might be chewed by children,' thus allowing the inclusion of lead dryers in such paints. The 'poison' wording was also modified."[132] They were particularly proud that "modification of the New York City lead paint labeling regulation was secured by means of American Standard Z66.1, prepared by a committee of the American Standards Association, sponsored by the Lead Industries Association."[133]

The industry's activities in New York paralleled its broader strategy throughout the nation. The National Paint, Varnish, and Lacquer Association was particularly concerned because "there is much agitation by various groups throughout the United States which could result in conflicting legislation by individual states and municipalities on methods of labeling paint products."[134] T. J. McDowell, of the NPVLA, proposed a "Suggested Course of Action" regarding labeling laws in which he reviewed the pressure that had been exerted on industry to become more responsible: "The legislators from various states are constantly being contacted by pressure groups to pass a law—any law will do—to eliminate this hazard to our children.... It appears that the best course to pursue from the standpoint of the industries interested in the use of lead as a pigment and otherwise is to launch a campaign of education directed at the legislators to forestall any further unnecessary legislation, at the pressure groups who are promoting the passage of these laws, at the user and sellers of these products so that the proper use is made of them and the hazards reduced to a minimum and most important of all at the general public to remove the false impressions from their minds and educate them in the proper use, the precautions to be taken and the real causes of these unfortunate occurrences."[135] Labeling was to be a last resort and then only on a voluntary basis.

But the LIA made it clear it would not concede any action it did not need to. Bowditch told Felix Wormser, now an assistant secretary in the Department of Interior in the Eisenhower administration, that he had made every effort to cultivate the "good will" of public health officials "and get them into a receptive frame of mind as to our viewpoint." Bowditch bragged that he believed that his efforts had "paid off, as, for example, in Chicago, where we have been able to stave off a paint labeling regulation like that here in New York."[136] (It bears mentioning that Wormser's allegience to the lead industry was unaffected by his new position in the Department of Interior. On receiving the appointment, he wrote to the president of St. Joseph Lead that in his new position he could "do more for the country, for the President, and for my company."[137] In 1957 he resigned under a cloud as it was revealed that St. Joseph Lead Company, to which he was returning, had benefited from government largesse during his tenure. In 1962 new charges were raised—that Assistant Secretary Wormser had unnecessarily bought huge quantities of lead and zinc for the federal government, although none was needed. The lead companies received a windfall while the lead market had been sagging.[138])

In 1958 New York City proposed a revision of its regulation of the use of lead paint containing more than 1 percent lead, prohibiting its use on interior walls, ceilings, or windowsills of any apartment or room, tenement, multiple dwelling, or one- or two-family home. (This was passed in 1959 and went into effect in 1960.) The reaction of officials in the NPVLA was predictably ambivalent. E. P. Hubschmitt, on the NPVLA's Subcommittee on Uniform Labeling, continued to maintain, despite the mounds of evidence, that the ingestion of lead was not a serious hazard. In a review of the proposed code he told members that "many persons of note, . . . question the hazardous effects of lead by ingestion. I can recall that there is in fact very little evidence, indeed, in the medical reports to support instances of death by ingestion of lead."[139]

Even though the proportion of lead in paint had been dramatically reduced in the early 1950s as titanium, zinc, and water-based vinyl coverings took over a larger share of the market, the industry continued to be vigilant to any attempts to label its product a danger.[140] When forced to accept the reality of warning labels on paint products, the association knew labels were better than other kinds of regulation: "Every effort is being made to confine . . . regulatory measures . . . to the field of warning labels, which, as applied to paints are obviously less detrimental to our interests than would be any legislation of a prohibitory nature."[141] In 1958 there was what the association called a "veritable wave" of precautionary labeling legislation proposals. The NPVLA maintained that "watching for adverse legislation in our many states is an important part of our work and one in which the help of our members . . . is again and earnestly asked."[142]

Even through the mid-1950s the industry continued to deny responsibility for a situation that had been developing for nearly a half century. Its long-term claim that the industry had done everything it could to be responsible seemed fatuous in view of the fact that the emergency wards and hospitals of cities and communities were treating more and more children poisoned by lead.

Nevertheless, the LIA still reacted to reports of sickened children by blaming the victims and their families. In 1956 Bowditch, in a private communication to Felix Wormser after an article appeared in *Parade* magazine, remarked that "aside from the kids that are poisoned ... it's a serious problem from the viewpoint of adverse publicity." The basic problem was "slums," and to deal with that issue it was necessary "to educate the parents. But most of the cases are in Negro and Puerto Rican families, and how," Bowditch wondered, "does one tackle that job?"[143] Bowditch was a bit more discreet in his statements to the LIA's general membership. At the association's 1957 annual meeting, he argued that "the major source of trouble is the flaking of lead paint in the ancient slum dwellings of our older cities"—though in saying this he obscured the fact that lead had been a major component of the paint applied to buildings as recently as a decade before. "The problem of lead poisoning in children will be with us for as long as there are slums," he argued.[144] But once again, as Wormser had done before him, he absolved the LIA of responsibility, arguing that the real problem lay with ignorant children and parents. "Because of the high death rate, the frequency of permanent brain damage in the survivors, and the intelligence level of the slum parents, it seems destined to remain as important and as difficult as any with which we have to deal."[145] But who was responsible for this condition and how could it be addressed? Bowditch was not optimistic: "until we can find means to (a) get rid of our slums, and (b) educate the relatively ineducable parent, the problem will continue to plague us."[146]

Despite the assertions of the industry that lead poisoning would vanish when "ancient slums" were replaced with newer dwellings, evidence that lead was still in new paint continued to appear. New York's Department of Health "disclosed [in 1973] that ten companies are selling highly leaded paints in violation of the New York City Health Code." In a survey that tested "one hundred and thirty-eight cans of interior paint from 23 companies ... for lead content, twenty-four cans from 10 companies were found to be highly leaded."[147] Even painted toys continued to have lead in significant quantities. In 1957, Robert Kehoe analyzed toys from a variety of companies, including Mattel and Marx, two of the nation's largest manufacturers, and found that the paints that one Chicago toy manufacturer used on its red trailer trucks contained over 34 percent lead pigment. Mattel's Jack in the Box was painted with red paint containing 10 percent lead, and Marx's red fire truck had 3.75 percent lead.[148]

It seems that no amount of evidence, no health statistics, no public outrage could get the industry to regard the fact that its lead paint was killing and poisoning children as anything but a public relations disaster. Until the end it wore moral blinders and obsessed over bad publicity rather than address the problem. By 1959, when childhood lead poisoning had clearly entered the popular culture through articles in *Parade* and television news programs on CBS, the LIA was still engaged in efforts to restrict public attention to the issue. When the LIA learned that a popular television program, *Highway Patrol,* had in one of its episodes a reference to lead poisoning in a young boy, the association's representatives convinced the producers to eliminate the offending reference. "We now have their verbal agreement to eliminate all reference to the toxicity of lead in an episode of the series which reflected no credit on the metal or on the producers themselves," the LIA proudly announced in its quarterly report.[149]

The negative publicity about lead paint was of concern because it "hurt our business" and had resulted in "thousands of items of unfavorable publicity every year," the industry association argued. Bad publicity "may even mean that your product won't be used at all because your potential customer doesn't want the problems that the use of lead may involve."[150] Yet the association continued to insist that childhood lead poisoning was (1) primarily a problem of the eastern slums, and (2) a result of the lack of education, racial inferiority, and inattentiveness of poor people. "This is particularly true since most cases of lead poisoning today are in children, and anything sad that happens to a child is meat for newspaper editors and is gobbled up by the public." The LIA's response to the crisis was to persuade government agencies to relax government regulations. "We were largely responsible for the increase of one-third in the maximum permissible concentration of lead dust and fumes that became effective a couple of years ago," the LIA trumpeted. They worried that a lawsuit brought by a tenant in Milwaukee, if successful, could lead to the banning of lead pipe and the loss of the sale of thousands of tons of lead a year, and therefore worked with the defense to defeat the suit.[151] Smaller cities began to test their own children and, as with the lead poisoning epidemic historically, the more they looked, the more poisonings they found. The LIA acknowledged that there had been "something of a change" in its understanding of the eastern and big-city nature of the epidemic as it began to find reports of childhood lead poisoning in rural communities and small cities as well. Lead poisoning was no longer just a problem of "the slums of our older and larger cities," but was now appearing also in Albany, New York, Springfield, Massachusetts, Covington, Kentucky, and Gastonia, North Carolina.[152]

The lead industry had lost its battle to preserve the image of lead pigment as harmless, especially as the Civil Rights movement and the beginning of the War on Poverty shifted public and professional attention to the rights of the poor and those exploited by industry. Community activists began to demand change in the way government reacted to the dangers of lead.[153] Throughout the late 1960s, in city after city, community groups demonstrated for screening programs, popular education, and housing reform in order to defuse the racially and economically charged issue of childhood lead poisoning.[154] Periodic high-profile deaths of small children who had ingested paint chips, and exposés such as Jack Newfield's *Village Voice* newspaper article, "Silent Epidemic in the Slums," heightened public and professional awareness.[155] In 1966 the U.S. Public Health Service published statistics showing that in the early 1960s lead was, outside of aspirin, the largest cause of poisonings of children under five years of age.[156] All this activity led President Richard Nixon's surgeon general, Jesse Steinfeld, to convene in 1970 a committee to set guidelines that would help cities define what constituted lead poisoning. At that time, as historian Christian Warren explains, there was no consistency among urban health departments about what constituted lead poisoning among children: "New York and Baltimore defined a 'case' of pediatric lead poisoning as a child whose blood-lead exceeded 60 μg/dL." Chicago used 50 micrograms and most others used 80 μg.[157] Steinfeld's committee established the following criteria: above 79 μg was viewed as "unequivocal cases of lead poisoning" and between 50 and 79 μg "were to receive further medical evaluation."[158]

In mid-January 1971, Nixon signed the Lead-Based Paint Poisoning Prevention Act (LBPPPA), which prohibited, in any housing built with federal funds or assistance, the use of paints containing more than 1 percent lead on interior surfaces or any exterior surface such as porch railings and windowsills, where children might chew the paint. It also created programs for federal grants to cities for lead paint abatement and screening and treatment programs and to evaluate the nature of the lead paint hazard and to develop programs to address it.[159]

By the early 1970s estimates of the extent of childhood lead poisoning were alarming. The National Academy of Sciences prepared a report for the Consumer Product Safety Commission that estimated that "600,000 children would show increased blood lead content if tested [more than 40 micrograms per 100 milliliters]." Studies of children in sample areas showed that "9.1–45.5% of children surveyed have blood lead concentrations above 40 μg/100 ml and that 12.5% have concentrations above 60 μg/100 ml."[160] Because of the growing public outcry, the industry sought to develop support for its views on the matter. In 1971, the LIA's

Environmental Health committee had the well-known public relations firm Hill & Knowlton produce a report on childhood lead poisoning and discussed whether it was possible for the LIA "to induce a recognized scientist to 'author' the Hill & Knowlton report."[161]

Despite administrative problems and inadequate funding, Warren concludes that "the programs administered with LBPPPA funds prevented thousands of deaths and reduced the consequences of lead poisoning in hundreds of thousands of children.... By the early 1980s, federal funds had established some 100 lead-testing laboratories, 4 million children had been screened, 250,000 at-risk children had been identified for treatment, and 112,000 homes had been cleared of toxic paints and plaster."[162] Amendments to the act in 1973 and 1975 "lowered permissible lead contents, first from one per cent lead in dried film to 0.5 per cent, and then to 0.06 per cent."[163] In 1977, the Consumer Products Safety Commission banned any paint above 0.06 percent in interstate commerce.[164] Warren observes, however, that as of 1981 25 states, predominantly in the South and the West, still were not using federal funds for lead abatement and screening.[165]

In the early 1970s, Dr. J. Julian Chisolm Jr., who had himself received research support from the LIA, began to be concerned about the "effects of sub-acute or asymptotic [lead] absorption." Chisolm had pioneered the use of chelating agents as a method for reducing children's blood lead level and was legendary in Baltimore for his documentation that lead paint was the overwhelming cause of childhood lead poisoning.[166] Researchers had developed new laboratory methods for measuring blood lead-levels with less expensive, quicker techniques. This allowed Chisolm and others to "measure directly the effects of lead on biological processes that were invisible to the clinician—distinct physiological mechanisms taking place inside the body."[167] Specifically, Chisolm was able to document "consistent relationships between blood damage and blood-lead levels well below those associated with clinical symptoms, casting doubt on the notion of a clear threshold for damage and raising questions about the effects of asymptomatic lead absorption in other body systems."[168] This work led the U.S. Public Health Service to progressively lower its definition of "undue lead absorption" in children from 60 μg/dL in 1971 to 30 μg in 1975 to 25 μg in 1985, and to 10 μg/dL in 1991.[169]

Up until the mid-1950s, the lead industry managed to keep information about lead poisoning among children largely out of public view. As a result, the industry thwarted attempts to regulate or ban lead in paint and thereby continued to reap enormous profits from the production of lead.

This all changed in the 1950s and especially in the 1960s as community activists took up the issue of lead poisoning, viewing it as a symbol of the assault that poverty constituted on the human body itself, particularly on poor African American and Hispanic children. Only when the market for lead paint began to dry up and the assaults on lead paint came from every direction did the industry turn its attention *away* from lead paint and *to* preserving the market for lead in what was the expanding gasoline and automobile industries.

OLD POISONS,
NEW PROBLEMS

In the face of overwhelming evidence of lead's dangers, the lead industry was reluctantly willing by the early 1970s to sacrifice lead in paint. Besides, lead paint was accounting for a smaller and smaller share of the lead market. This was not the case with lead in gasoline, and what had once been a limited crisis over workers and children would emerge as a concern about the health of the entire population. In the 1960s, lead researchers began to absorb the implications of the work of such writers as Rachel Carson, Barry Commoner, and Paul Ehrlich regarding the fragility of the environment and the dangers posed to humans through the introduction of man-made pesticides and other toxins. As growing cities like Los Angeles, Detroit, and Denver based their transportation systems overwhelmingly on the automobile, the dangers from smog (a term popularized in the 1940s to denote a combination of smoke and fog) brought to public attention the impact of leaded gasoline on air pollution and on the general population.

But even through the 1950s the Lead Industries Association (LIA) insisted that its product presented no problem to the public health. As environmental air pollution gained the attention of state and local governments, the LIA held that attacks on lead were absurd. One paper touted by the LIA claimed, "No theory as to the causation of lead poisoning is too crazy to be brought forward. . . . A group in Los Angeles had put forward the claim that lead from the exhausts of motor vehicles constituted a menace to the public health."[1] The LIA mailed out nearly 1,000 copies of the speech because they found it "a most useful means of disseminating sound common sense on this subject."[2]

Given that in the 1960s the press and the public health community were beginning to pay greater attention to chronic disease caused by long-term exposure to environmental toxins, however, it is not surprising that attention was drawn to the automobile. The burning of leaded gasoline was quickly pinpointed as a major contributor to smog and air pollution in major cities. The gas-guzzling engine that became a hallmark of the 1950s eight-cylinder tail-finned family car depended upon high-octane gas containing ever-increasing amounts of tetraethyl lead. As of the 1920s the U.S. Public Health Service had capped the tetraethyl lead content of gasoline at 3 cubic centimeters per gallon. But in 1958, under pressure from the automobile industry, that level was raised to 5 cc/gallon. This increase, however, was still below what the Ethyl Corporation and automobile industries' leaders had requested, in part because Surgeon General Leroy Burney and other officials noted that no good environmental lead pollution study had been conducted since the first tetraethyl lead crisis in the 1920s and that without good evidence it was difficult to make sound public policy. It was "regrettable that the investigations recommended by the Surgeon General's Committee in 1926 were not carried out by the Public Health Service," said the final report of Burney's ad hoc committee created to evaluate the scientific literature on leaded gasoline and public health. Given the attention focused on tetraethyl lead in the 1920s, it *was* amazing that independent environmental studies had not been conducted.[3] Robert Kehoe of the Kettering Labs, funded largely by Ethyl and auto industry grants, had controlled research and had continually declared that leaded gasoline presented no danger to the public. But in 1955, Kehoe acknowledged privately that the "concentration of lead in the atmosphere of various areas, including the streets and highways of American cities" was "the primary problem of the entire tetraethyl lead industry."[4]

This growing public health attention to the deleterious effects of leaded gasoline came just as tetraethyl lead was emerging as a major portion of the lead industry's market, replacing lead in paint.[5] In 1964, 224,000 tons of lead were used in gasoline alone in the United States (up from 85,000 tons twenty years earlier). That accounted for nearly a fifth of the nation's lead consumption.[6] Kehoe and others in the industry continued to maintain that lead was a natural ingredient in the human environment and that "the occurrence of lead in the tissues, body fluids and excreta of its human inhabitants is inevitable."[7] Kehoe did experiments on humans from 1937 to 1971 to document this. Supported by the Ethyl Corporation, DuPont, the International Lead Zinc Research Organization (ILZRO), the LIA and even the U.S. Public Health Service, Kehoe used sixteen of his employees as experimental subjects—among them his animal caretaker, laboratory assistant, students, record keepers, a shopkeeper, and even his accountant and personal assistant. Kehoe fed measured amounts of lead to his subjects or put them in a chamber into which lead fumes were pumped for periods ranging from three hours to 24 hours per day. He wanted to show that lead could safely be absorbed by the human body without the appearance of symptoms.[8] "In both the ingestion and the inhalation experiments, all subjects were instructed to collect daily duplicate portions of their food and all other ingested materials. Each fecal, and also each urinary evacuation was to be collected in a separate container over the 24-hour period. All samples were to be identified by date with fecal samples also being identified by the hour."[9] While human experimentation has a long and inglorious history in America and other nations, these studies were particularly pernicious because their objective was not the discovery of a therapy for those with lead poisoning but was to gather evidence that could be used by industry to prove that lead in the blood was normal and not indicative of poisoning by industry.[10]

The industry was forced to confront growing attacks on lead in gasoline. In 1961 Robert L. Ziegfeld, the secretary treasurer of the LIA, reported on a troubling situation in California that threatened to bring the lead industry bad publicity and would therefore have to be confronted quickly and decisively. The secretary reported that Donald G. Fowler, the new director of safety and health, had gone to Los Angeles, which had a terrible smog problem, for a "week-long series of meetings" on this subject. Aware that negative publicity might result in bans on lead, the secretary reported that "our primary interest is to prevent any prohibition of the use of lead additives in gasoline without proof of a hazard that probably does not exist."[11] A few months later, an LIA official visited the American Oil Company "in an attempt to prevail upon them to reduce their attacks on lead in their advertising for leadless Amoco gasoline." They received "assurances" that the advertising campaign "would be changed."[12]

Finally, after years without studies of the environmental impact of lead, the Public Health Service itself produced what was at the time the most extensive and expensive study of air pollution and lead—"The Three City Survey (1961–1963)." Studying human blood samples, along with the air and soil of Los Angeles, Philadelphia, and Cincinnati, the Public Health Service found that the populations of these cities had higher concentrations of lead in their blood than the populations of rural areas. While no human subject had more than the then accepted "safe" level of 80 μg/dl (i.e., 80 micrograms per deciliter), a small number had more than 60 μg/dl, raising concern among some members of the committee and other members of the medical and public health community.[13] (Note that a microgram [μg] is one millionth of a gram, and a deciliter [dl] is one tenth of a liter.)

It was at this time that Clair C. Patterson, a geochemist who had received his training at the University of Chicago and had worked on the Manhattan Project during World War II, wrote a damning indictment of industrial lead's adverse effects on the environment.[14] He and T. J. Chow took core samples of ice from the polar ice cap and measured them for metal content. They documented that the increase of lead in the core samples from Greenland paralleled the increase in lead smelting and, what was more telling, the consumption of leaded gasoline. The lead concentration of the ice rose 400 percent between the mid-1700s and the mid-1900s, and it rose another 300 percent between 1940 and 1965 as the tetraethyl lead market expanded. While the Greenland data indicated an overwhelming increase of lead in the environment, no such increase had occurred in the Antarctic since 800 BC. Patterson observed that the Northern Hemisphere was quickly polluting itself through its rapid industrialization and the rising consumption of lead.[15]

In the coming years Patterson would force the public health and scientific community to pay attention to the implications of this work, by writing in a variety of journals, particularly technical journals aimed at the occupational hygiene and environmental health communities. One article that Patterson submitted to the *Archives of Environmental Health* particularly outraged both Aub and Kehoe, the industry's experts, who were asked to review it before publication. Only Kehoe was willing to critique it directly. Patterson estimated that the average level of lead in the blood in the United States was about 20 μg/dl, well below the "danger point" of the 1960s, which was 80 μg/dl, but still startling; the kicker, for Kehoe, was Patterson's suggestion that the 20 μg/dl figure was 100 times higher than true "natural" levels. (Today, the Centers for Disease Control defines 10 μg/dl as "elevated.")[16] Far from it being "normal" for Americans to have such elevated levels, Patterson claimed, "the average resident of the United States is being subjected to severe chronic lead insult."[17] (Ten micrograms per deciliter "is equivalent to one teaspoon of lead in a large backyard swimming pool," according a watchdog group.[18])

Patterson, unlike earlier researchers, was coming at the issue of lead poisoning from outside the small world of lead toxicologists who had largely depended upon the industry to support their research. It was as important, from the industry's point of view, to undercut the credibility of this "outsider" as it was to rebut his argument. The lead industry had long controlled research and had undermined and obscured the work of those who suggested lead produced acute poisoning in workers and children. Now it would begin a campaign to undercut the findings of researchers who dared look at the subtle impact of low-level lead pollution on the general population's health and specifically on children's mental development. Kehoe worried that so many copies of Patterson's unpublished paper had already circulated that without a formal method for rebuttal, there was a danger that Patterson's position would gain greater and greater credibility through word of mouth alone. In the end, Kehoe supported the *Archives of Environmental Health's* decision to publish the piece, a move Christian Warren ascribes to Kehoe's recognition that its publication was inevitable and to his hope to thus obligate the journal to make room for a subsequent detailed critique.[19]

In addition to questioning Patterson's credentials, methodology, and interpretation of the data, his critics were most concerned about his conclusion that environmental lead pollution could produce severe chronic effects. Patterson undermined the accepted threshold levels, which allowed for harmless low levels of exposure. He was raising the possibility that the "threshold for damage concept," which held that workers were lead-poisoned only if they showed the classic acute effects of lead intoxication, was inappropriate when measuring the more subtle effects of neurological damage.[20] In the coming years Patterson's model would be embraced by those who pushed for the removal of lead from gasoline and, hence, from the atmosphere.[21]

At a 1965 conference sponsored by the Public Health Service to sort out the conflicting interpretations of lead toxicology, Robert Kehoe laid out the traditional view of lead's dangers. He once again argued that the intake of lead "is balanced for all practical purposes by an equivalent output," so that there was "an equilibrium with the environment." As to the question of whether the lead that people absorbed in the course of their daily lives constituted a risk, "the answer," he said, "is in the negative."[22]

Harriet Hardy, one of the nation's preeminent occupational health physicians, condemned the entire concept of the threshold limit, calling it inadequate as a means of protecting special populations outside the workplace. As coauthor with Alice Hamilton of the widely used textbook in occupational medicine, she argued that there was a possibility that children, the elderly, and pregnant women outside the workplace might feel the effects of lead at much lower levels of exposure than the levels established for workers. Hardy was especially precise in defining the inadequacies in earlier definitions of lead poisoning, arguing that lead poisoning produced a host of subtle and extremely difficult-to-define symptoms that could easily escape physicians. "It is necessary to emphasize that no harmful effect of lead is unique except perhaps the motor palsy of the most-used muscle group, as in the wrist drop," she wrote. This meant that the "identification of low-level damage requires a combination of epidemiological evidence, astute clinical observation . . . and new experimental evidence critically judged for consistency and repeatability." Hardy felt that "the growing child" was at most risk. Numerous experimental studies and clinical observations supported her opinion that lead was more toxic to the young than to adults.

In contrast to Kehoe, who used adult males in his studies and in his model of classic lead poisoning, Hardy conceptualized the problem completely differently. "Prevention of diagnosable Pb poisoning in healthy male workers is important but not enough in our society." Lead was a known toxin, and Hardy pointed out that there was "no available evidence that lead is useful to the body." In an early statement of what would become known as the "precautionary principle," Hardy quoted Bradford Hill's presidential address to the Royal Society's Section on Occupational Medicine: "All scientific work is incomplete. . . . All scientific work is liable to be upset or modified by advancing knowledge. That does not confer upon us a freedom to ignore the knowledge we already have, or to postpone the action that it appears to demand at a given time."[23]

As more attention was paid to environmental pollution, it became clear that lead was entering the human environment, and particularly the food chain through contamination of the soil by lead-bearing insecticides; through fall-out from lead-bearing compounds during smelting, mining, and fabricating processes; and through automobile exhaust. In addition, grazing cattle absorbed lead, which was then consumed by humans. Pots and pans, water pipes made of lead or joined by lead solders, and cans sealed with lead solder—once hailed by the industry as symbols of lead's role in creating the modern environment—were now suspected as contaminants of the human food chain. One Harvard professor at the conference found it "incredible that a 3-fold increase in lead consumption [over the past thirty years] would produce no apparent increase in average lead absorption in the general populations." He rejected the idea that there needed to be a correlation between the lead absorption of workers and that of the general population: "I am of the opinion that the majority of the population is absorbing somewhat more lead while lead workers alone are absorbing a great deal less."[24] Of particular worry was the rapid expansion of the interstate highway system through the heart of most American cities. Studies had found that much more lead was deposited from exhaust pipes when cars were moving at high speeds, thereby creating added threats to urban populations.[25] A study of the soot of New York's streets revealed the startling information that it contained 2,650 ppm (parts per million) of lead.[26]

For most of the 1965 meeting, the critique of the lead paradigm developed by Kehoe and Aub and the lead industry was essentially businesslike and respectful. The world of lead toxicology was still relatively small and dominated by a few recognized experts. Although there was criticism of virtually every element of Kehoe's model throughout the conference, it was only in the discussion on the last day that the extent of the critique became explicit. Harry Heimann of Harvard's School of Public Health, who had worked in the government's Division of Air Pollution in the Public Health Service, told the conference that he wanted to make some "comments based on my listening for the last two days, having some discussions with some people in and outside the room, and on my experience as a physician who has spent most of his life in public health work." While he did not "mean to get into any acrimonious debate" and was "not intending to impugn anybody's work," Heimann confronted Kehoe directly. He felt compelled to "point out that there has been no evidence that has ever come to my attention . . . that a little lead is good for you." He also pointed out that it was "extremely unusual in medical research that there is only one small group and one place in a country in which research in a specific area of knowledge is exclusively done." Specifically, Kehoe's long-standing assertion "with regard to the metabolism and the balance experiments . . . needs to be repeated in many other places, and be extended" before the scientific community should lend it such credence. He questioned Kehoe's model stating that no danger existed below a certain blood-lead level, 80 μg/dl. He called for studies that would help decipher what problems people who had lower blood-lead levels might develop over a lifetime.[27]

Kehoe was stung by Heimann's criticisms, claiming that the Harvard professor had distorted his remarks. Heimann's comments led Kehoe to recall his first foray into the professional debates over leaded gasoline in the 1920s when he was a junior faculty member trying to establish a reputation. Kehoe believed that at the surgeon general's conference in 1924 he was "suspected of making statements that went far beyond the facts elicited by clinical and experimental evidence."[28] (Certainly, as his career wound down he became introspective. A few years before the 1965 conference he had worried about his place in history, speculating that "the information which has been obtained in this [Kettering] Laboratory will be regarded as of dubious validity because the bill for obtaining it has been paid, largely, by Ethyl Corporation, with some additional support, in recent years, from DuPont."[29])

The conference clearly challenged Kehoe and the paradigm that he and the lead industry had carefully propagated for over thirty years; more broadly, it challenged the very basis of industrial toxicology. In the words of one of the participants, "the whole field of environmental health is . . . on trial in terms of defining the risks and benefits that we will derive from use of these materials, so that the public at large can be given a rational basis on which to decide, on political grounds or whatever, that lead should or shouldn't be taken out of gasoline, that pesticides should or shouldn't be used in various situations, that asbestos should be curbed."[30] Indeed, in the coming years, the field of lead toxicology would be transformed.

In the mid-1960s industry spokesmen were still repeating their mantra that the critical measure of lead's toxicity was the worker in the plant. It was the worker who was the guinea pig. Studies had shown that lead workers on average were absorbing less lead than earlier in the century, and industry touted this as proof that the public was protected as well. When Senator Edmund Muskie, a Maine Democrat, held hearings in mid-1966, the LIA, with the assistance of the public relations firm of Hill & Knowlton, prepared a campaign to undercut any criticism. In addition to preparing articles and news clips for use in the media in the hope of generating "positive stories regarding lead and its uses," it prepared testimony for the hearings.[31] Felix Wormser, now retired but still on retainer to St. Joseph Lead Company, testified on behalf of the LIA, asserting that "vast clinical evidence" showed that "the general public is not now, nor in the immediate future, facing a lead hazard." Leaded gas posed no harm at all, he argued, and a vast literature and much research confirmed this view.[32]

Kehoe's testimony reinforced Wormser's view. Muskie asked Kehoe if his claim that "no other hygienic problem in the field of air pollution has been investigated so intensively over such a long period of time and with such definitive results" applied to the exposure of the general public. Kehoe responded that "the evidence at the present time is better than it has been at any time and that [lead] is not a present hazard."[33] Kehoe's commitment to the 80 μg/dl blood-lead level blinded him to the possibility that, whatever the adequacy for protecting adults, children might be at much greater risk at lower levels because of the effect of lead on their developing neurological systems.

The industry took solace in the fact that although Kehoe's position aroused skepticism in the scientific and political arenas, it was still widely accepted among the general public. (In Ethyl's commissioned history, a company official noted that Kehoe had "bought us time." According to Ethyl historian Joseph C. Robert, Richard Scales, a long-time chemist and colleague of Thomas Midgley's at General Motors, believed that "Kehoe had the fate of the company in his hands; if he had wavered the company would have been faced with disaster."[34]) Kehoe himself had told Muskie's committee that his laboratory was "the only source of new information" about lead in the factory and the environment and had "a wide influence in this country and abroad in shaping the point of view and activities . . . of those who are responsible for industrial and public hygiene."[35] In 1967, the LIA commissioned Opinion Research Corporation to conduct a survey of "Public Knowledge and Attitudes on Lead"; it revealed that the public acknowledged lead to be a poison but did not perceive automobile emissions as the source. The survey showed that 42 percent of the public identified "lead among 10 substances as being harmful to health." Lead ranked second in Americans' perceptions of risk, following carbon monoxide, but well ahead of carbon dioxide and sulfur dioxide, other components of auto emissions. The LIA was reassured that "the question of lead being harmful seems to be associated primarily with paints," with only 1 percent of the population identifying "gasoline fumes as a reason for believing lead harmful to health." Still, few in the survey could identify any positive uses for lead, the LIA learned, a point that didn't augur well. That so many people believed that lead posed a health problem meant "they could be expected to be receptive to—or are, in effect, preconditioned for—suggestions that lead emissions into the atmosphere may constitute a health hazard." That the general public was "not now aware" that lead in gasoline was a threat "should not lead to complacency that they will not be made increasingly aware of leaded gasoline, as the official and mass media publicity campaigns on air pollution intensify."[36] The LIA understood the test it faced: "Our industry is now, and will be in the foreseeable future, facing a most serious challenge. The challenge of pollution. The challenge that is being directed against all industry and industrial products and must be met."[37]

As was the case with lead and paint, the industry made it its business to question any assertion that lead was dangerous and to promote lead as good for society. The industry challenged any reference that associated lead in the atmosphere with danger. In a letter to its members in 1968, the LIA extolled the importance of its new pamphlet, *Facts about Lead in the Atmosphere*, which it described as "one phase of the LIA's efforts to refute the many claims made in the technical journals and the lay press that lead in the ambient air is reaching dangerous levels." It argued that such claims were "entirely without foundation."[38] Just as the early Na-tional Lead ads bragged about the numerous uses that lead played in the early part of the century, the LIA called lead "an essential metal that is too commonly taken for granted by the public." But the uses to which lead was being put were now of a decidedly more modern and technological nature. It was used as "the basic ingredient in the solder that binds together our electronic miracles and is the sheath that protects our intercontinental communications system. It is the barrier that confines dangerous x-rays and atomic radiation. It is sound-proofing for buildings and ships and jet planes." And, it was, of course, the major component of batteries and in the gasoline that ran the nation's automobiles.[39] A year later, the LIA board of directors, with the help of Hill & Knowlton, established its "Policy and Program on Childhood Lead Poisoning," an ironic "primary objective" of which was "to keep attention focused on old, leaded paint as its primary source and to make clear that other sources of lead are not significantly involved."[40]

The catalytic converter, invented in the late 1960s and introduced into new automobiles to cut back on pollution by converting carbon monoxide to carbon dioxide and water, was fouled by leaded gas. That destroyed the long-standing alliance between the lead and auto industries and created a deep fissure between the Ethyl Corporation and major car manufacturers. The lead industry found itself increasingly isolated as the movement for the removal of lead from all gasoline gained power and scientific authority.[41] Even one of its oldest allies, General Motors, abandoned the lead industry, leading to deep resentments within the Ethyl Corporation's management.[42] Despite the lead industry's efforts to keep the public's attention off gasoline, the first EPA administrator, William Ruckelshaus, accepted in 1971 that tetraethyl lead was "a threat to public health."[43] The lead industry's authority had been so seriously eroded by 1971 that even Kehoe admitted privately, "I am still suspected all over the public area of being committed to defend the lead trades."[44] Still, the acknowledgment of the dangers of lead in gasoline led to reduction of its use but not a ban. In December 1973 the EPA called for a reduction over five years from 2 grams per gallon to 0.5 gram per gallon by 1979.[45] By the early 1980s the industry sought to protect its gasoline market for lead by blaming the widespread low-lowel childhood lead poisoning that researcher Herbert Needleman had identified on "old paint," the battle it had already lost. Jerome Cole, executive vice president of the ILZRO, argued that "easing the present lead-in-gasoline regulations would make no measurable difference in the blood lead of children and, of course, would make no difference in the number of cases of pediatric lead poisoning. The real problem with lead," Cole asserted, "is old lead paint."[46] In 1986, nearly 40 percent of all gasoline sold in the United States still contained small amounts of lead. It would not be until late in the 1980s that lead would finally be removed from all gasoline.[47]

As the distinction between occupational and environmental health became less rigid, an interesting thing happened. Not only were dangers once seen in the factory now seen in the environment, but also the awareness of the dangers to the environment seemed to reopen the question of how safe factory conditions really were. The new attention to environmental lead poisoning spurred NIOSH and OSHA, which, like the EPA, had been established in 1970, to reevaluate the long-standing assumption of the industry and the industrial hygiene community that occupational lead poisoning had been largely, if not completely, eliminated as a serious threat to the workforce. In 1973 NIOSH, the scientific arm of the federal occupational safety and health effort, published a criteria document that largely acceded to traditional assumptions about the threshold of blood-lead levels below which workers were safe. The 80 μg/dL blood level was accepted as safe, but in response to the growing attention to environmental lead, NIOSH made one major recommendation that would become the focus of a heated dispute for the rest of the decade. Rather than depend upon blood-lead levels as the sole measure of safety in the factory, NIOSH argued that air monitoring of the workplace for lead content should become standard. NIOSH proposed turning away from routine blood tests and installing air monitors that could more sensitively measure the long-term exposure of low levels of lead. By this recommendation NIOSH challenged industry's insistence that the only significant measure of lead's toxicity was the blood-lead levels of the workers themselves.

In 1974, based upon the NIOSH recommendations, OSHA called for air lead levels to be reduced from the 200 μg per cubic meter that the American Conference of Governmental Industrial Hygienists (ACGIH) had established in 1957 to below 150 μg per cubic meter. (In 1957 the LIA trumpeted to its members that its representative had played a critical role in raising the threshold limit for workers' exposure to lead in the air from 150 μg to 200 μg per cubic meter. The LIA asserted that the ACGIH's increase of 33.33 percent "followed recommendations of an American Standards Association subcommittee of which our Health and Safety Director [Bowditch] is chairman."[48]) OSHA quickly revised this standard downward, proposing a preliminary standard of 60 μg/dl blood level and a

100 μg per cubic meter air standard. By the end of the decade, when OSHA adopted a final standard, it was generally accepted that low-level, long-term exposure was dangerous to workers. This fundamentally reshaped the occupational health community's understanding of danger for the workforce.[49]

In 1977, eighteen months after OSHA's proposed standard was published, the agency held hearings and called for comment. In the succeeding months, tens of thousands of pages of testimony and written comments flooded the OSHA office from labor, industry, women's groups, and the scientific community. It became clear that the alarm sounded by environmentalists in the 1970s about the dangers of low levels of lead had deeply affected multiple constituencies.

Labor in particular, long assured by professional industrial hygienists and industry that the health of the workforce was protected to the extent technically feasible, now sensed that there was a new opportunity to address an age-old industrial hazard. Over the course of the 1970s, labor argued that the accepted measure of safety, 80 μg/dl, was inappropriate for measuring danger in light of the growing evidence of subclinical renal, neurological, and reproductive damage caused by prolonged low-level lead exposure. Further, the new standards developed for air pollution convinced labor that blood-lead levels might be not only inadequate but completely irrelevant as a means of evaluating danger. Labor leaders charged that industry was not living up to even its own minimal standard and that workers were being poisoned just as their fathers and grandfathers had been. Scores of occupations—brass founder, brickmaker, cable maker, dental technician, enameler, artificial flower maker, glass polisher, insecticide maker, imitation pearl maker, tilemaker, and typesetter among them—regularly exposed workers to lead as did the more traditional occupations of miner, smelter, solderer, printer, plumber, and petrochemical worker.[50]

The OSHA hearings were like few other industrial hygiene meetings in the twentieth century. While there had been earlier meetings where labor, women's groups, and consumer groups had participated, by and large technicians and specialists had set the agenda. Coming at the beginning of the new Carter administration, when Dr. Eula Bingham, an industrial toxicologist at the Kettering Institute and the University of Cincinnati who had long been sympathetic to labor's health concerns, was appointed OSHA's assistant secretary, the conference attracted the attention of activists, labor leaders, and public interest groups who sensed a unique opportunity to broaden the dialogue about lead and frame a whole new agenda. In the course of these hearings, which had the support of a federal agency whose new leadership appeared to be committed to flexing its regulatory muscle, questions of social equity, sexism in industrial policy, and sexism in science itself became the subtext, and often the overt text, of many of the participants. In a sense, technical questions were framed through the lens of the previous decade's social struggles over equity and women's rights. Here technically trained labor advocates and women's groups challenged the supremacy of industry and the dominance of technicians hired by industry.

Struggles over chronic and low-level lead exposure raised a host of issues that called into question the very definition of disease itself. The silicosis controversies of the 1930s and 1940s had similarly challenged prevailing notions of what constituted an occupational disease, but industry closed down that issue by arguing that silicosis was not a disease until it produced disability. The environmental issue of lead poisoning in children in the 1950s and 1960s reawakened arguments about the effects of low-level exposure and biological change as a harbinger of disease. But in the 1970s, these environmental arguments re-entered the discourse over occupational disease itself. The thorough and heated discussion of the meaning of "subclinical findings" or "low-level exposure" or even the meaning of the terms "biological" and "disease" augured a revolution in the understanding of danger and risk.

Despite industry's assurances that it had eliminated nearly all the risks that had plagued the dangerous trades in decades past, lead was still poisoning many workers. One worker at a National Lead company plant said that he had lost all strength after exposure and that he, unable to straighten his legs, often had to lie in bed all day with his knees up to his chin. Another spoke of terrible intestinal cramping that he ascribed to his exposure to lead: "Last September I more or less blacked out at the plant. I got sick to my stomach, throwed up and everything...I couldn't hold nothing down." Turner Chandler, who had worked for National Lead in Indianapolis for twenty-three years, explained that lead had "affected my brain, speech, mood, and what has got me living now, obviously the doctors, or the pills." Recounting the names of workers who had died from what he suspected to be lead poisoning, he said, "the company, I mean, they don't care anything about it. The only thing they care about is your work."[51] A United Auto Workers representative from Georgia, Frank Nix, spoke of workers at various soldering jobs throughout the plant and whose blood-lead levels had risen well above the danger point. He described the inadequate protection given to workers, even those who worked in enclosed booths and wore air-fed helmets: "Management says things like 'he chews tobacco in the booth and raises his helmet to spit,' or 'he works in a body shop outside' [the plant] or 'he drinks moonshine whiskey.' It's anything but the booth." He noted that "the booth sure doesn't keep all the lead inside—particles come flying out both ends."[52]

Workers complained that "companies still continue to parade a series of excuses designed to suggest that causes other than occupational exposure to lead are responsible for the sicknesses of its workers." They pointed to one company doctor who suggested "that the lead problems of the workers ... in western Pennsylvania were really the result of those workers' affinity for Budweiser beer in cans rather than from exposure to lead in the plants."[53] Louis S. Beliczky, the director of industrial hygiene for the United Rubber Workers, told of his visits to Eagle-Picher chemical plants in Joplin, Missouri, where 83 percent of workers had "blood lead levels in excess of 60 μg" and more than a third had levels above 80 μg/dl of blood. He suspected kidney and nerve damage as a result of high exposure to lead.[54] Some locals were forced to strike to get decent working conditions. Strikes against the National Lead plant in Indianapolis and an ASARCO facility in Glover, Missouri, were aimed at forcing industry to meet the relatively lax OSHA standards.[55] Labor maintained that the impact of lead was clear: "Workers are in fact dying as a result of the effects of lead intoxication and those deaths can be laid squarely at the doorstep of OSHA's inactivity."[56]

The pattern in the industry was that workers who became lead poisoned would be laid off with virtually no protection outside very limited workers' compensation insurance. Labor sought to include in the lead standard an explicit statement that management could no longer engage in such tactics[57] and that the company would guarantee that workers who had blood-lead levels above the action point would be transferred to safer jobs and not lose their wages, seniority, or other employee rights. Unless these protections were guaranteed, labor said, workers would be reluctant to report excessive lead exposures.[58]

Labor had some reason for optimism about setting these standards because OSHA's new assistant secretary, Dr. Eula Bingham, did not believe that the economic impact of setting standards should be considered when establishing exposure levels.[59] Labor also believed that much of the rhetoric of economic feasibility was a smokescreen for general opposition by industry to any government regulation of the workplace. At the time, Sheldon Samuels, the director of health, safety, and environment in the Industrial Union Department of the AFL-CIO, asserted that the lead industry's argument that these regulations would lead to impossibly high costs and the loss of thousands of jobs was a sham.[60]

While the traditional issues of chronic exposure and severe clinical symptoms were high on labor's agenda, unions and their allies were paying increasing attention to the impact of low-level chronic exposure.[61] Labor turned to Sidney Wolfe of the Public Citizens Health Research Group and Irving Selikoff at Mount Sinai Hospital in New York City to counter the experts who worked for industry. The Steelworkers union argued, "The distinction between clinical and sub-clinical effects of lead exposure is an artificial one, perpetuated by observers who either lack the expertise or the interest to document the presence of changes at blood lead levels below 80μg/dl."[62] The United Steelworkers were drawing on a new breed of researchers trained in the 1960s and 1970s. Not only did the younger investigators have new tools for measuring low levels of ambient lead and subtler effects of lead on humans, but also many of them, coming to maturity during a time of social turmoil, sought to put their technical skills at the service of disenfranchised workers, minorities, and women. These young investigators eagerly challenged industrial hygienists like Robert Kehoe, who had for so long been the favorites of industry. They were eager to transform the field of industrial hygiene and of lead toxicology in particular. Quoting one younger researcher, the Steelworkers maintained that "we must assure ourselves that the development of this standard will not crystallize the techniques of diagnosis to those of ancient Rome or even to those of 1950, 1960, or 1970."[63]

For the most part, the new generation of industrial hygienists and occupational specialists turned to a small group of neurologists, toxicologists, nephrologists, and other specialists to document the danger of low-level exposures to workers. One physician documented a "statistically significant reduction in motor nerve conduction" among workers in one plant whose blood-lead levels were below the allowable limit. Another physician related that "enormous and irreparable damage" to the kidneys had occurred by the time the effects of lead could be "detected by usual clinical procedures."[64] Still another noted that cerebral hemorrhage as well as chronic nephritis was the result of damage from extremely low lead exposure.[65]

Herbert Needleman, then an associate professor of psychiatry at Harvard Medical School and the director of the Low Level Lead Exposure Study at Children's Hospital in Boston, provided some of the most important testimony in support of a lower blood-lead level. Despite the fact that he presented his evidence with "modesty and some trepidation" because he had little experience with occupational lead exposure and was trained as a pediatrician, he believed that some of his evidence of the effect of low-lead levels on children was relevant to OSHA's deliberations. He said that he had found evidence that low lead levels created "neuro-psychologic dysfunction in schoolage children" and that he also had "insights" on the impact of lead on developing organisms. Such observations, he maintained, were important for understanding the dangers of lead to the "worker and his or her progeny."

Needleman believed that the sponsorship of research and the nature of individuals doing that research in large measure determined how they evaluated danger. When public health specialists and pediatricians were freed from the constraints placed on them by industrial sponsors, he said, they generally concluded that low levels of lead were hazardous. "Industry and its spokesmen maintain that the evidence for low dose effects is faulty and far from persuasive," said Needleman. He countered that the evidence from the pediatric lead poisoning literature, beginning with the Byers and Lord study in 1943, established that there were long-term intellectual deficits in children who had once been poisoned by ingesting lead paint, even though their blood levels had subsequently gone back to normal. He also quoted from a series of studies by J. Perino and Ernhart, De la Burde, and Choate of African American preschoolers and other children without pica. They found that children with higher levels of blood lead (though not lead poisoned) did significantly worse on IQ tests, school performance, and speech. Needleman also related animal studies showing that lead affected fetal development of mice, rats, sheep, and dogs. He concluded that "the level or dose at which one finds a health effect depends on the avidity and sensitivity with which one looks for it."[66]

Some of the most provocative and troubling testimony at these 1977 hearings came from women and women's groups who submitted extensive documentation of the teratogenic effects of lead. A number of well-known industrial hygienists—Andrea Hricko, Jeanne Stellman, and Vilma Hunt—testified at the hearings. Hricko, who had worked with Sidney Wolfe's Public Research Group and was at the University of California, Berkeley's Center for Labor Research and Education, was explicit in laying out the "monumental" problems posed by lead to reproduction. She asked: Does society have any responsibility to future generations of children or "is this solely a 'women's' problem"? If this were defined as a woman's problem, would lead be eliminated or controlled in the work environment or would "susceptible groups" of workers, like women, be banned from the workplace?[67]

Hricko next turned her attention to sex discrimination laws, sterilization, pregnancy testing, sperm damage, and equal rights to a safe job. She argued that the decisions by OSHA on these issues would dramatically affect "many more than the estimated 1.3 million workers exposed to lead."[68] Her detailed report pointed out evidence suggesting that lead damaged chromosomes, impaired sperm and egg cells before conception, passed through the placenta during pregnancy, and was a danger to babies being breastfed. Marshaling a huge recent literature detailing the teratogenic effects of lead, Hricko provided a social analysis that discussed the policy and legal implications of differential hiring practices between men and women, which led her to conclude that industry's focus on women as a susceptible group must be simultaneously discriminatory *and* based on scientific ignorance. There was little scientific rationale for treating women and men differently, because men as well as women were harmed by lead. Sperm as well as ova were damaged. "The combination of already existing studies of damage in both males and females is enough evidence that serious detrimental effects on reproduction can occur in either sex. Enough is now known to constitute a clear call to preventive action."[69]

Hricko believed the principle of industrial hygiene was that the workplace should be made safe for both men and women; women, who had only recently won the right to work in jobs previously reserved for men, should not be fired, moved, or selected out.[70] While an assistant professor at Yale Medical School in the mid-1960s, Vilma Hunt (in 1977 a professor at Pennsylvania State University) had been involved in community lead poisoning studies that concluded that there was "no evidence . . . that women of child bearing age themselves are more susceptible to the adverse effects of lead." It was the fetus in utero and the children of workers, both male and female, "with blood lead levels high enough to alter their genetic integrity" that were at risk. Since both men and women were affected, the workplace had to be made safe for both.[71]

Jeanne Stellman, then the scientific advisor to the Coalition of Labor Union Women and the author of *Women's Work, Women's Health: Myths and Realities,* published the same year as the hearings occurred, agreed with Hunt that there was no scientific rationale for singling out women for special protection or job removal because lead damaged the germ cells of men and women alike. She sought to refute the assumption in the OSHA standard that lead represented a particular hazard to women. "It will be shown that many of the generalizations made by OSHA in its proposed standard with regard to the 'Effects of Lead on Reproduction' are unfounded." Stellman was particularly concerned that the very science that OSHA had depended upon for its singling out of women was itself shaped by unexamined assumptions that "are based on judging female biological parameters with male norms." Anticipating a critique of science that feminist scholars would develop in the coming quarter century, Stellman identified language in a variety of studies that incorporated scientifically skewed statements, revealing the influence of gender assumptions. The sexism of industrial hygiene was deeply rooted in the historical literature. Thomas Oliver and others at the beginning of the century had promulgated the myth that "females contract lead poisoning more readily" than men, and this had been incorporated and repeated continually over the course of the century, despite virtually no data.[72] Stellman's primary focus was on the effect of relatively low lead levels on the genetic material of men *and* women. She concluded that if it was "the intent to protect all workers from the negative effects of lead to themselves and to their potential offspring, there is no justification for considering women as a susceptible sub-group of the population."[73]

If science was incorporating outmoded and culturally bound models, then OSHA as well was using a dated idea of the make-up of the workforce and their responsibilities to male and female workers. Over the course of the previous decade, the nature of the workforce had been radically transformed. Organized labor, which had formerly been the preserve of white men, was seeing a measure of racial diversity in its ranks. In the wake of the black migration to the North during and after World War II, African Americans now accounted for a significant and growing portion of union membership in major unions such as the United Auto Workers in Detroit and the United Steelworkers in Pittsburgh. In the 1960s and 1970s there was a general increase in women-headed households dependent on female wage earners. It had also become increasingly necessary for middle-class women to enter the workforce in order to maintain their family's standard of living. These factors significantly changed the makeup of the industrial workforce. While those involved in the labor movement and in women's groups understood the implications of this change, it was still unclear whether OSHA had incorporated it into the new policy recommendation.

Samuel Epstein, a leading occupational and environmental health specialist at the University of Illinois Medical School and the author of *The Politics of Cancer*, to be published a year later in 1978, joined Herbert Needleman and Donald Johnson in accepting the idea that women were at special risk, although he broadened the argument to include African Americans. Testifying on behalf of the AFL-CIO, the men said that women were at special risk because of the effect of lead on the number of abortions, premature births, stillbirths, sterility, neonatal mortality, and congenital malformations. They argued that African Americans and certain other ethnic groups (such as Jews and Sicilians) were at special risk of lead poisoning because of genetic disorders such as sickle cell anemia and glucose-6-phosphate dehydrogenese deficiency. In light of this, they believed, it was even more important to provide protection for the entire workforce because such a large portion of the workforce was already, and would become ever more so, composed of women and African Americans. "The only proper way to protect susceptible 'sub-groups' is not to exclude them from the work place, but to promulgate standards which adequately protect such 'sub-groups.'"[74]

They also challenged the very terms that OSHA had used to define subgroups in the industrial workforce. They began by pointing out that women and African Americans were hardly "a specialized small population" but rather were "an important and large element of the total working population at risk." The size and significance of these subgroups were not reflected in the recommendations that OSHA was proposing. Rather than allow employers to reserve jobs in lead industries for men alone, the workplace had to be made safe for everyone.[75]

The UAW concurred, pointing to these increased risks for many of the ethnic groups in their workforce as proof that all workers, not just women and African Americans, had to be protected from the ravages of lead. The UAW was particularly sensitive to this issue because in December 1975 the General Motors Corporation in Canada had fired women of childbearing age from a storage battery plant because of possible exposure to lead. Odessa Komer, a vice president of the UAW, worried about the implications of GM's policy, which required women to establish that they would not be getting pregnant before they could qualify for the higher paying jobs traditionally reserved for male workers.[76] The UAW objected to OSHA's acceptance of a management technique of removing susceptible groups from dangerous jobs, arguing that "the degree of increased risk for these groups of workers is not known" but that "in any case, job selection on this basis would inherently result in job discrimination along racial or ethnic lines."[77] The UAW argued that "the government should take into account the susceptibility of all workers to set a lead standard that will protect everyone. Industry representatives have instead urged the exclusion of susceptible groups, specifically fertile women, from the work force."[78]

While the UAW and other labor and industry groups may have accepted the view that women were particularly vulnerable to lead, feminists in and out of the labor movement challenged the language of industrial hygiene. Even the term "susceptible" was seen as problematic when applied to women in their childbearing years. Claudia Miller, an industrial hygienist who worked for the UAW, objected strongly to OSHA's incorporation of the term when describing such workers. "For OSHA to apply the label of 'susceptible' to women who are fertile is, in my judgment, inappropriate." She maintained that "the word 'susceptible' should be confined to cases of individuals who have 'predisposing pathology.'" Reflecting the contemporary arguments regarding natural childbirth and the objections to the pathologizing of pregnancy, she pointed out that "the capacity to bear children would hardly fall under the heading of 'predisposing pathology.'" She concluded that "our very way of thinking about susceptibility [has been] turned around—rather than talking about certain groups or individuals as being 'susceptible,' should we not instead describe their counterparts as 'superimmune'?"[79] Anne Trebilcock, also of the UAW, argued that OSHA's mandate was "not to 'protect' one sex out of certain jobs, but rather to make those jobs safe for all."[80]

The Lead Industries Association had initiated a policy that "no fertile, gravid [pregnant] or lactating female be employed in lead industries until such time as adequate information has been developed regarding the effect of lead."[81] Stellman blasted this policy as incorporating a set of inadequate or inaccurate presumptions about the special susceptibility of women to lead. As researchers going back to Alice Hamilton had documented, lead was a threat to men as well as women.[82] Stellman, like Miller, argued that the evidence of women's greater susceptibility that had been repeated for decades was not credible and merely reflected scientists' gender biases. For example, women's lower hemoglobin levels had often been depicted in the scientific literature as "'a relative insufficiency of iron' among females." This view came to be regarded as absurd because it pathologized a normal state. "It makes good scientific sense to assume that females have enough hemoglobin for female functioning, and males have enough for male functioning. There is no justification for using male norms for females, and vice versa."[83] If women and children were used as the norm, then the standard for lead exposure would have to be set at a level below which men, women, and children could not suffer harm. Because OSHA had accepted the prevailing assumptions about the pathological definition of women's lower hemoglobin levels, it implicitly legitimated industry's long-standing practice of removing women in their childbearing years from jobs in the lead industries.[84]

What the Steelworkers now proposed for a standard was a 50 μg blood level with an action level of 30 μg; this standard implicitly accepted the assumption that men were the norm and that levels below 50 were usually safe.[85] Andrea Hricko took Stellman's argument a step further, maintaining that "no workers, male or female, [should have] a blood lead level above 30 μg/100ml [i.e., 30 μg/dl]," a level assumed to be safe for men, women, and the growing fetus. Hricko believed that any worker who was "seriously contemplating becoming a parent" or any woman who was pregnant or breastfeeding whose blood level went above 30 μg/dl "shall be immediately offered a temporary, voluntary transfer to a job without lead exposure, with retention of seniority, wages, and fringe benefits."[86] A consensus was slowly emerging among women's groups and labor that largely reflected women's call for equal opportunity in employment. Lead endangered all workers, men and women alike, and hence all should be protected from danger at the workplace. If industry had previously refused to hire or place pregnant women or women in their childbearing years in leaded workplaces, then the new feminist and labor position was to say that all men and women in their childbearing years were equally at risk. Neither men nor women should be exposed.

A major point of contention at the hearings regarded how to measure risk. The historical method had been that the blood-lead levels of employees were the true measure of safety and danger in the plant. Labor leaders strongly objected to what they termed the "philosophically repugnant" and inaccurate method of blood-lead sampling partly because it involved an "invasion" and violation of a worker's body. Labor argued that, in practice, the institution of regular blood drawings would engender enormous resistance within the workforce and tremendous antipathy toward OSHA, which would be held responsible for requiring this practice. In addition, the dependence upon blood monitoring would obscure the relationship between lead and physiological damage in a number of ways. The Steelworkers also maintained such monitoring was grossly inaccurate, generally underestimating the true level of lead absorbed by body tissue. Quoting numerous toxicologists, pathologists, and industrial hygienists, the Steelworkers noted that the understanding of lead's dangers had become much more sophisticated in the previous decade. Lead was no longer defined as just a threat to hemoglobin in the blood but was now acknowledged as a poison that affected the brain, the kidneys, and the nervous system in much subtler ways and at much lower levels. Testing the blood did not accurately measure the ability of the lead to affect these other organs or functions. Nor did it accurately predict the long-term damage that lead could cause.[87]

Part of the reason why labor objected to depending on the blood-lead level as an indication of lead poisoning was that lead was stored in the bone and tissue and only slowly released into the bloodstream. Since the 1950s industry and occupational physicians had used chelating agents, such as British Anti-Lewisite (BAL), to bind with lead in the bloodstream to produce less toxic compounds than the body was able to excrete. During the 1950s and 1960s other chelating agents such as calcium ethylenediamine tetraacetic acid (CaEDTA) were developed. The problem with this method was that the blood-lead level quickly returned to its elevated state shortly after chelation had been completed, as the blood reabsorbed more lead from the bones and tissue. Hence, only long treatment regimens had a significant effect, and the chelating agents themselves were dangerous. The AFL-CIO's Sheldon Samuels was greatly concerned that these toxic agents were being widely dispensed by company physicians when "leaded" workers were discovered. Treating leaded workers only obscured the basic problem, which was excessive exposure to lead in the plant. He believed that "the first step" in addressing the lead problem was prevention through engineering controls. The medical treatment of a poisoned worker was the last step, a sign of failure.[88]

Samuels pointed out that the problem of leaded workers was not simply that they absorbed lead in the plant, but that they also absorbed it in the general environment. There had been a "dramatic increase of community levels [of lead] especially since 1945," and he worried that "half of a lead worker's body burden may derive from the air he breathes, the water he drinks and the food he eats." Hence, "the solution to our problem lies as well in the jurisdiction of EPA as it does in OSHA." Removing lead from gasoline would allow industrial hygienists to more accurately gauge the lead workers absorbed in the plant. But until the time came when environmental lead would not be a factor, it was necessary to directly measure the lead in the air of the plant. Because biological monitoring could not differentiate between lead absorbed outside or inside the plant, it was only through workplace air monitoring that one source of lead poisoning could be specifically identified and controlled.[89]

Labor stressed that it was immoral to depend upon elevated blood-lead levels as the measure of good or bad industrial hygiene practice because it was an "after-the-fact" methodology that measured only damage and not risk. "We would prefer elimination of the crime rather than calling a policeman after the crime has been committed," the Steelworkers maintained.[90] The refusal of the lead industry to depend on air monitoring

130 / Deceit and Denial

echoed the historical arguments over responsibility for risk. The Steelworkers suggested that industry had avoided costly engineering controls in favor of blood monitoring because it allowed industry to blame workers' personal hygiene practices for any elevated blood-lead levels. The industry had long faulted personal habits such as fingernail biting, unwillingness to shower, general slovenliness and particularly a resistance to hand washing, and an affinity for dirty clothes among the industrial workforce as the "true" source of lead poisoning.[91] But labor countered that the high levels of lead that workers and the public were encountering were so pervasive that they could not be the result of personal idiosyncrasies.

Industry spokespeople and especially the LIA continued to work from older assumptions about lead's toxicity. In the face of assaults from an independent public health movement and labor and women's groups, they simply continued to repeat the old mantra—threshold limits protected workers, and if those levels did not produce symptoms, the public was safe. By and large, they were content with prevailing conditions both within the factory as well as in the broader environment. For Jerome Cole, the director of environmental health for the LIA, "normal" lead exposure was exactly what was occurring in the 1970s and "blood lead concentration up to 80 μg/dl can be tolerated with safety." Workers in the lead trades had to accept the fact that it was "for all practical purposes, impossible to keep blood lead concentrations in the lead industry with[in] the normal range" of those outside the factory. But this was not a problem because, Cole said, there were "no ill-effects... from exposures sufficient to produce blood leads in the 40–80 μg/dl range." While workers with these blood-lead levels should be watched, there was no necessity for extraordinary measures. Cole maintained that the lead industry was not unique. "Any industrial worker is exposed to the material with which he works to a greater extent than the general population. This is why the fields of occupational medicine and industrial hygiene exist."[92]

In industry's view, air monitoring was merely a redundant test that produced less reliable data information than biological (that is, blood) monitoring. A "leaded" worker was the best indicator of the need to clean up a plant, and an elevated blood-lead level was the best way to determine potential danger.[93] An air monitoring standard would be impractical because the lead industry was composed of so many companies producing so many kinds of products; one standard could not fit all.[94]

Industry then used its own failure to protect the workforce from lead poisoning to argue that there was no reason now for stricter government regulation. "Since few of the major segments of the lead industry appear to be in compliance with the existing standard," the LIA maintained, "no one knows what health improvements would be achieved were the existing standard to be enforced." Let's see, LIA officials said in effect, "what benefits, if any, would flow from the existing standard, properly implemented." Finally, the industry predicted economic disaster for the industry and the country if a proposed tougher standard were adopted: one of the nation's primary smelters was sure to close, and as many as 113 battery manufacturers would likely fail.[95] The industry claimed the science was in dispute, so economic considerations had to be in the forefront of OSHA's policy making.

Industry was particularly disturbed that so much of the controversy had centered on the "significance of the so-called 'sub-clinical' effects of lead exposure." For the most part, industry trotted out its old war-horse responses—principally that evidence was lacking to indicate that levels below 80 μg produced "clinical lead intoxication." Of course, this amounted to little more than a refusal to address the murky issue of subclinical effects.[96]

Industry representatives argued that the subclinical effects of lead were too inexact and based upon unproved and unprovable scientific reasoning, and were "almost by definition . . . outside the scope of the [labor] Secretary's authority," which is to set standards only with respect to 'material impairment of health or functional capacity.'" It was not the agency's mandate, the LIA argued, to eliminate all danger to the worker, and even if low-level lead exposure "may cause biological changes, not every biological change which occurs in response to an external stimulus is harmful." Like industry spokespeople in the 1940s who fought a broad definition of silicosis based on evidence of silica in workers' lungs, the lead industry argued that the fact that lead caused biological changes did not mean that the changes were pathological. "The fact that a biological change has occurred does not necessarily signal physical injury or even the threat of injury." They argued because even NIOSH had stated that "no one 'has all of the answers to at what point [sub-clinical changes] . . . become significant,'" the government should wait for more data and conclusive proof before imposing a standard that could disrupt the industry.[97]

While industry felt it was possible to turn to an old literature to buttress its claims that low-level lead was innocuous for the blood and neurological systems, at least for adult male workers, the new literature on the teratogenic effects of lead on male as well as female workers demanded a direct attack. At the 1977 hearings Vilma Hunt had quoted from a study by Ioana Lancranjan documenting a decrease in the number of sperm, a reduction of the motility of sperm, and changes in the form of sperm among men exposed to lead. The LIA was highly critical of what it called the research's "serious shortcomings," particularly "the fact that her biological determinations appear to be erroneous." She had argued that her subjects had exposures below 80 μg, but the industry reanalyzed her data and argued that they were well above this level. The industry also argued that Lancranjan had been unable to confirm or guarantee that her subjects had abstained from having sex for three days before the testing occurred. Making much of these issues, the industry noted that "had some of the test subjects not abstained, this would have materially affected...the number and motility of the sperm studied." They also objected to her use of the terms "poisoned" and "non-poisoned" as totally meaningless. They argued that her controls were completely inadequate because they were office workers and students, "people with sedentary occupations," rather than "persons engaged in heavy manual labor." They believed that "this difference may have influenced the results of her study" perhaps because of the effects of differences in class and social status on sperm motility and number![98]

The LIA paid special attention to the arguments of women's groups and industrial hygienists such as Andrea Hricko and Jeanne Stellman, who sought a reduction of permissible levels to those that would protect not only men and women but also fetuses. This dilemma, the industry maintained, could not be addressed by regulatory mechanisms alone. Women demanded equal opportunity for high-paying or highly skilled jobs, but in the lead industry these jobs came with inevitable risks. The LIA agreed with the goal of equal opportunity, but it maintained that the industry required some mechanism for guaranteeing that the industry would not incur liability for damage. From the industry's perspective there was no possibility of setting a standard so low that it would protect women, men, and unborn children alike. Quoting one of its senior executives, the LIA argued that "we can demand, demonstrate, and agitate all we wish but it will not change the basic facts. And if OSHA decides that it must set a standard so low that it is known to be fully protective of the fetus, then we all must bear in mind that there will be very few jobs, indeed, in the lead industry for either men or women."[99]

The final standard adopted by OSHA in November 1978 was ultimately a compromise, yet it incorporated many of labor's most important positions. Monitoring of air quality, rather than dependence on biological monitoring, became the standard for measuring pollution. It gradually lowered the exposure limit from 200 micrograms per cubic meter of air (or

200 μg/m³) to 50 μg/m³, and plants that had airborne lead levels exceeding 30 μg/m³ were required to begin biological monitoring of blood. OSHA lowered permissible blood-lead levels to 50 μg from the traditional 80 μg/dl of earlier eras. For those workers with elevated blood-lead levels, companies was required to place them in jobs with no exposure to lead, with full pay and no loss of seniority, until "their blood lead fell below 40 μg/dl."[100] No other standard "embodies this enlightened concept," Ellen Silbergeld, Philip Landrigan, and John Froines reported, that a worker was entitled to be removed from a dangerous worksite at full pay and benefits.[101]

The lead industry reacted vehemently, claiming that OSHA's standard was too stringent and could not be enforced. With the election of Ronald Reagan as president in 1980, the industry's position found a receptive audience. And no sooner did Thorne Auchter, a construction industry executive, replace Eula Bingham as OSHA's assistant secretary, but that agency joined a suit brought by the steel industry, automobile makers, and paint manufacturers to abandon its own recently passed standard. This was one of the more stark examples of the Reagan administration's policy of undermining standards set during the Carter administration. OSHA even withdrew its own publications on cotton dust, acrylonitrile (a raw material used in plastics), health and safety rights, and vinyl chloride, considering them too one-sided. Returning to a much older conception of the Department of Labor as a watchdog of labor rather than an advocate, OSHA abandoned more than 100 projects in 1981 and "recalled or weakened" eight standards.[102] The chief criterion in standard setting was now industry's concern about the costs of regulations rather than ascertaining the lowest feasible level that would protect workers from toxic substances. In 1981 the U.S. Supreme Court rejected the industry's and OSHA's position and upheld the 1978 lead standard. The court stated that "OSHA had a duty to protect workers from proven dangers, regardless of cost-effectiveness." OSHA ignored the Supreme Court, arguing that enforcement was impossible because it did not have the funds for the technology necessary to monitor the nation's lead industry.[103]

Despite Auchter's changes in policies to weaken enforcement of lead regulations, the lead standard stayed on the books and ultimately had a profound impact on the American workplace. Ellen Silbergeld, Philip Landrigan, and John Froines, some of the leading lead and occupational health researchers in the country, maintained that it was clearly "among the most influential actions [ever] undertaken by OSHA."[104] Yet, there were still numerous problems. In 1986 alone surveys of workers in New Jersey, California, and New York found that more than one thousand had blood levels above 40 μg and 200 above 50 μg/dl. Workers in smelters, foundries, construction, demolition, and automotive repair suffered from dysfuntion of "multiple organ systems," induced by lead exposure. Also studies in the mid-1990s showed that the 1978 "trigger level" of 50 μg, above which workers must be removed from the job, did not protect workers from lead's toxic effects. OSHA's standard for airborne lead often went unenforced, and in at least fifty-two industries using lead, exposure exceeded the OSHA standard. There were also tremendous gaps in coverage for workers "engaged in demolition, lead paint abatement and bridge repair," where many cases of lead poisoning were found over the fifteen years ending in 1997.[105] Finally, and perhaps most ominously, part of the "success" of the lead standard has been gained by the exclusion of entire groups of workers from dangerous workplaces. "Pregnant women and, in some cases, all fertile women," have been subtly and not so subtly denied skilled jobs in certain high-paying industries because of industry's fear of liability.[106]

For most policy analysts and historians, the lead standard and the controversies that surrounded it are understood in terms of victories and defeats for organized labor and the business community. The hearings, however, can be seen as an important transitional moment when the issues of workers' health and the impact of industrial toxins on the broader environment became more intertwined and complex. Women, the fetus, the economic life of the family, and work within the factory all became issues of debate.

The conference was a critical transition in the history of lead toxicology because it brought together two of the main themes that had dominated the field for fifty years. Since the late 1920s, childhood lead poisoning and workers' exposures were defined by the lead industry as two largely unrelated ends of the same toxicological problem. The LIA had sponsored Joseph Aub and others to look into the physiology of lead among an adult, predominantly male, population, and the petrochemical and automobile and gasoline industries had promoted the research of Robert Kehoe to establish that low levels of lead were a normal and essentially benign part of the human environment. Clair Patterson had challenged part of this paradigm by showing that people in the industrial world were subjected to much more lead in their environment and had absorbed much more lead than their historical predecessors. Now activists and younger industrial hygenists attacked another part of the prevailing view of the problem by suggesting that women and the unborn were at risk from far smaller amounts of lead than were harmful to the adult male. This argument owed a great deal to the women's movement, the environmental movement, the changing nature of the industrial hygiene community, and the reinvigorated health and safety leaders in the labor movement. It also owed a great deal to the ideas and research of Herbert Needleman.

Herbert Needleman was a young pediatric resident working in Children's Hospital in Philadelphia in 1957 when he found his first case of lead poisoning in a young child. A three-year-old girl presented to him the classic symptoms of acute lead poisoning: pallor, listlessness, headaches, stomachaches, anemia, and erratic behavior. After treating the girl with chelating agents, he determined that she had been poisoned at home by eating paint and absorbing lead dust. By the mid-1960s he had completed a residency program in psychiatry and was working in a community mental health center, where he regularly encountered poor children suffering from school failure, erratic behavior, and mental retardation. While the children did not show all the clinical signs of lead poisoning, Needleman connected their symptoms to those he remembered from a paper he had read some years earlier. It was Byers and Lord's paper, from 1942, that alerted him that these symptoms might well be related to lead. According to one account, Needleman was working at his office across from a Philadelphia school, watching children walk through car exhaust fumes as they traveled between their lead-painted houses and lead-painted school.

Beginning in 1971, Herbert Needleman began studying "the lead content in baby teeth collected from 761 Philadelphia school children" and was able to demonstrate a direct relationship between poor housing, environmental pollution, and lead content in the teeth.[107] By 1979 (Needleman was now on the faculty of Harvard Medical School) he had documented a profoundly more troubling relationship: the association between childhood lead exposure and lowered IQ and school performance in Boston-area schoolchildren in Chelsea and Somerville, Massachusetts. Although the 273 children studied showed no sign of acute poisoning and had blood-lead levels below 40 μg/dl, their IQs and teacher evaluations declined as their blood-lead levels went up. More than a decade later a reevaluation of about half of the original children showed "a seven-fold increase in failure to graduate from high school, lower class standing, greater absenteeism, impairment of reading skills" and other problems.[108] In 1984, Needleman published an extremely influential article, "Developmental Consequences of Childhood Exposures to Lead," in which he estimated that "about 678,000 American children under the age of 6 are lead-intoxicated."[109]

Both his research and his advocacy made him a target for others who questioned the accuracy of his results and the implications of his finding. In particular, Dr. Claire Ernhart, a developmental psychologist at Case Western Reserve University, directly challenged his results as they were contradicted by her own research, which showed that while low-level lead exposure was associated with low IQ scores, no long-term effects could be directly linked to lead exposure. Ernhart's findings quickly attracted the attention of the International Lead Zinc Research Organization (ILZRO), which later funded her research over a period of nine years. In 1981 she began a sustained attack on Needleman that culminated in her charge that Needleman should be barred from any role as an advisor to the EPA or any other government agency on the issue of lead. As a result, in 1982 the EPA convened a panel of experts to investigate these demands. The panel concluded that Needleman had failed to prove a connection between children's exposure to lead and their future intellectual development. Needleman's own review of the panel's findings, however, turned up several serious errors in their handling of his data. In 1983 the EPA rejected the panel's flawed report, confirming Needleman's original results and hailing his work as "a pioneering study."[110]

In 1991 Dr. Sandra Scarr, a developmental psychologist at the University of Virginia, joined Ernhart in filing formal charges of scientific misconduct, claiming that Needleman had distorted and deliberately manipulated data to accentuate the damaging effects of lead exposure to children. (Scarr, it should be noted, was a member of the panel that erroneously faulted Needleman's 1979 paper linking lead exposure and school performance.) The National Institutes of Health's Office of Scientific Integrity directed the University of Pittsburgh Medical School, where Needleman was by then on the faculty, to conduct an inquiry.[111] In December of that year, a three-person panel of inquiry concluded that there was "no evidence of fraud, falsification or plagiarism." More investigations followed, and in April 1992 Needleman's data were subjected to another inquiry, which again cleared him of any charges of falsification. While industry succeeded in dragging Needleman through endless investigations, it could not prevent his work from having a tremendous influence on the thinking of government regulators.

During the 1990s research by John Rosen, the head of the Division of Environmental Sciences at the Children's Hospital at Montefiore in New York, David Bellinger, at Children's Hospital at Harvard University, Bruce Lanphear, at Children's Hospital Medical Center in Cincinnati, and others documented troubling evidence that lead at lower and lower levels has important neurological effects on children. Lanphear, for example, demonstrated that school performance was adversely affected in children with blood-lead concentrations below 5 μg/dL.[112] Philip Landrigan argues that these findings "suggest that there is no safe threshold for the toxicity of lead in the central nervous system."[113] This is particularly true for children whose developing bodies take in more lead, pound for pound, than do adults and whose organs and nervous systems are developing and thus more susceptible to even tiny amounts of lead and other toxins such as nitrates, mercury, radiation, and PCBs.[114]

Today, even such conservative critics as the American Council on Science and Health agree that there is "a healthy debate as to whether a threshold or no-effect level exists for lead-induced effects, particularly those associated with effects on intelligence and neuro-behavioral endpoints."[115] While they argue that "claims of subtle neurobehavioral effects in children due to elevated BLL [blood-lead level] are not based on firm evidence," the shifting paradigm of lead toxicology has forever altered the debate.[116] By the turn of this century, investigators were listing reasons why models borrowed from occupational medicine were incapable of addressing environmental concerns.[117]

Lead, the mother of all industrial poisons, has to be understood as the paradigmatic toxin that linked industrial and environmental disease in the first two-thirds of the twentieth century. That link was always there, but it often was hidden by the intense political and economic interests that shaped industrial hygiene as a field and our understanding of industrial disease. Ultimately, the environmental, women's, and labor movements all changed the thinking of physicians, industrial hygienists, public health experts, and government officials, who were forced to confront the challenges of the world outside the laboratory and to question the language and assumptions of a science often sponsored by and indebted to industry. Similarly, the new breed of public health professionals greatly influenced the environmental movement itself, bringing new tools and attention to the pervasive problem of low-level lead poisoning. The slow loosening of the industry's stranglehold on Americans' understanding of the relationship between environmental and occupational health, however, was accomplished with enormous social costs measured in destroyed lives and diminished abilities for thousands upon thousands of people. Children, the most susceptible to lead as a poison, suffered most. Too many minds were destroyed and are still being destroyed across classes and across social groups. There are still twenty-five million homes that have lead paint, and they represent an ever-present risk not only to children who live in them today, but also to generations of children who will inhabit them in the future.

A great deal of good came out of the struggles over lead in the 1960s and 1970s. As popular awareness of the dangers of lead increased dramatically, lead was eliminated from paint, and tetraethyl lead began to be phased out as new cars designed to run on unleaded gas came onto the market. According to the Centers for Disease Control and Prevention, between 1976 and 1996 (when leaded gas was completely phased out) there was a 90 percent reduction in the average blood-lead levels of children.[118] Once lead became a concern for consumers as well as for factory workers, the discussion of industrial toxins never again focused solely on the workplace, but inevitably crossed the boundaries into discussions of the safety of the general population. Lead poisoning also raised consciousness about the subacute, subtle, and sometimes undefinable effects of industrial toxins on health. As the popular press exposed the insidious qualities of lead and its potential to cause serious harm to the public, citizens and environmental groups organized to limit lead's use and began to discuss industrial pollution issues in the language of class, race, and gender as much as in the language of science and medicine.

If lead was paradigmatic of the problems of industrial pollution in the first half of the twentieth century, plastics were emblematic of these problems in the second. Whereas lead had been understood to be a poison for centuries, the new synthetic materials produced by the chemical industry arrived on the scene without history, without "baggage." Whereas lead was considered a dirty industry and understood historically to be dangerous for those who mined it and poisonous for those who consumed it, the plastics industry seemed clean and had no toxic record. Plastics were generally viewed as benign and certainly beneficial in the production of consumer products. Thanks to a public relations campaign waged by the chemical industry, plastics continued to be viewed positively, even though workers in the petrochemical industry who came into contact with coal tar, benzene, and toluene were documented as suffering higher rates of bladder and other types of cancer. This erroneous perception of plastics ultimately allowed for such widespread production of them that by today plastics permeate every corner of the earth, creating what one sociologist has called "a carcinogenic environment."[119]

Better Living
through Chemistry?

Today chemicals pervade so many phases of man's environment we
might say the environment has been "chemicalized."
—Harvey F. Ludwig, "Chemicals and
the Environmental Health," 1955

In the 1940s and 1950s the chemical industry, much like the lead indus-try
earlier, undertook an extensive public relations campaign to promote
petrochemical products, particularly plastics, as materials that would transform the lives of Americans. Like lead, plastics were promoted as essential
to modern American consumer society—vital in the building and maintenance of homes and the production of automobiles, the development of
new styles of clothing and modern conveniences. Like lead, these products
and their byproducts persisted in the environment, not degrading, pene-
trating into the food chain, ultimately ending up in the human body.

But the story of plastics was different from lead in one significant way:
Lead had been used for centuries and was known to be dangerous to workers, while plastics, particularly vinyl, were new substances and their health
effects were unknown. This fact accounts for slightly different plots in these
stories. Because plastics were unknown substances and because industry
operated according to the notion that a product was to be considered safe
until proven dangerous, the industry was able to build huge plants that produced untold amounts of these materials for disposal throughout society.

This chapter examines the period from the end of World War II to the
establishment of the Environmental Protection Agency (EPA) and the
Occupational Safety and Health Administration (OSHA) in 1970. As we
saw in the last chapter this was a period of growing activism among environmentalists, labor unions, and civil rights groups. Because the late 1950s
through the 1960s was a period when Americans were both becoming
aware of dangers to the environment and growing increasingly suspicious
of industry's motives and trustworthiness, it was not long before armies of
environmental activists and labor unions joined to challenge the arguments of industry concerning industrial pollution. Unlike in the history of

lead, in which industry scientists, managers, and spokespeople held nearly absolute power before the 1960s, the chemical industry was quickly confronted by an environmental and labor movement that pressed newly created federal agencies to control the industry.

In the decades after World War II, the chemical industry argued that the pollution from its plants constituted a nuisance, not a health hazard, and that it represented the price the country had to pay for economic progress and the good things that chemistry made possible. But privately, industry worried that the stinging eyes and bad water might lead the public to believe that these chemicals were toxic. If the public did, the industry would see its growth and profitability greatly affected.

In the 1960s the environmental, consumer, and labor movements began to express their mistrust of the chemical industry. Rather than seeing the public and the workforce as allies who needed to be protected, the industry saw them as enemies. As in the case of lead, the industry believed that it had to keep the public unaware and, if the public learned of danger, the industry had to convince people to put their faith in the honor and integrity of an industry that was making their lives richer, more comfortable, and more convenient. While some within the chemical industry viewed environmental pollution as a very serious hazard that the industry ignored at its own peril, publicly the industry remained united in assuring the public that it could be trusted to protect community residents and the environment as well. The industry tried to convince the public that federal regulation should be kept to a minimum and that local and state regulators would work hand in hand with the industry itself. Despite the industry's assurances, most Americans moved from a generalized faith in industry's ability to look after the health of its workers and the well-being of communities to a conviction that there was no alternative to the federal government's taking on this responsibility.

DARKNESS AT NOON

After World War II the chemical industry proclaimed for itself a special role in America's newfound affluence. DuPont announced that the American century was made possible by "Better Things for Better Living... through Chemistry." For over fifteen years, despite particular environmental crises and increased scientific concern about pollution, Americans were fairly hypnotized by a parade of technological advances and remained largely unaware of the ecological and health costs of progress. Most eagerly incorporated the products of the chemical industry into their lives, never thinking that the synthetic chemicals in these products could possibly pose a danger.

Industry understood during the 1950s that the anxiety most Americans felt about the threat of nuclear war and the reality of fallout from atomic testing had the potential to translate into a fear about the toxicity of chemicals. Americans listened to Civil Defense advertising, watched the building of fallout shelters, and participated in air raid drills and "duck and cover" exercises in schools. The vaguely understood effect of unseen radiation on human health raised the specter of unknown dangers posed by human manipulation of the natural environment. The testing of atomic bombs in the Nevada desert destroyed the immediate environment and threatened children—both immediately downwind and thousands of miles away—as dangerous levels of strontium 90 were found in milk sold in upstate New York supermarkets. At any moment these general fears might cause people to wonder about the possible toxicity of chemicals.

Americans remained largely indifferent to pollution from the chemical industry[1] until a tragedy occurred in 1948 in Donora, Pennsylvania. This small factory town near Pittsburgh was enveloped in "a poisonous mix of sulfur dioxide, carbon monoxide and metal dust . . . from the smokestacks from the local zinc smelter where most of the town worked" as an air inversion turned the street dark at noon. "Twenty residents died and half the town's population—7,000 people—were hospitalized over the next five days with difficulty breathing."[2] Donora was home to a number of smelters and steel mills, including the American Steel and Wire Company's zinc works. For five days, a cloud of toxins sat over the town. It was estimated that the air contained between 1,500 and 5,500 micrograms per cubic meter of sulfur dioxide emissions, whereas today's Clean Air Act mandates 80 mg/m^3 as a maximum average.[3] For a brief moment, Americans were shocked and forced to confront the dangers of air pollution.

The following year, undoubtedly in reaction to Donora, the Manufacturing Chemists' Association (MCA) formed the Air Pollution Abatement Committee. (The MCA, the major trade association for the chemical industry, was established in 1872; by the second half of the twentieth century it represented one hundred seventy-four U.S. companies, responsible for "more than 90 percent of the production capacity of basic industrial chemicals" in this country.[4]) Dudley A. Irwin, representing the Aluminum Company of America, argued in January 1950 that "the repercussions of the Gauley Tunnel episode on silicosis [America's worst occupational health disaster, which occurred in the early 1930s] probably will be dwarfed by the effects of Donora on air pollution. The Donora incident," he continued, "has not only made the public air pollution conscious and unduly apprehensive, but also it has advanced opinion with regard to the imposition of restrictive measures by many years." The implications of this for the legislative arena were clear: "The politicians have not been slow to sense this changed attitude of the public."[5] But, as *Modern Industry* magazine put it, "smart plants are cleaning up their exhaust gases right now—before laws or lawsuits start to pinch."[6] Decrying the lack of information, Irwin reviewed what was known and not known about the effects of industrial air pollution.

While the industry had argued throughout the twentieth century that if you could protect the worker, the public was safe, Irwin wasn't so sure. Industrial workers "are usually healthy individuals, while the general population includes those who are infirm or chronically ill." Furthermore, in the factory, workers were "usually exposed to a single contaminant while city air is a mixture of many contaminants, some of which may act synergistically." Finally, workers were only exposed to toxins "on a part time basis in contrast to the full-time exposure of ordinary citizens." Even so, Irwin was unwilling to acknowledge that "ordinary air pollution has any significant adverse effect on the health of the general population."[7]

The MCA developed a program that incorporated its view of nature and the environment as another resource at the disposal of industry. In its "Basic Principles of Legislation," the association laid out its vision in 1950: "the atmosphere should be regarded as a useful natural resource." According to the MCA, nature "should be utilizable for dispersion of wastes within its capacity to do so without harm to the surroundings." Rather than envisioning the atmosphere as a *national* resource to be protected for the people as a whole, it was simply considered a *local* resource. Therefore, "air pollution is a local problem," and the state should only interfere "to enable a particular locality to take action."[8] This reasoning was part of the industry's efforts to prepare for fights over threats to its sovereignty. Of particular concern was the U.S. southwest, where the chemical industry had experienced "unprecedented growth."[9] Similarly, the rapid growth of Los Angeles and its dependence on the automobile raised new worries about smog and its long-term effects on American health and therefore new worries for industry.[10] Smog, in the words of one trade journal, "cease[d] to be a joke to industrialists."[11]

Throughout the 1950s the MCA developed a keen awareness of the air pollution issue, closely monitoring national and state legislation. When New Jersey considered a bill to put the state Air Pollution Control Commission in the Department of Health, the MCA's Air Pollution Abatement

Committee sought to have the legislation altered to place it in the Department of Law and Public Safety. Understanding that health was a potent political issue, the MCA sought to depict air pollution as "a nuisance problem and not a health problem."[12]

When the MCA became concerned about federal air pollution legislation, it met with the Public Health Service "to impress upon the officials that we feel control of air pollution is largely a local matter." If the purpose of legislation was the "collection of information," then the MCA would have no objection, but there was to be no federal regulation.[13] Arguing that there was "no basis for the fear that health is endangered by air pollution" and that air pollution was only "a nuisance," the MCA believed that the industry should begin a determined program as an "investment in good will."[14]

In 1956 the MCA participated in a federal-state study of air pollution in Louisville, Kentucky. The industry needed to be on top of information about pollution if it were going to be prepared to counter challenges to its control. Monitoring the study for the MCA were technical personnel from the B. F. Goodrich Chemical Company, the same plant that would, in less than two decades, become the site of the first cancer deaths linked to the plastics industry. It was clear to the study organizers that emissions from the plant were escaping into the general population; the study was designed to identify the frequency and types of emissions that were escaping. As part of the project, "several school children in Louisville's West End," a predominantly poor, African American community, were given "sniff-kits," which were "small bottled samples of many materials used in Rubbertown processes." The children were taught how to use the kits to identify odors they noticed in the air.[15]

The MCA's state affiliates were less attentive to the looming issues of environmental and air pollution than the national organization. When the MCA approached the Louisiana Chemical Association (LCA), whose state was emerging as a center of the petrochemical industry, about holding a workshop session on air pollution abatement, the LCA declined: "they felt no pressing need for technical assistance on air pollution problems at present." Even the Air Pollution Abatement Committee believed that such attitudes were "all too typical of the 'let sleeping dogs lie' philosophy, likely to lead to frantic 'too little and too late' efforts when the pressure for action mounts."[16]

In 1960, as the MCA's Medical Advisory Committee considered what kind of public face to present, it was clear that its members understood that the field of environmental health had come to encompass both the environment of the factory as well as the outside world, into which companies were pouring pollutants. Pollution, particularly smokestack emissions and groundwater contamination, were real problems that industry was "doing an improved job" of addressing. The industry's dilemma was that emphasizing such claims would simply call attention to what had not been done to protect the environment in the past.

Monsanto's representative, Dr. R. Emmet Kelly, said, "If we claim we are keeping pollution down to low enough levels, we will be asked how we know such levels are low enough." Unfortunately, he candidly admitted, "there is bound to be pollution." H. H. Golz, American Cyanamid's representative, agreed that "it is difficult to prove that certain levels of pollution are not harmful to people. Absence of evidence of harm was not acceptable" in the contemporary social climate. The Enjay Chemical Company's representative pointed out that "so long as people die from unknown causes, pollution will be blamed." One way of proving that industry acted responsibly outside the plant, according to Union Carbide's representative, was to "show what a good job we are doing in industry to prevent the exposure of workers" inside the factory. But this, in turn, would pose other dilemmas. As DuPont's spokesman noted, critics would "tell us we protect our workers by pumping the pollutants out into the atmosphere and thereby exposing the general public." Golz worried that any statements made by General J. E. Hull, the MCA's president, could be used as an excuse to increase government regulation of the chemical industry and that any admission of responsibility for "a public health problem" should be accompanied by a "go-slow policy by government."[17]

The very success of chemicals in altering America's environment was accompanied by a growing sense of unease about the chemical industry's link to the military, about the possibility of nuclear war, and about radiation. President Dwight Eisenhower would soon warn America of a spiraling interdependence of investment and armaments—the military-industrial complex. DuPont's representative on the MCA's Medical Advisory Committee, Dr. A. J. Fleming, argued that the industry had to begin to change the terms of the debate. Rather than addressing the solutions to the hazards that industry posed, the chemical industry itself had to "work in some propaganda" that emphasized the "benefits to mankind through chemicals" such as the notion that "feeding the world will depend on the use of chemicals." "Chemicals," he maintained, "are important for both protection and production of food. Industry should set its own safety factors." Furthermore, American Cyanamid's Golz proposed that the MCA be more active in shaping legislation and ideas: "We should suggest liaison between MCA and the Public Health Service in an attempt to solve problems. MCA could have representation on government committees." He even envisioned a scenario in which "industry and the public health services should get together to prevent harmful legislation."[18]

The American Petroleum Institute (API), the trade association of the portion of the chemical industry that was primarily concerned with petroleum refining, directly addressed the growing fear that the industry's air pollution was linked to serious diseases. Seeking a way to reconceptualize the health issue as one of annoyance and nuisance, John C. Ruddock, a former lead researcher and the chair of the API's Sub Committee on Atmospheric Pollutants, argued repeatedly that with the exception of Donora, London, and Meuse, Belgium (where air inversions resulted in many deaths), no one had been able to prove "aggravation of such diseases as asthma, tuberculosis, bronchitis, etc., nor does air pollution particularly affect the aged or very young." He agreed that air pollution should be reduced. And he was "sympathetic with all those who do not like 'smog.' As true Americans, we do not like our rights infringed upon, whether it is the inability to see as far as we desire, or whether it is the discomfort and eye-smarting that occurs with air pollution." Certainly, there were many "poisonous and noxious fumes" in polluted air. But, they were dangerous only when they exceeded "a certain density and are either inspired or ingested." The API members assured themselves as well as the government that whatever the claims about the effects of air pollution, "we have found no single case, nor have we found any pathological effect attributable to atmospheric pollutants per se."[19]

Until 1960, the MCA hoped that most Americans would accept the industry's line that any general anxiety about the environmental impact of chemicals was generally overblown or based upon a few dramatic instances. Old-line industries such as steel and coal production had led to seemingly bizarre ecological disasters such as the one at Donora. Industry representatives argued that isolated ecological incidents were largely a result of unique local meteorological or local geologic characteristics.

EVERY VENTURE INVOLVES SOME RISK

In early 1962, coinciding with the impending publication of Rachel Carson's *Silent Spring,* the MCA's Public Relations Advisory Committee expressed a sense of "urgency of the situation confronting us." There was a "steadily intensifying assault on the right of business management to manage." While this assault came in part from organized labor, management believed that the more general impetus came from the federal government, which was pursuing "this line because it is the public's desire that it do so." The committee recommended a campaign to "educate," "inform" and "persuade" the American public about what industry was doing for them. They believed that without such a propaganda campaign government would adopt policies that would "result in the constriction and ultimate strangulation of the economic and social systems under which our free institutions have survived and prospered." They worried that "once the abyss [of government interference] has been reached" it would be too late to change direction.[20]

The MCA introduced into its argument the issue of acceptable risk. "Whether public health officials will admit it or not," Dr. E. O. Colwell of the Aluminum Company of America told the Air Pollution Abatement Committee, "there is a place for the term 'calculated risk' in this human health business." To the question "What price were we willing to pay for absolutely clean air?" he answered that it was both impractical and unnecessary "to make the air so clean that the most sensitive individuals will be comfortable if such is not economically sound." He argued that "the public we must satisfy would better risk a few cases of bronchitis or even emphysema than to risk mental and physical ills that would accompany the economic failure of an industry, a community, or a country." For the industry, as well as Colwell personally, public health could not be the paramount concern of the industry. The economic interests of the chemical industry were synonymous with the interests of the country.[21] The next year industry was pleased that the Clean Air Act encouraged states to initiate air pollution controls, permitting the federal government to act only at the state's request. Environmental historian Hal Rothman suggests that a "lackluster enforcement record followed," with "only eleven abatement cases filed between 1965 and 1970."[22]

Rachel Carson's *Silent Spring*, published in September 1962, sounded a loud alarm over the chemical industry. Carson's biographer, Linda Lear, has written that industry and others recognized *Silent Spring* as "a fundamental social critique of a gospel of technological progress." Some quarters were so threatened by Carson's book that they felt the need to attack her personally. Ezra Taft Benson, the secretary of agriculture in the Eisenhower administration and later a leading elder of the Mormon Church, is credited with barbed remarks about Carson. He asked "why a spinster with no children was so concerned about genetics," suggesting that it was because she was "probably a communist."[23] But it was the National Agricultural Chemicals Association, the trade association for pesticide manufacturers, and the MCA that led the attack on Carson and her writings, "sending out a steady stream of brochures and bulletins denouncing things that Carson had never said and circulating 'fact kits' to members."[24]

Almost immediately, the MCA began organizing to get a firmer hold on the broad issue of environmental pollution. Recognizing that an attack on Carson was not sufficient to regain public confidence, the board of directors voted to join with the National Agricultural Chemicals Association to wage a public relations campaign that emphasized the "constructive role played by chemicals in the field of environmental health."[25] As one of the board's officers stated in a general review of the MCA's program, the "public relations program on environmental health . . . is currently concerned with the problems created for the industry by such books as Miss Rachel Carson's 'Silent Spring.'" They feared that the public would accept "the implication that the chemical industry has no sense of public responsibility and is motivated solely by a desire for profits."[26] The MCA set up an Ad Hoc Technical Committee, developed contacts with other trade associations concerned about increasing environmental consciousness, and produced a "large volume of informational material" for consumers, scientists, politicians, and educators.[27] An Ad Hoc Planning Committee on Environmental Health was established in April 1963 to coordinate the defensive and offensive measures to carry out the "proper responsibilities for chemical industry leadership in this increasingly significant area."[28] The need to "get going" was essential "in light of mounting pressures for action, with the strong likelihood of a greatly accelerated program with or without industry cooperation."[29]

In June 1963 the Ad Hoc Planning Committee on Environmental Health, chaired by D. D. Irish of Dow Chemical, restated industry's long-held belief in its own beneficence and its role in improving on nature. "Man's environment has always been hostile, for it is from the environment that two of the traditional regulators of man's numbers—namely, famine and pestilence—have arisen," the committee posited. "Technological advances" were largely responsible for taming much of nature, resulting in longer lives, higher standards of living, and growing populations.[30] The panel argued that "the chemical industry has made major contributions to many of today's labor-saving, illness-retarding and wealth-producing elements of the total environment" and made possible "our way of life." It wrote, "Every venture involves some risk."[31] "The net gain has been tremendous," it boasted, but technology also had had some unintended consequences that industry had to address.[32]

The coming year brought a host of these "consequences" to the attention of the MCA. The Mississippi River, the drain for industries in the country's breadbasket, became the focus of congressional hearings after the U.S. Public Health Service blamed pesticides for the large number of "fish kills" in the lower Mississippi.[33]

By the mid-1960s, the chemical industry understood what it had taken the lead industry three decades to learn: it had to do something to stave off regulation. The political and social environments that chemical companies were operating in were substantially different from those of the 1920s and 1930s, when the lead industry could virtually ignore the government's presence. In November 1963, shortly after President John F. Kennedy's assassination, the Environmental Health Advisory Committee (EHAC) was established by the board of the MCA.[34]

"The environmental health problem, then, is simply this," summarized John Logan of Olin Mathieson and vice chair of the EHAC. "To what extent can the *increasing* population load up the *fixed* environment before the environment is so modified that it produces adverse effects on health?" "Nature," he pointed out, "has a solution to this problem. . . . When a population gets out of balance with its environment . . . the population is simply cut down to size . . . until balance is restored." This solution was clearly unacceptable. The gist of the problem was "that the environmental health problem should be taken seriously" for "it will not go away," he wrote. "If we do nothing, I am sure that the Government will tell us what to do."[35]

The MCA had to develop a program aimed at gathering information, cleaning its own house, providing knowledge to its own members about pollution, and helping the public with information needed to deal with the growing recognition that industrial wastes, whether in the air, soil, or water, were potential problems. "The program of the MCA [in the area of environmental pollution] has been largely defensive," but new action was needed to gain control over the pollution issue "before situations become acute."[36]

Again, as in the case of lead, the industry chose voluntarism as the method for reducing, not eliminating, risk from industrial pollutants. "Voluntarism" entailed two complementary components. First, the industry was to be left to itself. Whatever reform was to take place in the manner of production was to be done by the industry through its own initiative. Government was to have as minimal a role as possible. Second, communities and individuals had to recognize that the largest measure of responsibility for pollution resided in their own acts. "Effective action requires a high level of individual responsibility."[37]

The early meetings of the industry's Environmental Health Advisory Committee certainly underestimated the growing concerns about environmental pollution. It appears from committee documents that members believed that an effort to shape legislation, calm public worries, and provide the scientific base for decision making could quiet the rising cacophony of voices. "Handling of minor problems at the 'grass roots' could significantly reduce the hazard of a major conflagration" over pollution and chemical hazards, the MCA maintained. The MCA believed, as did the LIA in the case of lead, that industry's largest problem was public relations. "The greatest need in this area is for a strong program of education of customers and the general public in the *appropriate use of products*," members believed.[38]

Some in the committee were not so sanguine about the possibility of easily assuaging public fears with a propaganda campaign. Cleveland Lane, the representative of Goodrich-Gulf Chemicals, pointed out that for years the industry had been trying to address public unease by mounting a public relations offensive. "The subject is not new," he reminded his audience. "As far back as 1937 or '38, Louis Bromfield" had "attacked chemical fertilizers claiming they . . . were dangerous in food." The view "that chemicals caused cancer was being spread as early as 1946 and possibly earlier," Lane recounted. "In 1949, DDT was banned as a cattle spray because some cattle had died and because of high concentrations of DDT found in milk."

William Longgood's "*Poisons in Your Food,* the cranberry scare [of 1959, in which pesticides were suspected of causing cancer], the Donora, Pennsylvania, smog deaths, [and] various ammonium nitrate explosions," Lane noted, all preceded the recent uproar over *Silent Spring*. Public relations could not be the sole answer to the industry's crisis; in fact, public relations could be effective only if the industry maintained a reputation for honesty and reliability. The industry's most successful public relations efforts, Lane argued, occurred when "factual, scientifically accurate information" was made available. "This reliability may be our most precious weapon in meeting new criticism and must be jealously guarded."[39]

Lane admonished the committee members to ground their responses to the public's fears in "honest" science. He pointed out, "We have no control as to when or where these incidents [environmental crises] may arise, therefore, while planning and anticipation is very important, the Environmental Health Advisory Committee should always be prepared to deal with emergency situations." The Public Relations Committee has "developed very efficient means to combat public fear of chemicals and are ready to use these means in most cases. But no Public Relations operation, no matter how effective, can cover up acts of carelessness or neglect which do harm to the citizens, nor can such Public Relations operations prevent public corrective action in terms of legislation where our own control has been faulty." He admonished his colleagues to pay serious attention to the environmental effects of chemicals; relying on public relations experts was an approach fraught with danger. "As long as we produce products or conduct operations which can cause health hazards, public discomfort or property damage, we must do all we can to prevent these situations. This is a non-debatable condition of our doing business and should be a fundamental precept of this committee."[40]

Lane knew he was talking to a group that might very well see him as siding with kooks and environmental agitators. Therefore, he underlined his allegiance to the industry by depicting environmentalism as an effort by alarmists to cast doubt on his industry. "The Public Relations Committee," Lane concluded, "realizes that public fear of chemicals is a disease which will never be completely eradicated. It may lie dormant or appear from time to time as a minor rash, but it can flare up at any time as a major and debilitating fever for our industry as a result of a few, or even one, instance, such as the Mississippi fish kill, or the publication by some highly readable alarmist, or as an issue seized upon by some politician in need of building a crusading image."[41]

In June 1964, the MCA called on its Legal Advisory Committee to become more actively engaged in environmental matters, especially in "watchdogging legislative proposals" and to "offer advice on how to react to them."[42] The Environmental Health Advisory Committee pushed for the MCA to take the lead in maintaining a common front by industry against legislative and regulatory proposals.[43] Industry representatives had to follow "all matters in a given state or part thereof" and report activities to the air and water pollution committees "in order to ensure adequate depth of coverage of environmental health matters."[44] The MCA was determined to see that "regulation by government should be at the lowest effective level."[45] Three principles emerged as the basis of industry involvement in controlling the situation: self-regulation, support for local controls, and support for "appropriate" federal legislation.

Although self-regulation was clearly the industry's action of choice, it had its drawbacks. While there were responsible companies, the success of self-regulation would be "hampered by the fact that any effective industry effort" would be undermined by those in the industry "who will not fully adhere to the principles of self-regulation." Those who failed to act responsibly "in the absence of an enforcing power" could tarnish the industry's reputation. Although "moral suasion" was necessary to bring renegade companies in line, the industry realized that any industry effort to control "the careless or wantonly negligent few would run a serious risk of violating other statutory schemes governing intra-industry relationships."[46] The EHAC cautioned, "Industry should make the most of opportunities for self-regulation," but such voluntary efforts had "limitations because of recalcitrance by a minority and because other industry segments may have different objectives."[47]

The industry grudgingly acceded to the idea that federal legislation might be useful as a means of relieving the industry of the unpleasant task of trying to regulate its members. Industry leaders knew its reputation, and the political position of all the responsible companies could be jeopardized by the irresponsible few. Hence, "recognition should be given to the inevitability and desirability under certain circumstances for increased Federal participation in environmental health matters," the committee decided.[48] If the federal government could be used as an arbiter for issues that the industry itself was unable to handle internally, it could become a valued partner in negotiations among companies that had different interests and different internal cultures.

But still the MCA was deeply worried that government would develop standards for industry conduct in the area of environmental health that would be anathema to many of its members, renegade or not. Most particularly, the industry was worried that government would establish technical measures of accountability and would set standards that would be incredibly costly and burdensome. As a result, the MCA jealously guarded the historical role of letting the industry itself establish the measures by which it was to be judged. In the 1930s and 1940s the industry had sponsored and controlled groups like the Industrial Hygiene Foundation and the American Standards Institute, which had taken control of standards setting in industrial hygiene matters. Government had played a minor role, generally acceding to the presumed integrity and technological sophistication of the industries themselves.[49] "Government agencies are pressing increasingly for criteria and standards in environmental fields," the EHAC declared in its Overall Environmental Health Program of 1966. "It is vital that MCA assume leadership for the chemical industry in constructive participation in these efforts, both with respect to the establishment of standards by governmental bodies, and wherever feasible, to develop criteria for voluntary adoption by the industry to minimize the need for governmental controls."[50]

Given government's increasing activism in the 1960s, it appeared inevitable that some form of regulatory activity would come to pass. The industry had to be proactive, gathering information and developing an arm of the industry that could define the problems of industrial pollution and the boundaries between industrial, individual, and public responsibility. The industry first set out to develop a clearinghouse for data, to be controlled by and responsible to the industry. The committee contacted a management consulting firm, Booz, Allen & Hamilton. The MCA agreed to pay the firm $35,000 for a preliminary study of how to organize an institute on environmental health and how to gather, disseminate, and develop future research.[51]

Booz, Allen strongly suggested a research agenda to identify problems in the industry with the intention of providing information to the broader community about the impact of chemicals on American life. Almost immediately, a survey was conducted of the approximately two hundred companies that made up the MCA to assess their responses to the Booz, Allen proposal. The survey questions examined potential problems associated with gathering damaging information. Most companies strongly opposed giving the proposed institute any degree of independence from the MCA. In fact, it was "felt that such a staff and program should be directly under MCA control." While staff members could have "freedom of expression" within the organization, the member companies believed, they should not be able "to express their views or make statements publicly." In other words, the industry was intent on controlling the research as well as any findings that might be generated by that research. Only one member company representative surveyed "deplored what he felt might be a substantial loss of scientific objectivity (from the public standpoint) resulting from close identification [of the institute] with and control by MCA."[52] In November Booz, Allen provided its study report, *Environmental Health Information Organization—Feasibility Study*, with the recommendation that a small staff composed of "a director, two technical professionals, and a technical librarian" be brought in to organize the effort to gather together information about air pollution, water pollution, and the long-term effects of workers' exposures.[53]

From early on it is clear that the MCA faced a concrete problem in trying to reconcile its members' interests and perspectives on the seriousness of the pollution problem and the chemical industry's responsibility regarding environmental dangers. Some of the larger companies, such as Dow and Eastman Kodak, talked about "corporate responsibility" and the need for an "objective" and independent research arm that could gain the public's trust. These comprised a distinct minority, however, that was unable to exert sufficient influence in an organization that represented all companies and needed to provide a united front to the public and government.[54] It is not surprising, then, that of the $150,000 in the EHAC's 1966 budget earmarked for the new environmental health initiative, more than half of it, $83,000, went to "public relations activities."[55]

Despite its efforts to quell negative publicity, the MCA found itself deluged in the coming years with complaints from the emerging environmental movement. But many in the industry still thought that "things aren't that bad." In a March 1967 meeting of the EHAC, the committee's chair, James Sterner, insisted, however, that the available data indicated that the problems would soon be approaching apocalyptic proportions. Given that sulfur dioxide contamination in some urban areas was already a serious problem, he suggested that in the future it was likely to become extremely dangerous. Water pollution had already caused the near death of such major rivers as the Cuyahoga in Ohio; some would "in another decade... have zero dissolved oxygen." While some in his audience might think him too extreme, he noted, "there is a growing procession of thoughtful and critical scientists and citizens whose initial skepticism has changed to concern and even alarm."[56]

Sterner recognized that many environmental issues depended upon the interpretation of necessarily incomplete and somewhat speculative data. He knew that it would be impossible to predict with certainty what environmental pollution would mean for the earth in future decades. Better data were needed, but, even with this data, estimation of the benefits and risks of technological change would entail "value judgments" that were "ultimately social and political in character." He wrote, "We will have to make increasingly difficult decisions, involving not only specific diseases associated with a particular product or pollutant but in addition... on longevity of man, and on genetic changes extending into future generations."[57]

Sterner noted that many within the MCA were still skeptical about the true extent of the problem, that several members had recently voiced the opinion that "this present environmental health kick is only temporary. If we wait awhile there will be some other thing to distract the public." But Sterner maintained that such beliefs were only "wishful thinking, and a dangerous delusion, for the longer we delay action, the more serious the whole problem will become with the certain result that our solutions, generated by crisis and emotion, will be more costly and less beneficial to everyone."[58] The industry was at a crossroads. It had to choose between delay and obfuscation on the one hand, and proactive, responsible corporate action on the other. Over the next few years the MCA, trying to balance the competing tensions among its member companies, often caved in to demands for the least action possible in addressing environmental concerns. Despite increased environmental consciousness and a "growing militancy" on the part of government, the MCA settled for public relations efforts rather than serious activities aimed at reforming industry practice.[59]

Not only were there differences of opinion regarding the extent and nature of the industry's responsibility, but there also were different opinions about how to handle joint government-industry-sponsored research. Historically, industry had seen government as a partner that provided legitimacy and credibility to industry research conclusions. The debacle of the 1920s tetraethyl lead crisis was a case in point: the government had allowed the industry to control the nature of the research and its timetable. By the 1960s this sort of overt manipulation of the process was less easily achieved. When the MCA embarked on a number of joint research enterprises with the Public Health Service and other government agencies to assess the effect of air pollution on public health in the 1960s, it accepted that it could not gain complete control over the research. Although the MCA was unable to control the release of data resulting from such joint research efforts, it did reach an agreement with the government not to "include 'interpretation of project findings'" in any such release.[60] While the industry was not given the right of final approval, as it had been in the 1920s, it was still able to stifle adverse interpretations of joint government-industry research.

In 1969 the MCA did finally acknowledge that air pollution was a health problem and not merely a nuisance, but still the industry downplayed the dangers. The association agreed that some people already suffering from respiratory disease could be "adversely affected" by air pollution, but it argued that people in good health, "even though temporarily discomforted," would quickly recover from acute exposure to chemical pollution "without residual damage." The MCA posited that it was "unlikely" that air pollution was "a sole or principal cause of any disease entity" and that at worst it could accelerate the death of those previously ill, particularly among older people. But the MCA conceded no clear health risk from long-term exposure, no relationship between allergic asthma and air pollution, and no clear relationship in the United States between bronchitis and air pollution. The association agreed with a statement in a Health, Education, and Welfare Department report that said, "The association between long-term residence in polluted areas and chronic disease morbidity and mortality is somewhat conjectural."[61]

In December 1969 J. S. Whitaker, the chair of the EHAC, wrote to its members to bemoan the decision of the MCA's board of directors to disband the sometimes difficult EHAC in favor of a committee dominated by board members themselves.[62] In January 1970, a week before the nation was shocked by a massive oil spill off the coast of Santa Barbara, California ("birds covered with sticky oil struggled for life; dead seals floated ashore."[63]), three months before the first Earth Day demonstrations occurred around the country, eight months before the Environmental Protection Agency was established, the EHAC was dissolved for sounding too much like environmentalists.[64]

In 1969 the federal bureaucracy included more than eighty agencies that dealt with air or water pollution and other problems of the environment. That year, Congress passed the National Environmental Policy Act, creating the Council on Environmental Quality to provide an "exhaustive study" of the environmental impact of any proposed federal project. The act required projects to pass a rigorous review, and each project "had to include possible alternatives."[65] The President's Advisory Council on Executive Organization, appointed by Richard Nixon and chaired by Roy Ash, the former chief executive officer of Litton Industries, recommended in the spring of 1970 that an Environmental Protection Agency be established as "an independent body concerned with pollution abatement and with jurisdiction over all monitoring, research, standard setting and enforcement."[66] In early July, Nixon formally proposed the EPA as part of a reorganization plan, thereby outflanking the Democrats, particularly Senator Edmund Muskie, a Maine Democrat and potential challenger for the White House who had staked out the environment as one of his major issues.[67] With little active opposition from industry, the EPA was established as a cabinet-level agency in 1970.[68] Nixon, rejecting Texas Congressman George Herbert Walker Bush as too "tainted with oil" to lead the EPA, chose William Ruckelshaus, a conservative lawyer who later achieved fame by resisting Nixon's "Saturday Night Massacre."[69]

Nixon's embrace of environmentalism owed much to the developing environmental consciousness, which had emerged in part from the turmoil and protest movements of the 1960s. In the short span of a decade, an industry that had been the symbol of the country's progress came to be viewed with suspicion. Sentiment grew for federal regulation of industry in general and polluting industries in particular. While in 1965 only one-quarter of the public told pollsters that they were concerned about air pollution and one-third about water pollution, by 1968 two-thirds of the public expressed concern about both.[70] Similarly, in 1965 Americans ranked environmental pollution near the bottom of the ten most important problems, but by 1970 pollution had become the second most pressing issue in public opinion polls, ranking just below crime reduction.[71]

In the late 1960s the chemical industry was tied to the military-industrial complex and the divisive controversies of the Vietnam War. When Dow Chemical Company produced napalm as a weapon used against civilian populations and created herbicides to defoliate the forests that hid North Vietnamese and National Liberation Front troops, college protesters across America linked "ecocide" of the chemical industry to the broader antiwar movement, sporting signs declaring "Dow = Death."[72] More generally, the prosperity of the 1960s derived from President Lyndon Johnson's Great Society programs had ironically led Americans to become far less naïve about the deleterious effects of modern technological and industrial progress. In fact, historian David Vogel argues, the strong "performance of the economy" was critical to the "upsurge of citizen activism during the late 1960s and early 1970s."[73]

During the 1960s, new conservation and environmental groups attracted younger, more politically active members. The more activist bent affected the entire consumer and environmental movements.[74] As historian Samuel Hays explains, this period marked a transition in the history of environmentalism in the United States. Older groups such as the Sierra Club, the National Wildlife Federation, and the Audubon Society, which had focused primarily on outdoor recreation, forest preservation, and the maintenance of open spaces now turned to a consideration of air and water pollution. In the 1970s, they looked at the conservation of energy and a consideration of the effects of toxic chemicals, radiation, and other threats to the environment and human health.[75]

LABOR JOINS THE FRAY

As the 1960s saw a trend toward greater federal involvement in environmental protection, aspects of labor and consumer activists joined to push for the passage of two significant pieces of federal legislation: the Coal Mine Safety and Health Act of 1969 and the Occupational Safety and Health Act (OSHAct) of 1970. Never before had the federal government established agencies with a mandate to protect the nation's workers. Before this, especially after World War II, an implicit labor-management "accord" virtually eliminated issues of workers' safety and health from the formal agenda in contract negotiations. While wages and hours were negotiable, safety and health issues were seen as a challenge to management's prerogative to maintain control over the work process. Although the labor movement of the 1960s was viewed as conservative on account of its identification with the military and its blue-collar disdain for the youth movement of the day, there was a more activist strain within it. It was the Vietnam War, in fact, that placed new pressures for production on American industry, resulting in speed-ups, long hours of required overtime, and an increase in the number of industrial accidents, all of which laid the groundwork for rank-and-file attention to issues of health and safety.[76] In 1966 and 1967 the number of strikes was the highest in a decade, and declining productivity and an increasingly militant labor force spelled trouble for business.[77]

When Anthony Mazzocchi became the legislative director of the Oil, Chemical and Atomic Workers International Union (OCAW) in 1965, he believed that radiation was the only major health and safety problem his union members faced. "Then I started getting tons of calls about other health and safety issues and I finally framed [a] questionnaire to find out what was going on in the locals."[78] At the union's convention in 1967, the delegates passed a resolution that dealt with the dangers that had arisen over the previous two decades from the production and use of new chemicals and radioactive materials. The results convinced Mazzocchi that "all of these hazards threatened not only people working in the plants and operations involved, but also the residents of surrounding communities."[79]

More than any other union, the OCAW understood the relationship between what happened to workers in the factory and the threats that chemicals posed to the broader community. The OCAW resolved that, in addition to developing a health and safety program, it would cooperate with the rest of the labor movement to support "legislation and regulations—federal, state or provincial and local—which protect health and safety and place human values above property values."[80]

Mazzocchi's understanding that the substances his workers were handling could not be viewed as a narrow concern of the trade union movement had a history behind it. In 1956 he had become the president of his union's local in Roslyn, Long Island, and, working with the Committee for a SANE Nuclear Policy (SANE), he met Barry Commoner, who was documenting the presence of strontium 90, a radioactive isotope derived from the fallout of nuclear tests, in children's baby teeth. "Our members contributed thousands of teeth," Mazzocchi recalled. "Every morning, someone would come into the local with a little package. . . . It was their kids' teeth and to think that these teeth had strontium 90 in them."[81]

The results of Mazzocchi's 1967 survey gave him the leverage he needed to talk about the issue of nuclear testing to his union members, many of whom were engaged in producing nuclear weapons. ("Without that," Mazzocchi later wrote, "I think I would not have survived politically in the union."[82]) In late March 1969, Mazzocchi opened the first of a dozen sessions nationwide for nearly two hundred workers and union representatives at a Holiday Inn in Kenilworth, New Jersey, not far from Elizabeth and its oil and chemical refineries, where the tetraethyl lead disaster of the 1920s had occurred. Mazzocchi briefly reviewed the worsening situation faced by most of the chemical workforce.[83] Unlike the steel mills, mines, and foundries, where the dangers from accidents, extraordinary heat, dusty air, and odious fumes were fairly obvious, the new chemical plants looked clean and modern. "But," he warned, "the industry we work in has a danger that most people are unaware of, and it's insidious. It's the danger of a contaminated environment, the workplace; something we don't feel, see, or smell, and of which most of us become contemptuous, simply because it doesn't affect us immediately."[84] He lamented the conspiracy of silence that seemed to exist among government, organized labor, and industry, all of whom failed to protect workers from dangerous chemicals or even inform them of the danger. Not only were workers exposed to traditional and known toxins, but also thousands of untested and unregulated chemicals were regularly introduced into the environment where workers labored. "We're meeting within the framework of a situation where no one really knows about the problem; out of the 6,000 or so chemicals in use in industry today, there are only standards for a little more than 400."[85]

In the coming months, Mazzocchi visited community after community, developing an argument for the need for occupational safety and health legislation. Mazzocchi asserted that "exposing a person to a toxic chemical that shortens his life is tantamount to murder, in my opinion." He maintained that the tradition of overlooking the industry's liability for workers' deaths had to end. Up to this point, he noted, the workplace had been off-limits to federal inspectors, and state inspectors had been unwilling to assert their prerogative to inspect or condemn dangerous sites. Overall, the workplace was considered private property, owned by people who felt they had the right to do whatever they wanted behind the factory's walls.[86]

Now, he insisted, it was time for the government to stop treating the workplace as a private preserve. Even though Americans spent major portions of their lives at work, "there's no disclosure and no accountability; no one can be held accountable and there are no criminal penalties for actions" that lead to workers' disease and deaths.[87] Mazzocchi saw collusion between state bureaucracies and private industries in perpetuating dangerous conditions in the chemical industry. To demonstrate how systematic was the denial of information, Mazzocchi pointed to Texas, where it was a criminal act for any government official to disclose information on industry processes to the public. Thus, to publicize industry's harm to workers was viewed as the crime of revealing industry secrets.

Tony Mazzocchi argued that the Texas Occupational Safety Act was pernicious and actually a misnomer, in reality being a "disease promotion" act. In a section titled "Confidential Information," it required that "no information relating to secret processes or methods of manufacture of products shall be disclosed at any public hearing or otherwise." The Texas governmental representatives who violated the law would be subject to fine and firing and their action would be considered "an offense against the state." Mazzocchi pointed out that "here the state is certainly protecting the industries that they're going to be investigating, and making sure that there are criminal penalties for those who would even disclose what they might find out." Corporations suffered no penalty at all for "fail[ing] to disclose formulas that might be killing you."[88]

In these early days before the passage of the OSHAct, labor had been kept in the dark about safety and health statutes or uninformed about what was and was not covered by laws. In 2001 Mazzocchi talked about how not even he really understood the inadequacies of laws then in existence. When workers saw obvious danger they assumed that a law made such circumstances illegal. They believed that if they could uncover the relevant statute they could get industry to improve conditions. Even Mazzocchi was shocked to learn that the Walsh-Healey Act, passed in 1938 to enable the government to inspect the facilities of federal contractors employing more than 10,000 people, covered relatively few workers and that its provisions were not enforceable. He was further surprised to learn that the standards for some substances had been set not by government agencies but by private industries through organizations established by them or by voluntary agencies in which industry had a major role.[89]

At a 1969 meeting in Fort Wayne, Indiana, Mazzocchi questioned how the standards were set up. "Was an impartial investigating body set up? Were we represented on it? Was there public discussion? No." Instead, the standards were developed by the American Conference of Governmental Industrial Hygienists (ACGIH) through "consensus," which meant, Mazzocchi argued, "that if a large company had a representative on the committee, or objected to a particular standard, the committee raised it." The result was that standards were often set to allow higher levels of toxins so the least efficient, most powerful, or least responsible companies could meet them—what Mazzocchi called "the least common denominator, rather than strictly in accordance with scientific evidence."[90]

For Mazzocchi and most of the union delegates he addressed while touring the country, a major problem was that states were enforcing few of the environmental and occupational codes they had developed to protect the workforce, if in fact any enforcement provisions existed. Even in the industrial states, where the chemical industry was centered, codes were ignored. The "New Jersey safety program is an atrocity," Mazzocchi observed, to no objection, at the meeting at Kenilworth. "I think the fellows [i.e., the workers] from National Lead...would be the first to jump up and tell you, specifically" about the variety of problems in the plants and the complete lack of "response of the New Jersey State Health officials."[91] At the union conference in Fort Wayne, Mazzocchi noted that there were many times more game inspectors than state safety inspectors.[92]

Mazzocchi likened his union's sad experience with industry oversight of occupational health to the tragedy of Gauley Bridge, West Virginia, the site of the worst industrial health disaster in American history. In the early years of the Great Depression (1931–32), a Union Carbide subsidiary drilled a tunnel through a mountain that was virtually 100 percent silica without providing the workers with respiratory protective equipment or without informing them of the danger. The tunnel was needed to create an aqueduct to provide power to a Union Carbide chemical plant that the OCAW later organized. Mazzocchi in 1969 told the workers that "600 miners died of silicosis" while drilling the tunnel and that union members should remember their suffering. "Most of us probably never knew that 600 human beings perished in building this particular aqueduct that would carry water to a plant where OCAW members are employed today." West Virginia alone had a sorry history of occupational disasters, including black lung and other pneumonicoses, which Mazzocchi estimated were a factor in the death of 80 percent of coal workers.[93]

Mazzocchi argued that the massive problems in the nation's plants and mines could not continue to be addressed by industry alone. Nor could the union movement depend upon scientists and technicians whose loyalties lay with the industries that hired them. Mazzocchi related his own story about when he was president of a local at a cosmetic plant on Long Island, New York. He admitted that he had never been concerned about the use of talc in the manufacture of the cosmetic powder, nor had he ever been informed about the existence of threshold value limits for talc. "I just never knew enough to raise a question.... We had a doctor who used to say that, if you drank enough milk, you didn't have a problem." Later, notes Mazzocchi, "when the cost of milk went up, he decided that milk was unnecessary."[94] There were too many questions, too many issues, too many competing interests, and too many costs for any one union or any one company to address. It also required scientists who were not beholden to a single, and powerful, vested interest. "It takes the type of scientific personnel that are not on the payrolls of companies."[95]

Mazzocchi saw workers as the true repositories of information about unhealthful workplace practices. Their active participation and testimony would be crucial in creating an incentive for government or industry to provide the necessary protection. Mazzocchi knew what many workers were saying privately: that industries were dumping the dangerous poisons that they worked with in the plant onto the ground, into the air, and into the waterways of the nation. Workers reported "being instructed to permit certain emissions, into the air and into sewers, after dark but not during daylight hours." They were also instructed to curtail dumping activities when journalists or inspectors were present. "Workers in some plants tell of being ordered to inject perfumes into exhaust gases going up the stacks so that people in the vicinity cannot smell the gases."[96]

"Very few of us would now swim in water that we once swam in as children," Mazzocchi lamented in 1969. "Very few of us breathe the same quality of air or get up in the morning and see for any distance without our vision being cut short by haze and smog." He argued that the OCAW was particularly sensitive to these issues "because these very pollutants that are contaminating our environment emanate from the workplace.... So if the community at large is getting a bad dose of pollutants, we are getting it in spades, in much greater quantities, triple fold."[97] Mazzocchi warned that the country would soon face serious problems given the abuse of the work and environment by industrialization. "The urban environment is such that it is constantly assaulting us.... Cancer will probably reach epidemic proportions in major urban areas within the next ten years; urban dwellers will become particularly vulnerable to various forms of cancer."[98]

Glenn Paulson from Rockefeller University in New York provided attendees at the OCAW meetings with a warning about gases one couldn't see and couldn't smell. These included carbon monoxide and chlorine, substances that workers frequently complained about. Exposure to chlorine could destroy lung tissue, leaving workers unable to blow out a match from a foot away and making them "respiratory cripples" for the rest of their lives.[99] Chlorine, one of the most widely used substances in the chemical industry, had a particularly gruesome reputation, especially among older workers who remembered its military use during World War I: chlorine was a constituent of poison gases that were subsequently banned by international convention. Paulson reminded the workers that the recent attention to air pollution in urban areas should alert them to the fact that "chemical plants are much, much worse." The chemical plant of 1960s America was a potent stew of dangerous substances.[100]

At an OCAW conference in Salt Lake City, Utah, union representative Robert Marsh related his experiences at an acid plant in Arkansas: "The company insisted [that the pollution from the stacks] wasn't an unhealthy situation, it was just uncomfortable. We suggested to them it probably was unhealthy too because . . . for about a mile and a half from this plant, the trees were all dead. We got the company people to go out and see all these trees and we said, 'Look, if it doesn't hurt you, how come all those trees are dead?' And the company had a very logical answer. 'Hell, those trees can't spit it out.'"[101]

The meetings that Mazzocchi organized in Tulsa, Fort Wayne, Kenilworth, Montreal, Baltimore, Atlanta, Houston, and Salt Lake City were aimed as much at gathering information as disseminating it. At every meeting, workers were asked to relate their own experiences with dangerous chemicals and to become the eyes and ears, the experts and epidemiologists, for the union. The testimony, transcribed in order to document workers' experiences in the chemical, atomic, and oil industries, provide a rich source of firsthand descriptions of the conditions of work in Vietnamera America.

John Dacey, the president of an independent union at Union Carbide in Boundbrook, New Jersey, spoke movingly of his plant, where asbestos was used in large quantities and where workers' exposure abounded. He related how it was only "since the militant group took over the union" that management was asking the workers, "after thirty five years of operation, to take x-rays, because they know that we're going to double check them." Dacey described how, even though the workers were confronted with "dust and fumes where you can't even see across the room," the boss would reassure the workers that "it won't hurt you. Look at so-and-so; he's been working here fifteen years. . . . This is the kind of attitude we have."[102]

Peter Mac Intyre, president of Local 8-3660, OCAW, at the National Lead plant at Sayreville, New Jersey, brought along an informal survey of some of the workers' experiences in various departments. One worker described being "gassed [by chlorine] ten times at least." Another worker described being overcome twice and, instead of receiving medical treatment, being given "just cough syrup." A third described being overcome: "Fumes were so bad that other operators could not get to me to help me. I managed to get down, trying to hold my breath and proceeded to cough and throw up in the street. The foreman went inside and brought out some cough medicine."[103]

James Orth, from the DuPont plant in Wilmington, Delaware, described his earlier work with silica: "Your nose would be drying out, your throat, just everything, just drying out. So we complained. So then they started to send us down to medical once a week... to get blood tests. Finally, after a year and a half, they came back and told us, yes, you can get silicosis from this. But before that, nothing, everything was fine."[104] One worker from the Woodridge, New Jersey, Chemical Corporation, described the effect of working with toxic chemicals on his family. His father had worked in a chemical plant right next door to the one he had worked for. "He's dead now." His uncle had also worked there and "died of cancer, this cancer in the throat." The uncle believed that "a certain chemical that he inhaled got in his throat and his throat was a mess and he died. I mean, I don't like the expression—he died like a dog. We're a small bunch, but we've got a problem. The chemicals are going to kill us all."[105]

While a few corporate leaders such as Ford's Henry Ford 2nd and Xerox's Sol Linowitz understood the need for reform and even government regulation, most trade associations followed the lead of the Chamber of Commerce, rejecting government regulation in favor of voluntary action. Notably absent from the coalition forming around the twin issues of workplace safety and environmental protection, as historian Charles Noble observes, were "the two preeminent liberal business organizations— the Committee for Economic Development and the Business Council— [which] failed to take any position at all on occupational safety and health." He notes that they "concentrated on economic policy in the mid-1960s."[106] But their inaction may also have been due in part to the general social crisis that existed in the late 1960s that distracted them.

Although the political impetus for the Occupational Safety and Health Act originated among labor activists and the Democratic Party, the Nixon administration quickly embraced the effort as part of its more general attempt to bring white working-class Americans into a new Republican coalition. Courting the "silent majority" in the years of the Vietnam War and capitalizing on "white backlash" against the previous administration's War on Poverty and civil rights efforts, Nixon embraced conservative blue-collar workers. But Nixon's vision for the new agency, one that would prove less threatening to industry, was quite different from labor's. His object was to sign an occupational safety and health bill, but to structure the resulting federal agencies in such a way as to have minimal influence on the way business was conducted. To that end, the Nixon administration was intent that the powers of standard setting and enforcement not be located in the same federal agency. Nixon devised a plan in which a new agency, the National Institute of Occupational Safety and Health (NIOSH), to be located within the Department of Health, Education, and Welfare, would do research and propose standards, while OSHA, in the Department of Labor, would handle enforcement.

Nixon also wanted a bill that had weak federal enforcement provisions. As the legislative negotiations proceeded in 1969 and 1970, Nixon was forced to concede more and more ground to the Democratic-labor plan but held firm to the concept of separate agencies for research and enforcement.[107] Even so, when the Steiger bill (which ultimately became the OSHAct) went to the Senate-House conference committee, Nixon still held out for a weaker bill. The prospects for passage seemed dim. OCAW leader Tony Mazzocchi remembers standing outside the committee room (which was closed to the public) and seeing Walter Mondale come out to say that the Democrats did not have the votes to pass it.[108] But then Nixon called the Hill and told the Republican leadership to bring the bill to a vote. In the aftermath of an assault by New York construction workers on antiwar demonstrators along lower Broadway near Wall Street, the Republican president saw the opportunity to steal traditionally Democratic blue-collar votes by supporting the OSHAct.[109] The bill passed in the waning days of 1970 "with varying degrees of enthusiasm" from business and labor; thus were OSHA and NIOSH established.[110]

The OSHAct established the principle that workers had a right to a safe and healthful workplace and that the federal government had a responsibility to ensure this through inspection, regulation, and standard setting. By authorizing the imposition of fines and even prison terms (a rarely used punishment) for managers and owners of renegade industries, OSHA brought an end to the long-standing principle that the workplace was immune from federal control. The act guaranteed workers access to information previously held to be proprietary trade secrets about the substances they worked with and the possible harmful results from exposure to these chemicals.

One of the most important features of the act was the rejection of the chemical industry's demand that the cost of protection be taken into account as a factor in setting standards. The act held that OSHA should "set the standard which most adequately assures, to the extent feasible, on the basis of the best available evidence, that no employee will suffer material impairment of health or functional capacity even if such employee has regular exposure to the hazard dealt with by such standard for the period of his working life" (section 6B[5]).[111] Over the next several years, industry would make much of the phrase "to the extent feasible" to reassert the argument that economic costs to industry must be considered in any occupational regulation.

The very first complaint that OSHA was asked to address, and the first citation it issued under the OSHAct, was for a chlor-alkali plant of the Allied Chemical Corporation in Moundsville, West Virginia. The plant produced chlorine by the interaction of brine with mercury in an electrolytic process. Since 1965, Local 3-586 of the OCAW had complained to management about the health concerns of workers and had appointed a health and safety committee that tried to work with management to lower workers' exposures to chlorine, mercury, and other toxic materials. For years, management had essentially dismissed the complaints, maintaining that the environment was safe and that no health threats existed.

A few months before the OSHAct was passed, Thomas W. Riggle, the local's president, wrote to Tony Mazzocchi, then the OCAW's legislative director, seeking help. Ellen Silbergeld, then a doctoral candidate in environmental engineering at Johns Hopkins University and later one of the nation's preeminent lead toxicologists, was spending the summer as an intern in the union's legislative office and responded to the union's query.[112] She detailed the health hazards posed by the production of mercury, chlorine gas, and hydrochloric acid and explained that "mercury is such a serious problem that Tony and I would appreciate more information from you on conditions in the plant and on any history of incidents which, in your opinion, might be related to mercury poisoning."[113]

As conditions deteriorated in the plant, with several men showing "symptoms of possible mercury overexposure," union complaints went unanswered. Finally, the union sent a letter to Mazzocchi with copies to the company, the Department of Health, Education, and Welfare, the Department of Labor, and other state and federal agencies and representatives, detailing the environmental hazards faced by the workers. The union's complaint stated that the plant used "mercury type cells to produce chlorine, caustic soda and hydrogen. There are 104 cells of this type, each cell containing approximately 3,600 pounds of raw mercury or a total of around 1.87 tons." The union charged that "these products carry the deadly methyl mercury vapors. . . . Employees work in and around these vapors constantly. . . . Free and exposed mercury can be found all around the building. . . . Various acids and alkalis are dumped to waste beds through a system of pipes and open trenches. Vapors created from this operation are strong enough to irritate the eyes and respiratory organs, and often blanket the area with a dense, choking fog."[114]

Upset by the inability or unwillingness of the state to protect the workers and the unwillingness of Allied Chemical to voluntarily clean up its operation, the local's leadership, in coordination with Mazzocchi and with the support of Sheldon Samuels, director of occupational health, safety, and environmental affairs for the AFL-CIO's Industrial Union Department, decided to be the first major test case under the new federal legislation. They requested an inspection of their plant under the "imminent danger" section of the law. Five days later, on May 19, 1971, OSHA representatives arrived at the plant, where they observed pools of mercury on the factory floor and other hazards. "In one area chlorine fumes were so heavy that [Charles] Benjamin [of the Department of Labor] wore a respirator."[115] On May 28, the Department of Labor received air-sampling results showing that mercury levels were dangerously high. OSHA issued its first citation—the first time, according to Mazzocchi, that a federal agency held a company responsible for health rather than safety issues.[116] Months later, even though the company had made some improvements, workers continued to complain of liquid mercury, mercury vapor, and excessive chlorine in the plant.[117]

In the succeeding years, health issues grew in importance in industry-labor contract negotiations, sometimes leading to prolonged strikes. In early March 1973, chemical workers at nine Shell Oil plants along the Gulf of Mexico and in California went on strike for more than three months over issues of health, not safety. In general, management opposed union demands to create health and safety committees that would make critical decisions about workplace organization and procedures. Giving unions "a voice" in work-floor practices amounted to, in the words of one Shell spokesman, "'just another attempt at featherbedding' since workers could then decide how long they can safely work in the refineries and chemical plants."[118]

Still, the Shell strike significantly broadened the national coalition that began to see occupational safety and health as a critical social, as well as labor, issue. Noted academics, scientists, and activists from around the nation quickly joined hands with the workers, bringing attention and a kind of broad, liberal legitimacy to workers' issues. Leading scholars, scientists, and social activists such as George Wald, Richard Lewontin, Linus

Pauling, and Barry Commoner joined public health advocates such as Samuel Epstein, Victor Sidel, Eula Bingham, Sidney Wolfe, Lorin Kerr, Jack Geiger, and Wilhelm Hueper in sending an open letter to the academic and labor communities.[119] Quickly, ten environmental groups, including the Sierra Club, joined with the OCAW to protest the terrible work conditions and the more general threat to the environment.[120]

This significant joining of labor and environmental groups was widely noted in both the national press and among environmentalists. Environmentalists had been tagged as "elitists who are more interested in conserving pretty vista and saving wildlife than in helping working people," while unions were alleged to be willing to accept any and all pollution "if it means higher wages for them." The strike was seen as marking "the beginning of a new awareness of the scope of environmental issues by both organized labor and environmental activists."[121]

But the true emergence of the environmental crisis in the plastics industry still awaited both labor and industry. It would not be until an industrial hazard of some magnitude occurred that the public would become alarmed. Not until there was a story that affected entire communities would newspapers and magazines report on it. Only then would public pressure begin to shape the response of government agencies themselves. Corporate liability would become virtually unlimited when damage was done to citizens who were not prevented from suing companies, unlike workers, who were usually constrained by workers' compensation laws from pursuing litigation against an employer. Only then would the press, the public, liability lawyers, and the new agencies of government charged with protecting the nation's air, water, and consumers' demand that industry give up its sovereignty over the workplace and its stranglehold on information about the dangers facing workers and community residents alike.

EVIDENCE OF AN ILLEGAL CONSPIRACY BY INDUSTRY

In the mid-1960s, as the chemical industry was struggling with how to respond to the general problem of pollution, it discovered a terrifying fact: vinyl chloride monomer (VCM), the basis for polyvinyl chloride (PVC), one of the most widely used plastics, was linked to acroosteolysis, a degenerative bone condition affecting workers in a number of its plants. In the early 1970s the Manufacturing Chemists' Association (MCA), the industry group representing close to 200 companies, received even more troubling news: secret animal studies performed for European chemical manufacturers showed cancers at surprisingly low levels of exposure to VCM as well.

Industry leaders became terrified. The industry was faced by the question of what would it mean if the public knew that vinyl chloride, the basis for Saran Wrap and hundreds of other consumer products such as hairsprays, car upholstery, shower curtains, liquor bottles, floor coverings, and wiring, was linked to cancer? Would the public begin to view all plastics as threats to their health? To avoid public disclosure of industry-sponsored research indicating cancers caused by vinyl chloride monomer, the chemical industry planned and executed an elaborate scheme to deceive the government and mislead the public.

The MCA closed ranks to protect the image of its product as safe and to hide information about its health costs. As more data emerged from European investigators, confirming and even extending the findings of cancer, the Manufacturing Chemists' Association (now the Chemical Manufacturers Association) privately expressed extreme distress though it continued to show a calm and reassuring face to the government and the general public. The industry considered such deceit necessary in light of the unlimited liability it could face from lawsuits that might be brought by millions of Americans who used vinyl chloride every day.

Plastics had emerged in the 1950s as a mainstay of the petrochemical industry. In 1953 the industry employed 200,000 people and boasted annual sales of over $23 billion. It produced 3.5 billion pounds of plastics and resins per year.[1] Polyethylene, polypropylene, polystyrene, and polyvinyl chloride among others were all synthetic materials. Some, particularly polyvinyl chloride, were unusual in that they were created from chemical combinations that did not exist naturally. Chlorine-carbon molecules do not exist in nature, so their effect on the environment and on human health was completely untested. Of all the plastics, PVC is the most persistent in the environment. Because of its stable chemical properties, chlorine chemistry became a major part of the plastics industry, and polyvinyl chloride quickly assumed a major role in the post–World War II world.

Polyvinyl chloride was first manufactured in the United States in 1928 at the Union Carbide plant in Charleston, West Virginia; commercial production began in 1933.[2] Production skyrocketed during World War II, going from 1 million pounds per year to 120 million pounds per year; by 1952, production had grown to 320 million pounds.[3] In 1973 27 billion pounds of plastics were produced. Polyvinyl and vinyl chlorides accounted for 5.4 billion pounds, behind polyethylene with 8.4 billion pounds and more than polystyrene with 5 billion and polypropylene with 2.2 billion pounds.[4] With the addition of plasticizers that increased flexibility and durability, polyvinyl chloride was extremely adaptable to a variety of uses, especially in construction (40 percent of consumption); in wire and cable (10 percent); manufacture of pipe (25 percent); film and sheet for packaging and coated fabrics (15 percent); and flooring (10 percent).[5] Because of its low cost and great durability, it became a widely used substitute for woods, metals, glass, rubber, ceramics, and other plastics.[6] By the 1960s, VCM gas was also used as an aerosol propellant in beauty aids and cosmetics, drugs, pesticides, and a variety of other products.

There are four broad stages in the production of polyvinyl chloride plastics. First, salt (sodium chloride) is broken down through an electrolytic process to release chlorine as a greenish gas. Inherently unstable, chlorine alone does not naturally exist; about three-quarters of all chlorine is presently used in the chemical industry as a feedstock (i.e., component material) in the production of plastics, pesticides, solvents, and other products unknown in the natural world.[7] In the second stage, chlorine is combined with a variety of hydrocarbons to produce vinyl chloride monomer. (In the late 1940s it was used as an anaesthetic, but it was ultimately discarded because of dangerous side effects).

In the third stage, the monomer is formed into a polyvinyl chloride resin. In the fourth stage, it is fabricated into finished products. Vinyl chloride monomer plants are often huge open-air complexes of metal and steel tubing connecting large and small tanks to one another, much like oil refineries. By and large they are located in southern and western states, especially Louisiana and Texas. PVC plants are somewhat more enclosed and are located in a variety of states, principally New Jersey, Ohio, and Massachusetts in addition to Louisiana and Texas.[8]

While relatively few workers are employed in the production of VCM and PVC, the consequent fabrication processes employ many more. In the mid-1970s only about 1,000 workers were employed by the vinyl chloride monomer industry and another 5,500 workers in the PVC industry. (In total, from 1939 through the mid-1970s, only about 30,000 were involved in VCM and PVC production.) But many more were engaged in the fabrication of finished consumer goods or construction materials. In the mid-1970s there were nearly 350,000 workers using PVC in the fabrication of the wide variety of finished products.[9]

Americans have always been ambivalent about plastics. On the one hand, plastics provided Americans with a wide variety of consumer products previously reserved for the upper middle class and wealthy. On the other hand, many Americans felt that plastics undermined the very quality of American life. Mass produced, affordable consumer goods with faux metal and wood-like finishes were offered to the new middle class at a fraction of the cost of the "real thing," yet they were still recognized as "mere imitations."[10] In the postwar decades, Japan was often identified by Americans as the source of cheap plastic toys "invading" the American consumer market. Yet at the same time the plastics industry was increasingly perceived as critical to America's own economic advancement. So it was that Dustin Hoffman, as a cynical 1960s college graduate in the film *The Graduate*, would sneer when a family friend told him that he had just one word for him: *plastics*.

THE HAZARDS OF VINYL CHLORIDE

For much of the twentieth century, Americans took solace in the notion that industry and science used refined methods to ensure that workers in dangerous trades were not exposed to harmful levels of toxins. Because Americans believed in the ability of technicians and scientists to understand what constitutes danger and how to guarantee safety, they did not worry much about the chemical industry. They felt assured that there were levels below which danger from exposure to chemicals and other substances did not exist—and that the industry observed these strictures. This concept of a maximum safe concentration can be traced back to the nineteenth century when K. B. Lehmann, a German researcher, ordered his laboratory servant to spend an hour inhaling a variety of volatile fluids that he released into the atmosphere. Observing the reaction of the servant to this exposure, he determined levels "just tolerable for short-term exposure."[11] During the first three decades of the twentieth century, lists detailed "harmful concentrations of contaminants," and in 1927 the American Chemical Society identified limits for exposure for twenty-five noxious gases. In 1938 the American Conference of Governmental Industrial Hygienists (ACGIH) was founded as a voluntary agency of industrial hygienists who worked for government rather than industry. In 1941 it began to establish exposure limits for a wide variety of industrial toxins and to use the term *threshold limit value* (TLV) for the levels that it recommended. In 1940 Manfred Bowditch published for the Massachusetts Division of Industrial Hygiene a "code for safe concentrations of certain common toxic substances used in industry."[12]

From the 1930s on, the establishment of safety standards was a central concern of an industry worried about liability suits. But the question of standards was misleading. Most of the established standards were only vaguely dependent upon experimentation and epidemiological study. More often they resulted from bargains struck between industry leaders and public health officials.[13] By the 1960s the chemical industry had privately determined that whatever level of safety was represented by the official TLV for vinyl chloride monomer, it was not adequate to protect the workforce. The industry knew that TLVs were a benchmark of what was achievable, although not necessarily what was safe. Still, the industry continued to rely on standards for which there was often inadequate information and that today look arbitrary.

Through the 1950s and 1960s and even into the early 1970s, vinyl chloride was said to present "no very serious problem in general handling aside from the risk of fire and explosion" but vinyl chloride monomer (VCM) was known to pose a potential danger when workers were exposed to extremely high quantities. It caused faintness, disorientation, drowsiness, and other acute, but passing, effects. In 1954 the MCA set an upper limit of safety at 500 ppm (parts per million), a figure that would stand for two decades.[14] Prior to the establishment of OSHA, most standards from chemical exposure were arrived at in the same loose and often arbitrary manner that vinyl chloride standards were set. As Henry Smyth of Union Carbide stated in an internal memo, the 500 ppm TLV for vinyl chloride was "based largely on single guinea pig inhalation studies by the Bureau of Mines" during the Great Depression.[15]

The producers of vinyl chloride had a sense that vinyl chloride could possibly cause chronic conditions for the workers even before it was linked to any specific disease in the mid-1960s. In May 1959, Dow Chemical's Verald K. Rowe, who would later become that company's director of toxicological affairs in health and environmental research, worried about the fact that there was "no good toxicological data . . . of the chronic toxicity of vinyl chloride."[16] A graduate with a master's degree in biochemistry from the State University of Iowa in 1937, Rowe joined the biochemical research laboratory directly upon leaving the university.[17] In a correspondence with William E. McCormick, manager of the department of industrial hygiene and toxicology at B. F. Goodrich, he admitted privately that the 500 ppm TLV "cannot be relied upon to [sic] strongly when considering chronic exposures." He had "been investigating vinyl chloride a bit and [found] it to be somewhat more toxic when given by repeated daily inhalations." It was "too early yet to tell what vapor concentrations will be without adverse effect." Although he did not inform anyone outside the industry, he expected that the current TLV would produce "appreciable injury" to full-time workers.[18]

This study indicated that "vinyl chloride monomer is more toxic than has been believed"[19] and that repeated exposures at 200 ppm resulted in micropathological changes in the livers of rabbits. As a result of these experiments, in 1961 Dow recommended a 50 ppm TLV, but the American Conference of Governmental Industrial Hygienists failed to change the TLV for more than a decade.[20] The inaction of the ACGIH in revising the TLV and the refusal of the chemical industry to take notice, despite hints of toxicity problems in the plastics industry, provide an insight into the way industry would handle problems in the future. Sometimes the industry would make a crass attempt to control and even suppress information by misleading the government about what it knew about VCM's carcinogenicity. Sometimes the industry would take action within the factory to hide from workers the dangers they were exposed to. Often the industry saw itself at war with regulatory agencies or environmental and labor groups and established a pattern of hiding information about vinyl chloride's dangers.

BRACKETING THE TROUBLE AREA

When the industry learned in the mid-1960s about vinyl chloride workers who suffered from acroosteolysis (AOL), a previously undefined condition, it developed a strategy regarding health issues that it would use over the coming decade. While privately seeking to understand the source of the problem and by funding research that would provide the information it needed to devise a response, the industry released only the information that would reassure people as to the essentially benign nature of the finished products. The industry would also work to forestall any regulatory action.

The industry learned that a few workers who entered the polymerizer vats, where polyvinyl chloride was synthesized from vinyl chloride monomer, in the Louisville, Kentucky, plant of B. F. Goodrich, were developing hand and systemic health problems. The problem was discovered in 1964 by Dr. John Creech, a physician who had grown up in the mountains of Harlan County, Kentucky. In addition to his private practice (surgical oncology) in Louisville, Creech conducted physical exams of the Goodrich workforce. One day a worker came to Creech in the dispensary "complaining about his tender fingers and asked me 'what's going on . . . with my fingers?'" Creech noticed that the skin on the man's fingers, as well as elsewhere on his body, was thickened. Creech asked him "if he knew of anyone else over at the plant [who] was having this type of problem." He learned that another worker couldn't even open up his lunchbox because his fingers were so tender. Subsequent x-rays and examinations showed that the two workers had similar conditions.

Over the next six weeks Creech accumulated a few more cases and reported his observations to the plant management. "If four people doing the same type of work in the same room, the same department," Dr. Creech recalled thirty-five years later, "they come down with a bizarre situation like this, it doesn't take a rocket scientist to link it to industry—to their workplace."[21] It may not have taken a rocket scientist, but it may have taken a physician like Creech, who was not dependent on the chemical industry, to discover this syndrome, which was called acroosteolysis. The syndrome involved "skin lesions, absorption of bone of the terminal joints of the hands, and circulatory changes."[22]

Shortly thereafter, Goodrich officials asked Robert Kehoe, now nearing retirement as director of the Kettering Laboratory, to commence an investigation for the company.[23] After studying some cases, Kehoe concluded that this was an "entirely new" occupational disease.[24] Meanwhile, Rex Wilson, head of Goodrich's medical department, asked the physician of another Goodrich plant "to determine as *quietly as possible* whether similar disabilities" existed at his plant. It was clear that he did not want the employees to know the reason for any examinations. He told the doctor, "I would appreciate your proceeding with this problem as rapidly as possible, but doing it *incidentally* to other examinations of our personnel. We do not wish to have this discussed *at all* and I request that you maintain this information in confidence."[25]

Monsanto sought to gather information about the extent of the disease in one of its plants without telling the workers the cause of the company's concern. The workers were to be x-rayed, but a Monsanto official wrote, "I am sure Dr. Nessell can prepare these people with an adequate story so that no problem will exist. Depending upon what happens following this x-raying, we will have to see what our next step is."[26] Noting that it was not just polymerization workers who were coming down with the disease, Goodrich and Monsanto worried that this issue could become public, to the detriment of the industry.

In an attempt to forestall any disclosures, a curtain of secrecy was lowered around the diseases appearing in polymerization plants around the country and the world. In January 1966, Harry Warner, corporate vice president of B. F. Goodrich, learned of a physician with the Solvay et Cie Chemical Company in Brussels, Belgium, who had reported seeing at least two workers who exhibited the same bone destruction that was seen in the Goodrich cases and who was planning to publish a report about them.[27] "Goodrich was concerned enough about the response to such a published article that Mr. Warner attempted to have one of [Goodrich's] representatives, who was in Europe, stop by and try to discourage or to influence the wording of such an article to be sure that it didn't condemn PVC in general." The attempt was unsuccessful, but Goodrich made plans to send a team to Brussels in another effort to "discourage or edit the publication." Monsanto, which had its European headquarters in Brussels, offered to "cooperate with Goodrich" in this effort.[28]

At the same time that they sought to hide information from the public and the workforce, Goodrich warned other companies to be on the lookout for workers suffering from similar symptoms. In June Goodrich presented its findings to representatives of six major U.S. and European companies at a private meeting.[29] At the conclusion of this meeting, the MCA was asked to organize a larger meeting of all the plastics companies to decide on a common course of action regarding the medical and public relations dangers that lay ahead. Goodrich revealed to the companies that "1% of all PVC plant personnel were found to be affected" with AOL and that not all of these were in manufacturing jobs. Fully 6 percent of those working in the vats were affected.[30]

The growing plastics industry was terrified about the effect any public disclosure of a problem with an essential ingredient would have on its market. At the meeting a representative from Airco noted what was obvious to all—that "any action at the plant must be properly handled to avoid labor relations and publicity problems."[31] The problem went beyond labor relations and union issues, however, and B. F. Goodrich hoped that other companies would "use discretion in making the problem public," because of the need "to avoid exposes like *Silent Spring* and *Unsafe at Any Speed*," which had publicized the worst kind of nightmare faced by major industrial executives in the mid-1960s.[32] Goodrich noted that the condition "may be a systemic disease" and, if so, Goodrich "worried about possible long term effect on body tissue, especially if it proves to be systemic."[33]

Union Carbide's Robert "Nick" Wheeler emphasized the need for secrecy in light of the "definite health problem related to polyvinyl chloride manufacture."[34] Wheeler, who graduated from Virginia Polytechnic Institute in 1943 with a degree in chemical engineering, had been employed by Union Carbide since then in the development and manufacture of synthetic polymers. In the 1960s, he was the area superintendent at the Union Carbide Company's South Charleston, West Virginia, plant and production manager for vinyl resins.[35]

While the PVC manufacturers were concerned about the potential dangers from VCM exposure to the workforce, they were more concerned about the negative publicity. In the words of Wheeler's follow-up memo relating to a meeting of the MCA's Occupational Health Committee, "the need for bracketing the trouble area was believed essential. Unfavorable publicity with regard to exposure of finished products to the human anatomy could be very damaging to the industry."[36] If plastic products, particularly those that wrapped or came in contact with food, were implicated, the industry would find itself besieged not just by workers and their unions, but also by the general public and federal authorities.

Even though there had been no study on the danger of this consumer product, the technical director of the MCA, Dr. Frank H. Carman, had already prepared a short press release, agreed to by all at the meeting, to be disseminated in the event that word leaked out about any problem. The statement "stressed that [the] condition probably is an occupational disease and there is no indication of any hazard whatever to [the] general

public."[37] The participants at the meeting also agreed to fund an epidemiological study of PVC workers to be conducted by epidemiologists at
the University of Michigan's Institute for Industrial Health. This study
would "hopefully be expected to ... confirm that the condition is purely an
occupational disease and in no way affects the general public using PVC
products."[38] Underlying the study was the assumption that in eight
months' time, the investigators would "have identified the offending agent
or agents" that was poisoning workers in PVC manufacturing plants.[39]

Meanwhile, at the end of the summer of 1967, almost three years after
vinyl chloride-related disease had been noticed in the Goodrich plant,
researchers from B. F. Goodrich published in the *Journal of the American
Medical Association* a report of thirty-one cases of acroosteolysis among
vinyl chloride workers.[40] According to John Creech, the draft of the article
that he first saw specifically identified the monomer as the cause, a piece of
information that vanished by the final version.[41] The study, the first public
acknowledgment of a hazard from working with vinyl chloride, reported
that less than 3 percent of these workers presented symptoms of AOL.[42]
Even so, Goodrich Chemical's president, Anton Vittone, instructed his
managers that the article "was and is intended for medical people" and
should "only be circulated to your key people." Vittone saw the article as a
fail-safe, in the event "the general press becomes aware of this problem."[43]

In the late 1960s, however, the media were not in the habit of following
up on revelations made in medical journals, as they are today. A year and a
half later, in February 1969, the results of the University of Michigan
study were presented confidentially to the MCA's Medical Advisory Committee. The report acknowledged that AOL involved connective tissue as
well as bony structures and that an assumption that AOL was a localized
problem involving just fingers was incorrect. It had been assumed that
only when workers could smell vinyl chloride was there a possibility of
overexposure. But the report indicated that the "odor threshold" of vinyl
chloride was about 4,000 ppm, not 400 ppm as previously believed, and
well above the threshold limit value of 500 ppm. More importantly, the
document noted that it should not be assumed that vinyl chloride workers
were safe from disease even at the 500 ppm TLV. The study suggested that
"sufficient ventilation should be provided to reduce the vinyl chloride concentration [to] below 50 ppm."[44]

The members of the MCA's Occupational Health Committee were particularly troubled by this recommendation. To propose reducing exposure
to 50 ppm implied that vinyl chloride was the direct cause of disease. The
members, by a vote of seven to three, refused to accept the report as writ-

ten and unanimously voted to accept the report only if it were changed to avoid any implication that the 50 ppm was "a threshold level for general safety when exposed to VCM."[45] The MCA's PVC resin producers agreed that the wording must be changed to read thus: "Inasmuch as the etiologic agent of the disease is unknown, a level of vinyl chloride below 50 ppm should be used as an index of adequate ventilation."[46] Their object was that there should be no implication that exposure to vinyl chloride monomer at such low levels could cause disease.

The industry's viewpoint was reflected in the final version of the report when, in 1971, the University of Michigan researchers published their findings in the *Archives of Environmental Health*. Even the whiff of a suggestion that the 500 ppm standard was inadequate had disappeared; nor did the published report recommend that the 500 ppm TLV for vinyl chloride exposure be reduced. In fact, it paraphrased the MCA's assertion that the etiologic agent responsible for the workers' symptoms was unknown: "Although this study provided no evidence to suggest that vinyl chloride per se is the etiological agent, the measurement of vinyl chloride concentrations may serve as a useful index to the adequacy of reactor ventilation."[47] The University of Michigan researchers made no reference to the information provided to industry representatives two years earlier about the odor threshold. This meant that workers who smelled vinyl in the air were exposed to levels far above, not slightly below, the TLV. The report, masquerading as objective science, was in fact nothing more than an obfuscation of the real truth that served industry's purposes.

As late as 1969, fully five years after the first cases of AOL were identified in Goodrich's Louisville PVC plant, the industry still sought to promote the view that there was no causative relationship between vinyl chloride and systemic disease. Goodrich executives also decided "*not* to accept any proposals for additional research into the causes of acroosteolysis at this time."[48] In effect, they were saying that they did not want to know more than what they already knew. Instead, the MCA agreed to establish a case registry to be run by researchers at the University of Michigan, who by now had well proven their willingness to play ball with the industry.

Although the MCA had agreed to establish the registry, the industry soon lost interest. Bertram Dinman, the University of Michigan researcher who had collected the data, believed that the maintenance of the registry was essential for future researchers and the industry to understand the extent of the problem. In May 1971, Dinman advised the MCA's Occupational Health Committee that the "submission of case registry data has been slow."[49] Two months later, Dinman wrote to one of the member company physicians that the AOL registry was in serious trouble. Unless it continued, he warned, "we will never be able to determine the extent of the problem and reply to contentions that the problem is under control."[50] The MCA confirmed that the registry was "perilously close to collapse in consequence of the failure of most of the PVC producers to submit requested case data."[51] The registry limped along for the next two years and then was abandoned.[52]

SECRET AGREEMENTS: THE EVOLUTION OF THE CANCER DEBATE

The reactions of the industry to the link between vinyl chloride and acroosteolysis were a mere preview to how the industry would react when faced with a much larger and uncontainable problem—the link between vinyl chloride and cancer. When cancer became an issue, the industry took more extreme and potentially explosive actions to cover up the danger. The industry moved from denial and obfuscation to outright deception. Motivated by money and power rather than health, the industry was largely successful in hiding its information about cancer from the government and in deflecting national attention away from the potential hazards of thousands of mostly untested new chemicals and of vinyl chloride in particular. In the years to come the nation would learn the serious pitfalls that result when regulation of an industry is left in the hands of that industry.

The fear that vinyl chloride or other chemicals would cause cancer among consumers had haunted the chemical industry. In November 1967 the MCA's Food, Drug, and Cosmetic Chemicals Committee suggested spending $20,000 to develop "a position paper on carcinogenesis in an attempt to refute the Delaney Clause philosophy," which prohibited the use of a suspected carcinogen in any food product. They acknowledged that such an effort "will be difficult, maybe impossible," but the possibility that the principle of no acceptable risk would extend "into other legislative areas, such as atmospheric pollution" made such an effort important. Specifically, the MCA sought to "retain the services of a group of experts on carcinogenesis" who would support their position that there were safe levels of carcinogenic chemicals to which the public could be exposed.[53]

The so-called Delaney clause was a piece of federal legislation that had been passed less than a decade earlier, in 1958, as part of the Food Additives Amendment to the Food, Drug, and Cosmetic Act of 1938 (itself a revision of the Pure Food and Drug Act of 1906). For virtually half a century the federal government had been grappling with the problem of how to protect the public from potential harm caused by adulterations to foods and cosmetics. Beginning in 1906 "poisonous or deleterious substances" were banned as ingredients in foods if government could show affirmatively that such substances were harmful under conditions of normal use. The burden of proof for proving danger rested with the government and its relatively limited laboratories and scientific establishments. In 1938 the Food, Drug, and Cosmetic Act modified the act modestly, essentially allowing poisonous substances into products if they were deemed essential to their production and within the "tolerance promulgated as safe by the Secretary [of Agriculture]."[54] This language made the process of proving additives dangerous much more difficult. Legislative attempts were made to revise the act to develop more absolute criteria for determining whether additives could be banned.

Between 1950 and 1953 Representative James Delaney, a New York Democrat, held hearings about the adulteration of the food supply, which led to three significant pieces of legislation: the Pesticides Amendment of 1954, the Color Additive Amendment of 1960, and the Food Additives Amendment of 1958, which included the Delaney clause. The clause was of special concern to the chemical industry during the 1960s and early 1970s because it banned from foods any additive that caused cancer in animals.[55] While the structure for evaluating all chemicals proved to be difficult to administer, the Delaney clause proved to be the most enduring and effective legacy of this midcentury attempt to implement a federal policy for food safety. It lasted virtually untouched until 1996, when Congress passed the Food Quality Protection Act, which eliminated it.[56]

Businesses involved with pesticides, preservatives, food colorings, and the like were most concerned by the Delaney clause. Throughout the 1960s, the trade literature was filled with attacks on the clause by chemical manufacturers who objected to the "no tolerance" principle upon which it was based. While other potentially toxic substances were deemed "safe" when present in small quantities below an established threshold, the Delaney clause banned *all* cancer-inducing chemicals, no matter how small, as food additives.[57]

In the late 1960s a growing number of environmentalists and public health advocates used the law to ban even small quantities of substances once thought harmless, like the artificial sweetener cyclamate. Cyclamates were discovered to induce cancer in rodents when given in massive amounts; because cyclamates were widely used as a sugar supplement in soft drinks and diet foods, the industry responded quickly. In light of a rapidly changing technology that was capable of detecting substances in extremely miniscule amounts, the industry felt called upon to argue that even though miniscule amounts could be detected it did not mean that these amounts would harm people. According to industry members, the Delaney clause was fundamentally misguided: carcinogens, they argued, were no different from other toxic materials, which had threshold levels below which no danger to humans existed. Following the logic of the Delaney clause, the industry argued, many obviously benign substances, such as common table salt, could be considered carcinogens if administered in massive amounts or under special circumstances.[58] One well-worn argument in the early 1970s was that even hard-boiled eggs, when fed to mice in sufficient quantities, produced cancers and would therefore have to be banned for human consumption. This argument finally lost steam when it was pointed out that those eggs might very well have been tainted with cancer-causing agents such as DES or DDT.[59]

This debate evolved within the context of the popular recognition that chronic illness, and especially cancer, was replacing infectious and acute diseases as the major killers of Americans. In 1971 President Nixon began a War on Cancer that, he promised, would find a cure for the disease in less than a decade. Americans were told that the infusion of money into research would enable the country to win the war on cancer just as money would win the War on Poverty, the war in Vietnam, and the space race against the Soviet Union. It was assumed that the model used to conquer polio, smallpox, and even measles and other infectious diseases would work again. Medical researchers in universities, government, and industry were to be given the money and time to find a virus, a germ, or another agent that "caused" cancer; it was expected that a means to a cure would emerge from the nation's laboratories.

Many environmentalists and public health activists were not convinced. They proposed a fundamentally different approach, focused not on the search for a cure but on prevention as the first line of defense. Since evidence was accumulating that foreign substances such as nicotine, food additives, pesticides, or pollution caused cancer, environmentalists surmised that the culprit was the chemicals produced by industrial and human institutions. While it was a precept of industrial hygiene that safe levels of toxins like lead or arsenic could be established, it was becoming clear to many industrial hygienists that it was impossible to establish threshold levels for carcinogens. Unlike traditional industrial toxins, which caused a variety of conditions, carcinogens "triggered" a biological process that was virtually impossible to stop. It was theoretically possible for a single exposure to a carcinogen to begin the process. Given this, no exposure could be deemed safe. Nor did removing the person from exposure to the carcinogen do anything to stop the growth of tumors. Thus, reducing exposure to "no detectable limit" became the goal of environmentalists, many occupational health advocates, and many industrial hygienists.

The industry had recently learned that an Italian researcher, Dr. Pierluigi Viola from the Regina Elena Institute for Cancer Research in Rome, had presented a paper on the carcinogenic effects of vinyl chloride exposure in animals at the 1970 International Cancer Congress in Houston. Viola reported that rats exposed to 30,000 ppm of vinyl chloride monomer gas developed tumors of the skin, lungs, and bones.[60] In May 1971, the same month that Viola published his findings in the journal *Cancer Research*,[61] he was invited to Washington by the MCA's Occupational Health Committee to present a summary of his work. While executives were upset by his findings, they hoped that his results would be deemed not applicable to other animals or to humans who were exposed to far lower levels of vinyl chloride. As a result of the meeting, the MCA began to develop a research protocol aimed at evaluating the carcinogenicity of vinyl chloride and to consider conducting an epidemiological study.[62] They hoped that because the cancers showed up in the rat's zymbal gland, an ear gland that does not exist in humans,[63] the cancer might not show up in humans. The industry decided not to revise the Material Chemical Safety Data Sheet, the document used by producers to establish safe practices in their plants.[64]

A few months later the MCA learned that "further studies [by Viola] on the toxicity of vinyl chloride have confirmed the carcinogenicity of this monomer" even though it "has not been confirmed in the human body." Viola suggested, on the basis of his research, that a safer TLV would be 100 ppm, for he found that the "danger of a toxic action of the monomer on nervous apparatus, bones and liver is negligible if vinyl chloride concentrations are no more than 100 ppm."[65] Viola also reported to the MCA that he had found tumors in 10 to 15 percent of rats at 5,000 ppm.[66] He suggested that animal studies of vinyl chloride's carcinogenic properties be conducted at low concentrations, down to 50 ppm.[67] Union Carbide's Robert Wheeler understood that "publishing of Doctor Viola's work in the U.S. could lead to serious problems with regard to the vinyl chloride monomer and resin industry." Wheeler was concerned about this link to cancer because "the Delaney amendment bans the use of any material in food that can cause cancer" and, more broadly, that "the present political climate in the U.S. is such that a campaign by Mr. R[alph] Nader and others could force an industrial upheaval via new laws or strict interpretation of pollution and occupational health laws."[68]

Viola's finding of tumors at 5,000 ppm and his recommendation that a 100 ppm threshold would probably avoid future problems were tough enough for the industry to swallow. But the reports of research done in 1972 by another Italian researcher represented a potential catastrophe. PVC was now central to the economic viability of a number of critical American chemical companies. Between 1966 and 1971, PVC production in the United States doubled, from 1.2 billion to 2.4 billion pounds; in the case of B. F. Goodrich, for example, the chemical division was replacing rubber as the most profitable sector, and PVC accounted for half of the chemical division's sales.[69]

Late in 1972 the American chemical industry received a series of reports from European vinyl manufacturers who had, in the wake of Viola's reports, hired Cesare Maltoni, director of the Bologna Centre for the Prevention and Detection of Tumors and Oncological Research, to investigate whether Viola's findings had any merit. During the summer of 1972, the Europeans began receiving preliminary results of Maltoni's confidential work, which indicated that cancers were appearing in rats exposed to lower levels of vinyl chloride than in Viola's studies and in sites other than their zymbal gland. Almost immediately, the European producers began to enlist their American counterparts in secrecy agreements aimed at preventing any public discussion of this work.[70]

According to the Americans, the European chemical companies were especially insistent on the need for a secrecy agreement. "Apparently, Dr. Viola's presentation at Houston about 2 years ago was made without Solvay's permission," reported Allied Chemical's William A. Knapp to his superiors.[71] The secrecy agreement demanded that "the members of our task group as listed on the attached sheet, are the *only* ones entitled to receive information about the European project. In turn, they should feel honor bound to make sure such information remains within their own companies unless and until formal permission has been granted for its release."[72] Dow felt "honor-bound to make sure that information received from the European producers remains within our own company until formal permission has been granted for its release." To accomplish this, Dow instructed that no one "discuss the European work" even within the company unless such persons "have a need to know." Even then, such discussion should be cleared in advance.[73]

While it is common practice for researchers to jealously guard their findings until they are published, in cases where human lives are at stake, most researchers accept that they have an obligation to share knowledge about potential harm. Further, the insistence on confidentiality was not coming from the scientific researcher, but from the vinyl manufacturers. The secrecy was not entered into at the beginning of the experiments, but only when it became apparent that vinyl chloride monomer was carcinogenic at half the accepted TLV. Secrecy, in this case, was not to protect product information, patent secrets, or even innovative experimental procedures. Rather, its sole aim was to avoid a public relations and legal nightmare.

In October 1972 Dr. Walter Harris, representing the MCA, visited Maltoni in Bologna and concluded that the MCA's plans to study high dosage exposure were irrelevant since Maltoni was already finding carcinogenicity at lower levels of exposure.[74] Maltoni's results were revealed to American producers of PVC and VCM at a confidential meeting at MCA headquarters in Washington on November 14, 1972. Members were requested not to take notes; in fact, a European representative, D. M. Elliott of the British vinyl manufacturer Imperial Chemical Industries (ICI), "insisted that the work tables be swept clear of paper for note taking before he would discuss anything regarding the European group's efforts. Such was done."[75] The most disturbing fact that Elliott presented was that Maltoni had discovered "the occurrence of primary cancers in both liver and kidneys with one positive at 250 parts per million," half the long-held 500 ppm threshold value that ostensibly protected workers from AOL and other toxic effects of vinyl chloride.[76] In January 1973, company representatives were given a chart that showed that angiosarcomas of the liver were reported at exposures as low as 250 ppm. Maltoni was finding cancers in a variety of sites and at very low dosages. The MCA did not doubt the accuracy of this data.[77]

By the early 1970s it was becoming more difficult for the industry to keep information about carcinogens secret within the industry. Previously, what happened in the workplace remained largely a private matter concerning the employer, the employee, and, perhaps, a union. Only when a problem escaped the private sphere of the factory and ended up as an issue in a liability lawsuit or on the front page of a newspaper did an occupational health issue become a source of potential harm to a company's well-being.

Growing environmental awareness among consumers in the late 1960s and early 1970s resulted in new liability issues. Because of workers' compensation, it was extremely difficult for workers to sue employers who had exposed them to dangerous chemicals. Workers' compensation had been enacted in the early twentieth century as a means of compensating workers for injuries incurred on the job—and, later, for work-related health effects. But it also was a means of protecting industries from lawsuits brought by injured or diseased workers. Workers were assured a small sum of money, but in return they gave up the right to sue their employer. Industry was not protected, however, from *consumers*, who could, under product liability laws, sue manufacturers for defective products. The need to protect industry from suits by *users* of vinyl chloride products was foremost in the minds of executives as they considered the implications of Maltoni's, Viola's, and even their own research. What was the potential exposure for their industry from possible suits by consumers? Which products were worth continuing to produce and which were too risky? Which products could be abandoned without financial loss to the growing plastics industry?

The minutes of a December 1971 MCA "planning group" reveal that this ad hoc body developed a set of "principles" for its research in which the search for truth was secondary to protecting the industry: First, there was "the need to be able to reassure the public that polyvinyl chloride entails no risk to the user." Second, workers needed to be reassured "that management was concerned for, and diligent in seeking, the information necessary to protect their health." Third, research had to serve the purpose of developing "data useful in defense of the industry against invalid claims for injury for alleged occupational or community exposure."[78]

In the aftermath of Maltoni's research discoveries, the industry had to do something about its potential liability if its products were proven dangerous. The industry's actions with regard to aerosol propellants are an interesting case in point. Vinyl chloride monomer was used not only to create polyvinyl chloride plastics but also as an aerosol propellant in a variety of consumer products. Vinyl chloride was first used as an aerosol propellant in Japan in 1958.[79] By 1959, the Dow Chemical Company was considering using VCM as a propellant in hairsprays, insecticides, room deodorants, and spray paints. Dow expected that its market for vinyl chloride monomer in aerosols to be about 10 million pounds annually and did not believe that the current TLV of 500 ppm would be problematic for them.[80]

Ten years later, however, it was becoming clear that 500 ppm could pose a danger. B. F. Goodrich, after the experience with acroosteolysis, acknowledged privately that "the people in the cosmetics trade have been concerned about the possible toxicity" of vinyl chloride propellants. Measures of vinyl chloride in the air of hair salons had indicated that the "average concentration of VCl monomer is 250 ppm by volume." While this was bad enough in light of earlier recommendations by Dow that the TLV be lowered to 50 ppm, Goodrich worried that "in some cases where the duration of spraying is long (3 minutes) the concentration may be as high as 1400 ppm." The implication was frightening. Both beauticians and their customers may be "exposed to concentration of VCl monomer equal to or greater than the level in our [polyvinyl chloride plants]."[81]

Nonetheless, vinyl chloride was used as an aerosol propellant until sometime in 1974. Only after learning of Maltoni's findings did the MCA's research coordinators argue that "serious consideration should be given to withdrawal from this [aerosol] market since value of the product was limited and potential for liability great."[82] One participant at the meeting stated the issue succinctly: "If vinyl chloride proves to be hazardous to health, a producing company's liability to its employees is limited by various workmen's compensation laws. A company selling vinyl chloride as an aerosol propellant, however, has essentially unlimited liability to the entire U.S. population."[83]

Awareness of evidence of the dangers of chemicals to the broader public was becoming more widespread, as reflected by actions on the part of the government. In May 1973, the Food and Drug Administration suspended approval of the use of PVC bottles for packaging whiskey and wine. Because of the Delaney clause, the FDA, which had previously not regulated the use of vinyl chloride in food packaging, was forced to address the issue posed by the Viola studies and their indication of carcinogenic and other health effects.[84]

In January 1973 the FDA learned that the Treasury Department's Bureau of Alcohol, Tobacco and Firearms, which had been testing liquor bottles since November 1968, had found that plastic bottles were leaching vinyl chloride monomer, creating an unpleasant taste in alcohol products. The FDA's more sophisticated tests confirmed that "vinyl chloride monomer migrates to alcohol in PVC bottles used to package distilled spirits and wine."[85] In the end, the FDA established a much more stringent safety standard for consumer food products than existed for the safety of workers in the factory or among community residents subjected to environmental pollution. The FDA's regulation placed the burden of proof on the industry to show that food additives were noncarcinogenic. In the case of the workplace and in the case of toxins released into the ground, air, and water, the industry was held to no such standard. Workers and neighborhood residents still had to prove a substance dangerous. The FDA ultimately banned the use of vinyl chloride for liquor bottles because it knew "of no studies which establish a safe level of consumption when this monomer is leached from containers into alcoholic foods."[86]

The chemical industry's commitment to objective science and public access to information was tested in January 1973 when NIOSH published in the *Federal Register* a "Request for Information" on the potential hazards of vinyl chloride. NIOSH was preparing a document on the appropriate and safe exposure levels to vinyl chloride and sought information about potential health hazards from all quarters, including scientists, corporations, and public health officials.[87] This request for information put tremendous pressure on the MCA members as they sought to develop a common position concerning the health risks of vinyl chloride. NIOSH was a relatively new government agency. Its mandate to establish "criteria documents" that would guarantee a safe work environment meant that safety and health standards, previously a private matter for individual companies and their trade association, were now in the public sphere.

The industry faced a serious dilemma over NIOSH's request for information. In order to maintain its influence with the agencies that regulated it, the industry would need to comply with the request but would be providing information that would lead NIOSH to recommend standards that were anathema to industry. In this context, Dow's vice president, George J. Williams, believed that the information should be revealed to the government because "it would be extremely damaging to the chemical industry reputation if someone should discover that we have this information and have not disclosed it to the Government."[88] The MCA, as an organization, even acknowledged in a detailed letter to all its management contacts that it had a "moral obligation not to withhold from the Government significant information having occupational and environmental relevance," specifically Maltoni's new findings. It also recognized that by taking the initiative in sharing information the MCA could forestall the scandal that would result if the information eventually became public.[89]

But the MCA also recognized that the confidentiality agreement it had recently made with the Europeans inhibited any free interchange of scientific findings with government. This posed a moral and political dilemma. Would the American industry be willing to fulfill what it considered to be its moral obligation by revealing Maltoni's findings to the United States government even if it meant violating the trust between the American chemical companies and their European brethren?[90] Or would it keep vital information secret and thus prevent public health authorities from having the information they needed to pursue a rational public policy?[91]

In the spring of 1973 the MCA's members agreed on a plan that would both maintain their secrecy agreement with the Europeans and give the appearance of responding to NIOSH's request for information. Rather than waiting for NIOSH to contact the organization, the MCA set up a meeting with Dr. Marcus M. Key, NIOSH's administrator, whose role was to provide OSHA with state-of-the-art scientific information that could be used to establish regulations to ensure safe and healthy working conditions.[92]

In May 1973 the MCA began to plan for its meeting with Key and the NIOSH staff, scheduled for July. The pressure on the MCA was enormous because at that moment OSHA was announcing emergency standards for fourteen other potential carcinogens, and the industry had sued to forestall its implementation.[93] From the first, its Task Group on Vinyl Chloride Research and the Vinyl Chloride Research Coordinators were aware that "a significant element for consideration . . . was the development of an alternate presentation in the event that the release of European data cannot be negotiated with reasonable dispatch."[94]

The MCA's lawyers briefed the members "on their responsibilities and obligations under the confidentiality agreements." The lawyers' "admonishments" were that the American companies "should not volunteer reference to the European project or substantive data derived therefrom," but if asked a direct question, they should answer it.[95] Given that the European experiments were not known to NIOSH, there was little danger that a question could be formed that required such an answer. The MCA Research Group also decided that the companies would not volunteer information regarding "potential hazards" that involved consumer safety since NIOSH was "concerned with employee health matters" alone.[96] It appears that all references to consumer safety issues, particularly aerosol propellants, were removed "at the insistence of UCC [Union Carbide] and Allied [Chemical]" because it was not "a worker-exposure problem except for beauticians and can-fillers."[97] As Robert Wheeler of Union Carbide explained: "Hazard to UCC's interests exists if vinyl chloride is declared to be a carcinogen or if vinyl chloride monomer is detected by FDA in foods exposed to vinyl chloride polymers as film, coatings, or gasketing."[98]

Perhaps most troubling to the MCA representatives was the realization that their letter "to Company Contacts," which acknowledged "a moral obligation" to inform NIOSH about Maltoni's studies, was a legal minefield. They feared the letter could be interpreted to indicate that the industry was planning to mislead the government. According to Wheeler, the memo "could be construed as evidence of an illegal conspiracy by industry if the information were not made public or at least made available to the government."[99]

The industry also planned not to tell NIOSH about its own information indicating that the threshold limit should be reduced well below the 500 ppm recommended in the Chemical Safety Data Sheet and even below the 200 ppm level recommended by the American Conference of Governmental Industrial Hygienists. The MCA decided to remove references to Dow's recommendation that the TLV be reduced to 50 ppm for fear that the government would reduce the TLV even further.[100]

The policy to keep quiet about Maltoni's studies influenced the plastics companies' public statements as well as their private preparations for the NIOSH meeting. As these preparations were in progress, *Modern Plastics,* the industry magazine, published an article about the potential problems that industry could face from NIOSH's program to develop new criteria for testing the dangers posed to workers by various chemicals. In a long review of potential problems for the chemical industry, the article noted that vinyl chloride monomer had come under new scrutiny as a result of "recent animal studies conducted in Italy (at an elevated exposure level of 30,000 ppm)" that had led the MCA to study VCM's "potential hazards." Nowhere in the article is there a reference to Maltoni's discoveries of angiosarcomas in animals at 250 ppm.[101]

Throughout the early summer of 1973, the Americans continued to meet among themselves and with the Europeans to plan the presentation to NIOSH, scheduled for July 17. On June 15, 1973, the Europeans met and "agreed that the MCA would be given permission to reveal to NIOSH data arising from the Bologna study." Three weeks later, however, Montedison, the Italian producer of vinyl chloride, let its European counterparts know that this was unacceptable. Dr. David P. Duffield of Imperial Chemical Industries came to the United States to inform the American producers that the Europeans had decided to keep the information secret.[102] The moral qualms afflicting some of the American vinyl producers evaporated.

The Europeans and Americans decided on a much more pragmatic plan for protecting the industry. They would "comply" with NIOSH's request for information but do so in a way that was less than thorough and diverted attention from the seriousness of what the industry knew. If pressed by the NIOSH people, they should "acknowledge Maltoni's data" but point out that "Maltoni had done his work only with rats, whereas [future research by] the MCA . . . calls for mice and hamsters as well." The American chemical industry planned to provide NIOSH only with information about what they were finding in their own animal and epidemiological studies "in very general terms without leaving any written information."[103] The goal of the meeting was to make sure that the agency would "take no precipitous action now." Furthermore, "We should recommend no shift in priority" and at the meeting "our people [should] get off the topic of animal work as quickly as possible."[104]

The July 17 meeting took place at 1 p.m. at the NIOSH offices in Rockville, Maryland. Five industry representatives met across the table from five government scientists. Dr. Verald K. Rowe of Dow, Dr. William E. Rinehart of Ethyl, Robert N. Wheeler of Union Carbide, and George E. Best of the MCA represented the U.S. industry. Dr. David P. Duffield of ICI represented the Europeans (Dr. Tiziano Garlanda of Montedison was unable to attend). Dr. Marcus M. Key, the director of NIOSH, and members of his staff—Dr. Keith Jacobson, Richard B. James, Dr. Donald Lassiter, and Dr. Frank Mitchell—represented the U.S. government. The meeting was polite, collegial, and seemingly open. The American and European vinyl producers presented an apparently complete and forthright description of the industry and any potential problems. In fact, only the industry knew how skewed, deceptive, and distorted the presentation was.

Rowe made the formal presentation, speaking from pencilled notes. He began by emphasizing the size and scope of the vinyl chloride industry and described the industry's efforts to address the health concerns about acroosteolysis and cancer. Duffield described the "exhaustive" studies of vinyl chloride and polyvinyl chloride workers at ICI's European plants that revealed no "indication of hazard." He also described Viola's published research that had identified cancers in the rat's zymbal gland—a gland that does not exist in humans—and in the lung; he reassured NIOSH that "none of the observed lung tumors were primary tumors." He also referred to other ongoing research that confirmed Viola's studies while pointing out that "the program is still in progress and no firm conclusions [were] yet drawn."

No mention was specifically made of Maltoni, and no mention was made of kidney or liver cancers. According to the MCA, when NIOSH's Lassiter asked about the lowest concentration at which tumors had been observed, Duffield answered that nothing had been found below 250 ppm.[105] According to the notes taken by NIOSH's Richard James, however, although the industry told of Viola finding cancers at 30,000 ppm, there was no mention of tumors at 250 ppm.[106]

Of special note was a question raised by Jacobson of NIOSH. Jacobson had received a phone call asking him why it seemed so hard "to purchase vinyl chloride for use as an aerosol propellant." Avoiding any indication that concerns about liability from its use in consumer products like hair sprays had led to its removal, Rowe of Dow and Rinehart of the Ethyl

Corporation simply stated they were "no longer selling it for this purpose." They implied that the use of VCM in aerosol cans was not very important because it had "been used in this way only in relatively small quantities in paint and lacquer spray cans" and that it was likely to be "discontinued altogether by the end of the year."[107]

In truth, vinyl chloride was used much more widely. At least 3.5 million cans of aerosol products, including drugs, pesticides, and cosmetics "containing VC [were] in the possession of manufacturers, distributors, and consumers" in January 1974.[108] Although the manufacturers did not admit it to NIOSH, they understood that the potential liability problem was truly immense. True to their earlier plan, the companies left little other than previously published or reported materials: a single sheet summary of the vinyl industry, the single-sheet American Conference of Governmental Industrial Hygienists TLV report, the MCA's Chemical Safety Data Sheet for vinyl chloride (an eighteen-page booklet), the condensed protocols for the MCA's animal and epidemiological studies, and the MCA's news releases on these studies.[109]

At the close of the meeting, Rowe went to a separate office and spoke with NIOSH's Key. According to Wheeler, "this private discussion of the carcinogen problem was worth the whole effort."[110] NIOSH asked "to be kept fully appraised of the on-going work both the U.S. and the European industries have in progress," believing that they had been brought up to date on the status of knowledge up to that point.[111]

At the end of the day, the MCA and its various companies were ecstatic about the meeting and reported that "the chances of precipitous action by NIOSH on vinyl chloride were materially lessened."[112] The word that spread to member companies whose representatives had not attended the meeting was that "*no* problems were encountered" and that the "presentation was well received and appreciated."[113] Leaving the government with the impression that the companies were on top of the issue and that research up to that point had not indicated any serious problem with cancers among workers, the industry had accomplished its most difficult objective. It had appeared forthcoming and responsible to NIOSH officials without violating the agreement of secrecy with its European counterparts regarding the Maltoni studies.

The industry had avoided the issue of environmental danger in consumer products, remained silent on the primary liver and kidney cancers observed in the European experiments, and not mentioned the industry's own concern that the 200 ppm threshold value for vinyl chloride exposure was not adequate, while raising questions about the significance and even the integrity of Viola's work and reassuring NIOSH that there was no indication of danger to workers. In short, the industry's trade association had succeeded in preventing NIOSH from learning about the dangers to workers and consumers from vinyl chloride.

Almost immediately after the meeting, however, the industry's position that vinyl chloride was safe began to erode. Newspapers in Europe, and later in the United States, spoke of a very different reality. An article published in an Italian newspaper quoted Dr. A. Caputo, one of Viola's collaborators in the original cancer studies, as saying that vinyl chloride was responsible for the recent concerns among 40,000 workers in European vinyl chloride plants. Caputo said that dozens of workers had already died as a result of exposure and that it was potentially a huge environmental as well as occupational hazard. Responding to the view that "only" 40,000 workers were at a small risk of developing disease, Caputo had replied that "the menace applies to everybody...and [is] particularly hazardous in containers for foodstuffs...in filters for artificial kidneys, in cardiac valves."[114]

The MCA translated the article and circulated it to its Task Force on Vinyl Chloride as a way to alert the industry to the fact that information about the dangers of vinyl was leaking out. In late November, *Chemical Week,* the trade journal, reported on meat wrappers who had developed respiratory problems as a result of breathing fumes created by the heating of PVC film. Recalling the earlier ban on PVC bottles, the weekly told its readers that the Environmental Protection Agency had also been concerned that "a substantial increase in the use of PVC in packaging would be harmful to the environment."[115]

Around this time the MCA, recognizing that the issues of occupational and environmental cancers were not going away and that it was only a matter of time before events might occur which could threaten the industry's careful management of the problem, wrote to its member companies that a greater level of coordination of the entire industry, both American and European, was necessary.[116]

PLASTIC COFFIN

In January 1974 the nation learned that vinyl chloride monomer had been implicated in the deaths of four workers. A rare cancer, angiosarcoma of the liver, had struck down the workers at the B. F. Goodrich plant in Louisville, Kentucky. Throughout the nation newspapers reported that polyvinyl chloride, a seemingly benign and inexpensive replacement for wood, metal, and even wax paper in the homes and workplaces of millions of Americans, was now a possible deadly threat. Joe Klein, writing on the discovery of angiosarcoma in *Rolling Stone,* called the PVC plant a "Plastic Coffin."[117]

Dr. John Creech, who was still doing exams at the plant where he first identified acroosteolysis, had reported his concern over employee liver problems to Dr. Maurice Johnson, Goodrich's director of environmental health.[118] (Johnson, a graduate of the University of Minnesota medical school, had been involved in occupational medicine since 1954 and had only recently joined B. F. Goodrich, in 1972.)[119] After reviewing plant records, Creech discovered that four workers had died from angiosarcoma of the liver, among the rarest of cancers, a disease previously associated with heavy metal poisoning and arsenic. Usually accounting for fewer than two dozen deaths in the United States in any given year, the occurrence of four deaths from angiosarcoma of the liver in a population of a few hundred workers at one plastics plant was truly alarming.

These deaths were especially worrisome because this rare cancer was "identical to that seen in the European rat feeding studies" conducted by Maltoni, something that the industry had failed to let NIOSH, or even Creech, know about. Creech and Johnson met with Dr. Irving Tabershaw of Tabershaw Cooper Associates, who was then in the midst of an epidemiological study of vinyl workers for the MCA.[120] The information that Creech had revealed was terrifying to Goodrich's management.

On a Sunday afternoon, top executives met in Akron, Ohio, in what was described as "absolutely [a] crisis." All day lawyers, management, and physicians discussed the vast implications of the medical findings, including the company's liability. Finally, at 7 PM, top executives of Goodrich decided that the only thing to do was to let the information out immediately.[121] According to a private memo by another company's official, "At the insistence of Dr. Creech, [they] decided to reveal the information [about the angiosarcoma deaths] to the authorities and the industry."[122] On January 22, Goodrich informed NIOSH of the deaths, and NIOSH then informed OSHA.[123]

In all, Creech and his associates documented eleven cases of hepatic disease, including seven cases of angiosarcoma of the liver identified among workers at the plant, with the earliest diagnosis dating to almost ten years earlier, in April 1964.[124] Four of the workers died between 1968 and 1973, the very period when the decision to mislead the government was taking shape.[125] All the victims had been "pot cleaners" in their careers at Goodrich. Pot cleaners climbed into tanks no more than six feet across and ten feet high "to chip polymer residue off the inside surfaces. Their only source of fresh air was a 2-foot opening at the very top of the deep tanks."[126]

The industry responded to the crisis by preparing "a low key statement for the press," to be released if pressed, and drafting a letter to Marcus Key of NIOSH "reaffirming industry support and cooperation as offered in the meeting with NIOSH last summer."[127] Initially, Goodrich reported that its practices at the Louisville plant were unexceptional and that the air in the plant and, hence, the exposures to vinyl chloride were "generally 15–20 ppm with excursions above 50 ppm," well below the existing TLV.[128] Later this estimate would change dramatically.

But within three weeks, the vinyl chloride producers gathered in Cleveland under the auspices of the Vinyl Chloride Safety Association to assess the problems facing the industry.[129] According to Goodrich officials, other chemical companies were not pleased with the company's decision to reveal the information to NIOSH. One official recalled that "Goodrich was not a hero in the chemical industry" and was "given a fair amount of harassment."[130] The companies discussed means to limit the amount of VCM workers were exposed to and to more closely monitor VCM levels in the air of its plants.[131] Only after the issue had become national news did the industry act to protect workers by reducing their exposure to vinyl chloride monomer. It would not be until months later that the hint of scandal and cover-up would be raised, and not until almost thirty years for the true dimensions of its history to emerge.

For most in the industry, the crisis at Goodrich's Louisville plant represented a major challenge to the hegemony of industry over the science of vinyl chloride toxicology. No longer would discussions about the dangers of plastics be contained among a small group of government and industry officials. Although most Americans believed that the crisis was about cancer in the workplace and not outside, environmental and labor groups knew differently. They took seriously the headlines about a link between vinyl chloride and cancer and vigorously pressured new governmental organizations like the EPA and agencies concerned with consumer protection to address the danger.

It would soon be suspected that VCM posed a threat to consumers. Even after polyvinyl chloride, a stable material, is produced, vinyl chloride gas is trapped within the finished product. The gas can escape, creating potential hazards to the consumer. Further, when it was burned, PVC produced dangerous fumes.[132] It was also feared that communities neighboring the plants were in danger. Cancer, birth defects, and other conditions were documented among populations living near chemical plants where vinyl feedstock was being leaked and spewed into the water, air, and soil. The crisis that loomed for the chemical industry was this: If such a seemingly benign product as plastic could prove so dangerous and far-reaching, then what of the thousands of new chemicals that were introduced every year?

Damn Liars

The cancer deaths of four workers at the Louisville, Kentucky, B. F. Goodrich plant demonstrated to the Occupational Safety and Health Administration (OSHA) that its current standard for vinyl chloride was clearly inadequate. In 1970, OSHA had been given the mandate to "set the standard which most adequately assures, to the extent feasible, on the basis of the best available evidence that no employee will suffer material impairment of health or functional capacity even if such employee has regular exposure . . . for the period of his working life."[1] After the deaths at the Goodrich vinyl plant were reported, OSHA immediately called a hearing to elicit testimony about what emergency standard should be established. Some in industry feared, and many in labor hoped, that OSHA would interpret its mandate to mean creating a no-exposure level for employees.

The stakes were enormous. Ten companies with fourteen plants and more than fifteen hundred workers produced vinyl chloride monomer. Another twenty-three companies with thirty-seven plants and more than five thousand production workers used that monomer to create polyvinyl chloride. Finally, it was "difficult to estimate the number of workers employed in converting, molding, and fabricating the polymers into finished products" although "it is in the order of tens of thousands working in thousands of plants throughout the country."[2]

In an atmosphere of crisis, scientists, industry, and labor representatives gathered in mid-February 1974 for a standing-room-only OSHA hearing in Washington to discuss what was emerging as the major occupational health crisis of the early 1970s.[3] They all came prepared for battle. Dr. Irving Selikoff, "white-haired, gracious," and incredibly energetic, was a leading occupational physician and director of the Environmental Sciences Laboratory at New York's Mount Sinai School of Medicine. In the words of *Fortune* magazine, he was "a crusader and reformer" who seemed "personally as well as professionally close to nearly everyone who matters in government occupational medicine."[4]

Selikoff, whose work on asbestos-related disease had gained him international renown in the late 1960s as an advocate for labor, posed a difficult question to the OSHA hearing: Why was it only now that the dangers of vinyl chloride were beginning to be recognized? Vinyl chloride–related disease was "not a new problem," Selikoff began. "There has been evidence of a potentially serious disease among workers engaged in vinyl chloride–polyvinyl chloride manufacture for 25 years."[5] Why was it, he asked, that the issue had "been incompletely appreciated and inadequately approached" by scientists and government?[6] For Selikoff, although definitive proof of cancer-producing effects were not yet established, controls over vinyl chloride should have been established earlier. "We have had ample warning that cells, tissues, and organs could be badly damaged during VC-PVC production. Despite this, our approach to the problem... seems to have been somewhat leisurely."[7] Had industry and the state acted earlier this conference would not have been necessary.[8]

Now that cancer had appeared, he had a number of recommendations. First, there was no question that "vinyl chloride–polyvinyl chloride exposure should be added to the list of carcinogens promulgated by the Department [of Labor]," since "no threshold is known that would serve to prevent cancer among exposed workmen."[9] Second, it was necessary to "rapidly study whether health effects will be associated with end-product or consumer use."[10] Finally, he stressed the broader implications of the vinyl crisis. The substance was emblematic of "'invisible pollution,' associated with... [the] 'new industrial revolution, based on the chemical-process industry.'" Workers were paying for the rapid expansion of this industry, and their sacrifice was "becoming visible in terms of disease and death." Those who worked with new chemicals had "every right to expect that scientists, industry, and governmental agencies would protect them against known or suspect hazards. This we failed to do." Selikoff concluded, "Our task here today is to address this and insure that it go no further. No effort should be spared and no control considered too rigorous."[11]

Tony Mazzocchi, legislative director of the Oil, Chemical and Atomic Workers Union (OCAW), emboldened by the new influence labor appeared to have with the creation of OSHA and by his sense that labor could dramatically influence scientific decision making for the first time, challenged the very idea that safe doses could be established for carcinogens. He reminded the audience of the principle embodied in the Delaney clause, saying it was "impossible ... to establish any absolutely safe level of exposure to a carcinogen for man."[12] He demanded that OSHA set a no-detectable-limit standard for vinyl chloride. "Today, somewhere in the United States a worker is being exposed to vinyl chloride that will someday cause him cancer and a slow, painful death."[13]

The presence of recognized experts and professionals speaking on behalf of labor was extraordinary. Scientific meetings were generally dominated by industry scientists, whose arguments prevailed. Now, it appeared, the tables had turned. Dr. Thomas Mancuso, a professor in the Department of Occupational Health at the University of Pittsburgh, spoke on behalf of the Industrial Union Department of the AFL-CIO. He described a pattern of denial on the part of industry when a hazard was uncovered in the workplace. "Invariably, whenever a new occupational cancer is discovered, it is played down for fear of alarming the workers and the general public. . . . Nevertheless, from past experience, what happens is that as further work is undertaken and information obtained, the problem gets broader and broader with more implications." Mancuso argued that neither OSHA nor industry should wait for danger to appear before taking a course of action, especially given the extraordinary and rapid growth of the chemical industry. "The chance recognition of an occupational cancer by a unique combination of circumstances, clearly demonstrates what is not known about the carcinogenic potential of thousands of industrial chemicals that have been in use for decades." The case of vinyl chloride "focuses attention on the total absence of a national concerted study of occupational cancer in this country."[14]

THIS COMPLEX PANDORA'S BOX

Mancuso raised the specter of broader environmental disaster. "The serious national question that is raised and not resolved, because it is either too shocking to contemplate or because the agencies responsible for the protection of the public are reluctant to open this complex Pandora's box, is, in essence, that a national study directed at the industrial environment might uncover a whole series, a succession of occupational cancers, which in turn would implicate in the distribution of these chemicals a larger and larger portion of the population exposed to the risk of cancer." He also raised the question of chemicals interacting with one another. There was not sufficient knowledge since the "real carcinogenic potential of these chemicals acting alone or in combination with each other has never been established."[15]

The industry, as might be expected, vigorously disagreed with this version of the history of the problem of vinyl chloride, as well as with the proposed OSHA emergency standard. The industry's representatives argued that the vinyl producers had acted responsibly. Albert C. Clark, vice president and technical director of the Manufacturing Chemists' Association (MCA), and Dr. Kenneth E. Johnson, the association's assistant technical director, suggested that the MCA "as a regular and continuing service to its members, has long had active programs in occupational health and safety." They portrayed their response to the acroosteolysis (AOL) problems encountered in the 1960s as a sign of corporate responsibility. When cancer was suspected, the industry invited the Italian scientist who conducted the research, Dr. P. L. Viola, to the United States to give them ideas on how to design a research protocol to answer outstanding questions regarding the carcinogenic properties of vinyl chloride.[16]

These industry representatives failed to mention that the goal of their research was not to gather information in order to protect workers but to "reassure the public," to "assure the employees...that management was ...diligent...to protect their health," and "to develop data useful in defense of the industry."[17] They maintained that the industry had been seeking to test Viola's conclusions using "vinyl chloride of a source and quality characteristic of a U.S. industrial product," honorably trying "to determine, if possible, whether a no-response level exists."[18] In contrast to Selikoff's and Mazzocchi's position, the industry clung to the notion that any substance could be used safely if exposure levels were low enough.

Given that industry documents remained secret, there was no way to understand that the industry had acted to hide from the government information about vinyl as a carcinogen. As a result, the companies could still pass themselves off as working openly and cooperatively with the government. It would take decades for researchers and lawyers to shed light on industry documents and to learn of the cover-ups, denials, and lies. Until then, the industry could maintain that its desire to protect the workforce had led the MCA to initiate contact with NIOSH and to be completely forthcoming in providing information. The MCA officials pledged that its member companies would reduce exposures to the lowest possible levels. The hint of MCA's less honorable intentions was that it opposed OSHA's proposal to issue an emergency temporary standard. Even after the Louisville revelations, the MCA suggested that OSHA should take its time and begin a regular rule-making process, which could take years.[19]

Dow's representative, V. K. Rowe, countered Mancuso's alarmist position by calmly maintaining that industry had cleaned up its act and that the vinyl problem was an isolated incident, not representative of the workplace practices in the entire industry. Like representatives of industry today, who claim that the past is irrelevant,[20] Dow argued that "rulemaking should not be based on conditions that existed in the past, but should be based on conditions as they exist now." Because of the "widespread voluntary actions by industry, . . . we believe a temporary emergency standard would result in polarization rather than constructive definition of areas of concern and constructive problem solving."[21]

Management, having argued earlier that companies had never exposed workers to dangerous amounts of vinyl, now reversed course, arguing that the deaths from angiosarcoma of the liver resulted from "very high exposures years ago when . . . firms were 'much more cavalier' toward vinyl chloride's hazards."[22] Industry members assured the government that the angiosarcomas that had been found at Goodrich were a product of past, not current, practices.

Shortly after the hearing, Robert Wheeler of Union Carbide notified NIOSH that the company had discovered a case of angiosarcoma of the liver in a worker in its plant in South Charleston, West Virginia. Dr. David Duffield, of Imperial Chemical Industries (ICI), a British vinyl manufacturer, reported as well on the death of one of ICI's employees in December 1972, and Dr. William E. Rinehart of Ethyl reported that a worker had died on December 28, 1973, in Ethyl's Louisville bottle manufacturing plant.[23] Pressure began to mount on the industry within two weeks of the OSHA hearing after the MCA's Technical Task Group on Vinyl Chloride Research learned that 50 ppm would not necessarily protect the worker. As a result, the MCA's Work Practices Task Force decided not to recommend a threshold level for VCM.[24]

Very little information exists about the reactions within the industry to the gathering storm concerning exposure levels. But the records of Pittsburgh Plate Glass (PPG), a major producer of vinyl chloride, indicate that its medical director, Lee B. Grant, objected strongly to PPG's statement to OSHA in support of the MCA position that work practices be established under Section 6(b) of the OSHA Act: He pointed out that in OSHA's three-year history not one health standard had been issued under the regular process for "the procedure is very time-consuming." Instead, Grant argued, OSHA should use Section 6(c) of the OSHAct, which permitted the issuance of emergency standards when there was "a grave danger to persons from a newly recognized hazard." He worried, "The delay as 6(b) requires in developing a standard, in my opinion, is unwarranted when considering the significant degree of the hazard for human carcinogenesis potentially represented by permitting a continuation of exposure of persons to the present OSHA Standard for Vinyl Chloride Monomer of 500 ppm." He supported the use of the mechanism that "permits the emergency standard to become effective the day of publication in the *Federal Register*."[25]

NIOSH officials, still believing that the MCA was being candid with them, invited the trade association to provide industry experts as consultants in establishing new work practice guidelines, a request that the MCA quickly and gladly embraced. From a list of candidates provided by the MCA, NIOSH named Zeb Bell of PPG, Maurice Johnson of Goodrich, Mayo Smith of Air Products, and Robert Wheeler of Union Carbide to its panel of consultants.[26]

Before meeting with NIOSH, the MCA's Sub-Task Group on Work Practices held its own meetings to formulate a common industry position. Bell, the manager of environmental control and industrial health for PPG, privately expressed concern that the industry was not taking seriously enough the link between vinyl chloride and cancer. He admitted that "there [was] little doubt that VCM [was] a 'cancer suspect agent'"[27] and worried about industry's resistance to being forthright about the seriousness of the vinyl chloride cancer problem. He felt that the MCA's draft of what it hoped OSHA would adopt as its work practice standard for vinyl chloride workers reflected the industry's attempt to minimize the danger. The term *cancer suspect agent* had first appeared in the *Federal Register* when OSHA issued work practices for the first fourteen carcinogens in January 1974. According to Bell, "the industry did not like it" and proposed instead to call it a "hazardous chemical agent," even though Bell believed the prior term was more accurate.[28] Nonetheless, in a public statement to *Chemical Week*, Bell proclaimed that industry was a responsible corporate citizen. Bell claimed, "We were complacent before January, but we insist on strict compliance with work rules now."[29]

In March, shortly after the industry made assurances that the sloppy practices and high exposure levels that had been responsible for the angiosarcoma deaths were now corrected, a meeting of high-level vinyl chloride industry managers learned some surprising news. Richard Fleming of Air Products revealed that the industry was actually doing better than it had suspected in terms of keeping exposure levels at its plants relatively low. It was quite common for most companies, he told the executives, to keep VCM time-weighted average levels below 50 ppm. Rather than taking pride in this fact or congratulating themselves, the company representatives at the meeting found the news quite worrisome. Fleming warned that the "current low levels could jeopardize [the industry's] case [before NIOSH and OSHA] if not presented properly." He reasoned that if NIOSH and OSHA understood that the exposure level "[had] always been this low"—when angiosarcomas appeared at their plants—then it would mean that reducing the TLV to 50 ppm was inadequate and the TLV would have to be lowered even further.[30] A day later, on March 22, Goodyear announced in another press release that two more workers had died from liver angiosarcomas.[31]

THE EVOLUTION OF A NEW SCIENCE

The vinyl chloride crisis was raising complex problems about how to determine the potential dangers of the thousands of new chemicals that were being produced in factories and introduced into the environment through air and water emissions and consumer products. As Italian cancer researcher Cesare Maltoni, whose work on vinyl chloride finally appeared in print in the early spring of 1974, put it: "In the past 10 years, the number and amount of oncogenic agents produced and scattered in the working environment have increased and continue to increase in a distressing way. ... As a result of this situation, an increase in occupational tumors and of environmental agents in a broad sense is recorded."

Maltoni argued that although the recording of workers' diseases and deaths provided information, it was an insufficient way to address the problem and that the industry needed to find a way to predict what chemicals and levels of exposure would cause cancer. Retrospective epidemiological studies, which identified toxins long after they had harmed individuals, were a case of too little information too late. "Epidemiological proof should be avoided. For all new agents produced and used, systematic experimental tests should rather be carried out to predict their possible oncogenic potential." He acknowledged that a lack of standards and other methodological problems had caused skepticism about how animal data could "be extrapolated to man." But Maltoni believed that his results showing the carcinogenic effects of vinyl chloride in animals represented "the first time that an oncogenic hazard ... [had been] predicted with absolute accuracy by means of an experimental test."[32] In other words, animal experiments could help predict which substances would be dangerous.

Industry found this position untenable and maintained that evidence of human disease, not animal studies, should be used for regulatory purposes. Industry spokespeople had maintained until the human deaths "no special significance could be attached to the types of tumors observed by Maltoni."[33] Public health practitioners, labor leaders, academics, and government administrators disagreed. The American Association for the Advancement of Science had established the Committee on Scientific Freedom and Responsibility and had already identified the reliance on epidemiology as a major concern in the study of carcinogens.

John T. Edsall, a professor at Harvard University and a member of the committee, worried that industry was seeking refuge rather than information when it ignored animal studies and waited for evidence of death and disease among workers. "The extremely ominous findings in the animal studies did not trigger any major alarm" among industry officials, Edsall observed, "until cases of cancer in factory workers exposed to vinyl chloride began to be reported." What he did not know was that the animal studies *had* caused alarm, so much alarm, in fact, that the industry had hidden the results from the government so NIOSH would not move to regulate the industry. He believed that the lesson of the vinyl chloride crisis was that "new reagents introduced into industry on a large scale should be regarded as dangerous until proved safe."[34]

The dilemma for the government however was that it might take years, even decades, to prove a substance dangerous and it might not be possible to ever prove to the scientific community that a substance was completely safe. Nevertheless, the government had to develop guidelines that would protect the public and not paralyze industry.

Joseph Wagoner of NIOSH was more direct in his assessment of the relative values of animal bioassays and epidemiology. He maintained that animal studies "and in vitro studies should be the 'front line' of the attack on job-related cancer." He noted that vinyl chloride was not the only case in which human cancers had been accurately predicted, and he outlined the numerous times in which animal evidence had alerted the scientific community to a problem that was ultimately confirmed by epidemiological research. Epidemiology, while "a powerful qualitative tool," was "weak or inadequate" in identifying carcinogenic risks. By studying death from cancer and "not induction of cancer," epidemiology could only underestimate risk. Because it was "post hoc in nature," it could only record, not address, the "failure of government, industry, and society to . . . control chemical carcinogens introduced decades ago." Animal and microbial tests, in short, could be a more powerful and usable tool in assessing carcinogenesis and mutagenesis.

Louis Beliczky, director of health and safety of the United Rubber Workers, supported the use of animal studies, asking "will it take human deaths" to establish a substance's toxicity? "The only sane policy," he argued, "is to be conservative, to err on the safe side."[35]

While objecting to the government's use of animal studies, the industry privately considered animal studies a perfectly appropriate source of data. Before the issue of regulation arose, the industry had been properly sobered by the animal studies of Maltoni and Viola, which pointed to the carcinogenic properties of vinyl chloride. This was why they were so anxious that NIOSH not learn of them. Yet in the months following the exposé of the angiosarcoma deaths at Goodrich and other companies, the industry's position regarding the usefulness of these animal studies went through a metamorphosis. It was more a change in tactics than a change in attitude. Industry was now interested in delaying government regulation. By arguing that animal studies were inadequate for assessing the effect of their product on humans and demanding more long-term observational data, they could buy time. By maintaining that only epidemiological studies could accurately gauge the true danger of chemicals to humans, the industry could continue to claim that their products were safe until these laborious studies were done.

The industry maintained that there had been no "quantitative data that provides a basis for extrapolation of animal carcinogenesis to man."[36] Unlike Selikoff, who traced the vinyl chloride issue to 1940 studies among Soviet workers, or Mancuso, who saw vinyl chloride as a broad-based environmental issue, B. F. Goodrich officials argued that animal studies had proved of little value and that there was no reason to suspect that vinyl was a carcinogen. (Goodrich was arguing this after the MCA knew of Maltoni's studies and had accepted the implications for humans in them.) They held that only Viola's paper had previously reported on a relationship between cancer and vinyl chloride and that the cancer identified was not located in the liver.[37]

Robert Wheeler of Union Carbide also argued, "Data from animal toxicology studies cannot be directly applied to forecast human experience since laboratory animals, such as mice, tend to develop angiosarcomas spontaneously, they metabolize vinyl chloride differently, their lifetimes are shorter, and their rate of metabolism is higher. For these reasons, safe-exposure limits for workers must be based on human data and experience."[38] Paul Kotin of Johns Manville Corporation even argued that "some cancers will heal if the victim is removed from exposure." He said, "There are very few chemicals that produce malignant tumors exclusively. In some cases a heavy dose may produce a malignant tumor and a light dose a benign tumor."[39]

Public health experts and even industry placed such importance on Maltoni's findings of cancer in animals because finding cancers in such studies was statistically quite improbable. Carcinogens were known, even in the 1970s, to affect a very small percentage of any given population. For instance, if a substance affected only one out of two hundred animals, in a study of one hundred animals there would be a 60 percent chance that not even one cancer would appear. Even if two studies of such magnitude were conducted, there was a 30 percent chance that no animal would be affected. Such a "serious limitation on the validity of animal tests" made it economically unfeasible to conduct animal studies large enough to provide results that could reliably prove danger.[40] Thus, as scientists understood, most animal studies dramatically understated the potential harm that could result from exposure to a particular substance. That Maltoni found multiple cancers in multiple sites at low exposures at one-half of the human TLV was very alarming.

On April 4, 1974, OSHA issued an emergency temporary standard setting a permissible exposure limit (PEL) of 50 ppm of vinyl chloride rather than NIOSH's recommended level of 1 ppm.[41] The MCA's Sub Committee on Work Practices was greatly relieved by OSHA's action. Because this standard was already the usual practice within plants, it imposed no new economic hardships on industry. The MCA Work Practices group stuck to its position that anything below a 50 ppm "working level concentration" would be "uneconomic and all but impossible to meet" and that anything below this would be "simply a requirement for liquidation of a major industry." But they did not tell OSHA that the 50 ppm level did not satisfy Maltoni, who did "not wish to be quoted that 50 ppm is safe for man."[42]

The industry sought to maintain a common position. In early May the director of packaging service of the Society of the Plastics Industry wrote to PVC producers about the data they were gathering to present to OSHA about a permanent standard for VCM. "We must show that significant numbers of people are involved and that these people have been exposed long enough for the disease to become evident," the letter began. OSHA would certainly want to know what levels of exposure workers were already experiencing, and the industry data "must at least derive the implication that TWA [time weighted average] exposure levels were at least 50 ppm and possibly higher."[43]

If the industry could not show that the levels had previously been higher, OSHA might conclude that its proposed standard of 50 ppm was not low enough to protect workers. Indeed, the industry had already changed its claim that the plants in which the workers died had low exposure levels, now arguing that they worked in plants where exposures were high. Union Carbide's Robert Wheeler said that in the past "exposures at the affected plants were ten times" the current level. He concluded, "a maximum exposure level of 50 ppm TWA" was the proper standard.[44]

Shortly after OSHA issued its emergency standard, Industrial Bio-Test Labs, the company conducting the industry's animal tests, phoned the MCA with more troubling news. Preliminary results suggested that mice exposed to 50 ppm VCM were developing angiosarcoma. The MCA immediately forwarded that information to NIOSH, OSHA, and the EPA.[45] The MCA's Vinyl Chloride Research Coordinators met with representatives of the government to discuss the ominous implications of this finding. Shell Oil Company's representative, Howard L. Kusnetz, reported, "The consensus of the group was that despite these minor discrepancies, the tumors were real and they confirmed Maltoni's findings." One OSHA person, Donald Lassiter, "felt that the results reported would support the NIOSH recommendation of 1 ppm."[46]

A split emerged between the MCA and its constituent vinyl chloride manufacturers as the intense scrutiny of the plastics manufacturers threatened the public's perception of the entire chemical industry. The MCA leadership, as representatives of the broader industry, sought to insulate itself from the furor by withdrawing from all but the most technical aspects of hazard identification. When the vinyl industry asked the MCA to convene a meeting of the vinyl chloride and polyvinyl chloride producers "for the purpose of exchanging information and coordinating efforts to establish a safety standard," the MCA Executive Committee shocked the manufacturers by denying their request. The MCA claimed that such a meeting "would involve a standard-making activity concerning a single product which is potentially sensitive from an antitrust viewpoint." Such an activity, the MCA claimed, would be "beyond the approved purpose of the vinyl chloride research project MCA is administering," which they asserted was limited to animal and epidemiological research.[47]

The MCA, long the public face of the plastics industry, now sought ways to lessen its exposure. A. C. Clark of the MCA's staff was dispatched to the MCA's Technical Task Force for Vinyl Chloride Research to clarify for its members the new face that the MCA wanted to show. The MCA, he stated, would "not concern itself or become involved in non-technical or non-scientific items such as profit, return on investment, feasibility or lack thereof, or other industry problems that cannot be solved by scientific or technical studies." Nor would the MCA become "involved in any controversy or litigation whether of industry benefit or not."[48]

Meanwhile the public image of the plastics manufacturers continued to take a beating. The MCA staff learned that "Jane Brodie [Brody] of the New York Times" called about results of a meeting and that "CBS was preparing a one hour special on vinyl chloride" that would include film of Goodyear's plant in Niagara Falls, New York, and an interview with industry's nemesis, Dr. Irving Selikoff.[49]

Robert Wheeler of Union Carbide expressed his own and other vinyl producers' frustrations with the MCA's actions. "At the week's end, my own reaction as well as many other PVC industry representatives was first to question the value of being an MCA member and, second, to question whose side MCA was on besides its own."[50] It was felt that the MCA was not focused enough on the plastics industry to be a reliable spokesman for vinyl manufacturers. What was needed was another body whose interests were synonymous with plastics to lobby legal challenges against OSHA, NIOSH, the EPA, and the FDA. Such lobbying could forestall what the industry feared would be crippling regulations.

On April 16, shortly following the disastrous meeting with the MCA, "the VCM/PVC Industry Management Committee held an Ad Hoc meeting in Washington DC . . . and decided to form a permanent action group within the Society of the Plastics Industry where Bylaws of the SPI are compatible with present industry needs."[51] In the end, the MCA and the Society of the Plastics Industry succeeded in dividing their work and reinforcing each other's positions. "A considerable overlap of committee members has made this a very workable relationship."[52] The plastics manufacturers would "form a single, unified group to deal with all of the phases; actions to be taken with OSHA, NIOSH, EPA, FDA, and other agencies will be on a groups [sic] basis rather than each producer acting as an independent agent."[53]

Because the Society of the Plastics Industry, unlike the MCA, was an association of the plastics producers alone, it was not forced to address the multiple agendas of the entire chemical industry. It represented 1,400 member companies that accounted for 75 percent of the plastics industry sales in the United States. The Society's Vinyl Chloride and Polyvinyl Chloride Resin Producers Committee represented "more than 90 percent of the U.S. capacity for the production of vinyl chloride monomer and polyvinyl chloride resins."[54]

The SPI group expected that within days the MCA would publicly announce its findings that angiosarcomas were appearing in animals with exposure to VCM of only 50 ppm. They fully believed that this would result in OSHA's adopting NIOSH's 1 ppm standard and that "none [of their members] could operate if the NIOSH Work Standard were imposed on the industry."[55]

The vinyl industry was faced with a dilemma. On the one hand, it maintained that a threshold limit could be developed that would both protect workers while allowing the industry to maintain production. On the other hand, evidence indicated that there was no known safe level of exposure. Every time a new level of exposure was tested on animals, cancers appeared. The MCA, still responsible for gathering the scientific data, reported to industry representatives in early May some more discouraging news. "[M]ice in the 50 ppm exposure group were experiencing malignant tumors, including angiosarcomas of the liver, [and thus] industry was left without any exposure level of vinyl chloride that it could identify as a one at which there was no direct evidence of adverse effects.... [A] new series of experiments [should] be undertaken in an effort to show a no-effects level in a sensitive, rapidly-reacting species, i.e. mice."[56]

In mid–May OSHA published in the *Federal Register* its long-awaited "Comprehensive Proposal on Vinyl Chloride" and called for comment and criticism. The proposal included a "no detectable level" of 1 ppm permissible exposure limit for VCM. Two sets of public hearings were held in the summer, and enormous controversy arose as industry, labor, public health practitioners, and the academic community weighed in with advice. Simultaneously, a conference on the "Toxicity of Vinyl Chloride–Polyvinyl Chloride" at the New York Academy of Sciences learned that both Maltoni and the MCA had discovered angiosarcomas in animals at 50 ppm.[57]

Just as the OSHA proposal was announced, the industry held a meeting at which members decided, as they generally did when faced with a threat, that whatever their different success in reducing exposures, they would maintain a common front against OSHA and other agencies in the escalating battle over vinyl chloride. While most of the companies could live with an exposure limit well below the emergency standard, one company warned "against a company accepting a low VCM level that the majority could not live with." Furthermore, what was possible for the companies was not necessarily what they considered desirable. Goodrich had proposed an exposure level one-tenth the emergency standard. But this caused *"serious consternation among many of the members and warnings against such low levels within the short time period."*[58]

As scientific and popular consensus about the dangers from vinyl grew, the industry developed a sophisticated public relations campaign aimed at shaping regulatory decisions. The MCA staff feared that the vinyl chloride revelations were threatening the whole chemical industry, not just the vinyl producers. A staff report made to the association's board of directors stated: "A recent story by a leading newspaper in the Nation's Capital discussed the health dangers which have been associated with the manufacture of vinyl chloride and went on to criticize the inaction of Congress in failing to pass a toxic substances control law." If, as this article suggested, the growing attention to the vinyl deaths might result in increased regulation by Congress, the industry had better take charge. Recognizing that the public's concern about toxic substances would not go away, the MCA staff suggested that it might be beneficial to pass toxic control legislation in the present Congress, rather than to await a new session in which public opinion could force an even more stringent law.[59]

The carcinogenicity of vinyl chloride, seen as a problem solely for workers before the B. F. Goodrich angiosarcoma deaths, was now the subject of a heated national debate about carcinogens; the efficacy and role of animal biological studies in understanding and regulating chronic illnesses; the definition and identification of carcinogens; and the roles of OSHA, NIOSH, the EPA, the FDA, the Consumer Product Safety Commission, management, and labor in controlling industrially produced carcinogens. Aerosols, meat wrappings, PVC tubing, spills, tank car accidents, and plastic liquor bottles all came under suspicion for posing a long-term threat.

Within weeks of the crisis at Louisville in January 1974, Sidney Wolfe's Health Research Group, a consumer advocacy organization, called for a ban on the use of vinyl chloride as a propellant in spray cans and for a regulation requiring the publicizing of the brand names of products using vinyl chloride as an aerosol (a year earlier various VCM producers had quietly stopped selling VCM for aerosols but had done nothing to warn consumers of the danger). Shortly after Wolfe's action in late February, the FDA and the EPA asked for the recall of "over 100 hair sprays, insecticides, footsprays and deodorants, and other products which were determined to contain vinyl chloride as a propellant."[60]

In April, Clairol pulled 100,000 cans of hair spray from store shelves.[61] The EPA issued an "Emergency Suspension Order Concerning Registrations" under the Federal Insecticide, Fungicide, and Rodenticide Act for "all pesticide spray products" containing vinyl chloride "for uses in the home, food handling establishments, hospitals or in enclosed areas." A notice of intent to cancel registrations was published in the *Federal Register* in part because tests showed that "a 30 second release of the aerosol could result in a concentration as high as 400 ppm in the air" and that "a detectable concentration of vinyl chloride could still persist for several hours after spraying."[62] During the summer of 1974 the FDA, EPA, and the Consumer Products Safety Commission initiated or took final action to ban vinyl chloride's use in bottles and certain other consumer items.[63]

At a private session organized by the National Cancer Institute with representatives from ten federal agencies, including OSHA, NIOSH, the FDA, the CDC, the EPA, National Institutes of Health, and the Armed Forces Institute of Pathology, Nancy Beach, the coordinator of the EPA's efforts concerning vinyl chloride, told the group that estimates showed a 6 percent loss of vinyl chloride monomer during the production of PVC. She commented, "It sounds small, but if one considers that the annual production of PVC in the U.S. is well over 5 billion pounds a 6% loss figure is on the order of 250 million pounds, which is somehow getting out of the workplace." Preliminary studies by the EPA indicated this was a significant problem, especially for those living near a plant.[64] In monitoring environmental pollution around vinyl chloride plants the EPA had found that although the average exposure was less than 1 ppm, outside one plant there were readings of 33 ppm and even of 3.4 ppm three miles away from another plant. Russell Train, the administrator of the agency, acknowledged that "there is no scientific evidence to indicate that these emissions pose an imminent hazard to people living near these plants." He thought it "prudent" that "reasonable steps should be promptly taken to reduce vinyl chloride emissions to the lowest practical level."[65]

While the discovery of various kinds of industrial pollution had led the EPA to begin pressing for passage of a Toxic Substances Control Act (TSCA), the publicity and seriousness of the vinyl crisis would become the impetus for more assertive efforts to get TSCA passed, with a view toward regulating more chemicals than vinyl chloride. One report noted that "many of the considerations and uncertainties that have punctuated the vinyl chloride/polyvinyl chloride deliberations undoubtedly characterize a far broader swath of concerns over high volume industrial chemicals in general, and plastics in particular." TSCA "would provide a mechanism for addressing those products using vinyl chloride not now subject to regulation under other laws."[66]

In December 1974, the FDA "received from the [PVC] industry research findings showing that vinyl chloride residues had also migrated from bottles and packages into vinegar, apple cider, vegetable oil, mineral oil and packages used to wrap meats."[67] It would take another two years for TSCA to be passed. TSCA gave the EPA the authority to test chemicals for toxicity before they were introduced into the market and the right to test the toxicity of those already being used.[68]

The vinyl chloride crisis substantially blurred the line between occupational and environmental dangers. No longer could the field of occupational medicine be segregated from the emerging field of environmental health. In the coming years, with the disasters at Love Canal, Times Beach, and even Bhopal, what had been a side issue in the extraordinary battle over occupational exposures to vinyl chloride would become a national preoccupation. The SPI Producers Group knew that industry was in for bigger trouble and set out to hire the firm of Ruckelshaus, Beveridge, and Fairbanks as "counsel on EPA matters."[69] Because William Ruckelshaus had been the past administrator of the EPA, the very agency the chemical companies were seeking to influence, getting his firm on board would provide the industry with legitimacy as well as important contacts.[70]

As all this was unfolding, the industry was faced with the immediate problem of what to do about OSHA's call for a permanent standard of "no detectable limit" and the impending hearings planned to begin on June 25, 1974. The industry contracted with Hill & Knowlton, a major public relations firm, to refocus public and congressional attention and to reshape the national debate about the effect of plastics on American society. Shortly before the OSHA hearings, the SPI's Vinyl Chloride Public Relations Committee received a report from Hill & Knowlton outlining the dangers that awaited the industry at the hearings and proposing a public relations campaign that would focus on four points: the "important role" that vinyl played in American industry, the number of jobs that could be lost if the industry were to shut down, the unfeasibility of meeting the strict standards that had been recommended by OSHA and NIOSH, and the fact that "it has not been demonstrated that a health hazard exists at the levels recommended by SPI." This formulation shifted the burden onto government to prove danger and away from industry to prove safety. This was important to do, the industry noted, because "it has not been scientifically demonstrated that the SPI recommended levels are truly safe."[71]

The authors of the public relations campaign were acting with full consciousness of the nightmare that the asbestos industry had lived through over the past few months. In late October 1973, the *New Yorker* magazine had published the first of a series of sensational articles by Paul Brodeur that were seen as an indictment not only of the asbestos industry but also of American industry in general. The articles, according to a publication of the United Rubber Workers, detailed "how the medical-industrial complex hides the facts [about occupational disease], prevents real action and makes the key decisions in OSHA and NIOSH."[72] During the controversy about asbestos, which had proven disastrous to Johns Manville and other asbestos companies, the industry had been completely outmaneuvered by Irving Selikoff and his union allies, who were now at the center of the vinyl debate.

Control of public perceptions of the vinyl crisis was no easy task for industry. Even within the vinyl chloride producers' inner circle anxiety about the health risks of VCM had mounted. Lee Grant, the medical director at PPG who had earlier called upon the industry to support an emergency standard, now objected to the companies' position that "significant exposure levels be permitted without the use of respiratory protection."[73] He believed that although from an engineering standpoint it might make sense to slowly reduce exposure levels, doing so was inadequate "from a health standpoint." He believed that employees should not be exposed to concentrations above 1 ppm TWA and that "respiratory protection should be recommended until such time as the air concentrations of VCM are so reduced," which he thought could be accomplished in short order. Dow Chemical, he pointed out, had already accomplished this.[74] Grant, however, never told the government or the public about his misgivings.

Far more damaging than Grant's internal dissent was public criticism of the chemical community by its own members. In mid-July 1974, *Chemical & Engineering News* reported that the American Chemical Society (ACS), a professional organization representing chemists in a variety of industry and academic settings, "entered the vinyl chloride dispute ... coming out, in essence, in support of the Government's proposed 'no detectable level' permanent standard for worker exposure to the chemical." Testifying at the OSHA hearings, Howard H. Fawcett, chair of the ACS Committee on Chemical Safety, and Dr. Stephen T. Quigley, head of the Society's Department of Chemistry and Public Affairs, argued that such a level was attainable.[75]

The ACS's action brought an immediate response from Union Carbide's A. B. Steele, who wrote to the ACS's executive director that the director and members of the ACS had overstepped their professional mandate. He complained that their testimony before OSHA represented the point of view of a limited group of committeemen and was not the consensus of the organization. He also maintained that it was unclear whether "even continuous exposure to vinyl chloride monomer in high concentrations over a period of time will necessarily result in any deleterious effects in humans."[76] Steele made his statement despite all that was known within the industry about the dangers of vinyl chloride.

In the midst of this dissension the industry was faced with a much bigger potential threat. Government officials came forward with information that they had been deceived by the industry. NIOSH Director Marcus Key reported that he had personally been misled by the MCA at the critical July 1973 meeting set up by industry to appear compliant with NIOSH's request for information. The MCA had led him to believe that the only information it possessed regarding cancer was that derived from the Viola studies, which indicated that tumors had been induced only "at very high levels of vinyl chloride" and primarily affected the Zymbal gland, which does not exist in humans. "At this meeting," Key asserted, "there was no mention of angiosarcoma of the liver in humans or animals, no reference to production of liver tumors in animals by another Italian investigator, and no reference to Professor Cesare Maltoni by name."[77]

The industry leadership knew that Key's statement could mean that the industry would lose any influence it had in the controversy over the angiosarcoma deaths. The statement implicitly accused the MCA of having conspired a year earlier to deny critical information regarding vinyl's toxicity to NIOSH, the federal agency responsible for establishing safe work practices. Although members of the vinyl industry wanted to refute and argue with Key about the meeting, they feared such a debate would bring attention to the issue. They decided to avoid a fight and hope it would just go away. A. W. Barnes of British producer ICI told other industry representatives that he did not want "any more public commotion over this."[78]

But NIOSH officials were unwilling to let the matter drop, for with the Watergate scandals and the impeachment hearings of President Richard Nixon playing out in the background, the public was more than ready to see corruption and scandal at every level of government. According to J. William Lloyd, NIOSH's director of occupational health surveillance and biometrics, there was a pervasive "questioning [of] the integrity of our public officials and scientists who are deeply dedicated to protecting the health of the worker." Lloyd believed that industry took advantage of the public's heightened skepticism about government to attempt to deflect attention from themselves by circulating rumors that government officials had kept secrets.

In an angry letter to Barnes of ICI, Lloyd accused the chemical industry of misstating the facts regarding the meeting with NIOSH on July 17, 1973. He was particularly irked that the British chemical trade association maintained in a press release that "American industry and government

(NIOSH) were told" of Maltoni's work. He argued that "as best as I could determine no representative of NIOSH was ever made aware of these findings prior to January 22, 1974, and even on that date, they were transmitted with the stipulation that they be kept confidential." He believed that the British chemical industry release had been "intentionally misleading since it was at variance with the facts as I knew them." Further, he believed that the MCA was also trying to avoid responsibility by releasing a "chronology of events that also inferred that NIOSH had been given the same information." He was, "to say the least, very upset," and when asked by a British television interviewer his "reaction to the [British] statement that NIOSH had been informed," he responded, "I would characterize those making such statements as 'damn liars.'"[79]

Because of continuing pressure from Key and Lloyd, Barnes finally responded privately to Lloyd with a long, convoluted argument. He acknowledged that the industry had not revealed the critical information from the Maltoni studies, but he insisted it had acted in good faith. He asserted that the British had gone to the NIOSH meeting fully intending to reveal any information they had about Maltoni's studies, but since NIOSH had not asked about the studies, the British assumed that NIOSH was not interested. Barnes maintained that David Duffield, the European representative at the meeting, "was a guest at a formal meeting between NIOSH and MCA and, as such, it would have been improper to force the meeting into detailed discussions which it appeared not to want."[80]

Barnes rejected Lloyd's assertion that anybody had knowingly misled the U.S. government and insisted it was all a big misunderstanding. Barnes asserted that the Europeans had "attempted to get the right actions taken throughout Europe and the USA as soon as the possible significance of Maltoni's findings were appreciated,"[81] although he offered no explanation of what the Europeans had done to accomplish this. Whatever his intent in sending this response to Lloyd, Barnes's letter was an admission that the vinyl industry had failed to mention at the meeting with NIOSH what it knew from Maltoni's studies—that primary angiosarcomas and other tumors had been caused by vinyl chloride.

While NIOSH officials were fuming over the MCA's deceptions, in the summer and fall of 1974 industry, labor, and public interest groups were battling over OSHA's proposed "no detectable limit" standard.[82] The industry made two arguments: first, that the epidemiological and scientific evidence regarding the dangers posed by vinyl chloride was ambiguous and that sacrificing a crucial industry by imposing untenable and unreachable standards would be irresponsible; and second, that the costs of initiating unnecessary workplace reforms would be so economically unfeasible that it could wreak havoc with the national economy.

The general counsel of the Society of the Plastics Industry, Jerome Heckman, told the OSHA hearing that "much of the scientific data obtained by researchers to date is quite inconclusive" and that "misplaced reliance on mere suspicions rather than proven data, or precipitous and emotional reaction to such incomplete information . . . could lead to major economic consequences." Heckman relied heavily on a recent decision of the United States Court of Appeals for the District of Columbia, *Industrial Union Department, AFL-CIO, vs. Hodgson,* which declared that the secretary of labor and OSHA were "required to consider feasibility of proposed standards" during their deliberations.[83] Interpreting this to mean not just technical or engineering feasibility, but also feasibility in terms of the costs of meeting these standards, the industry argued that greater emphasis on the economics of change should be critical to any OSHA decision.

Hooker Chemical and Plastics Corporation, which would soon become infamous for the Love Canal disaster in Niagara Falls, New York, also voiced its concerns. Its representative, Raymond J. Abramowitz, stated flatly that "it is the firm opinion of technical experts in our engineering and production departments that we could not continue to operate our plants and contemporaneously meet the proposed OSHA standard of 'no detectable level' of vinyl chloride." To do so would result in the loss of fifty thousand jobs, including both Hooker employees and those using their PVC to produce finished products, he maintained.[84] In sum, the industry believed that it was unfair to impose a "no detectable" limit because there had been no evidence of angiosarcomas at levels of exposure below 50 ppm.[85] For the industry a reasonable compromise would have been to establish a standard somewhere between the industry's and labor's position, "say 25 ppm."[86]

The industry's companies were counting on the likelihood that, despite their reckless deceit, they would still be seen as responsible partners in the decision-making process and that the delay in reporting Maltoni's findings would be viewed as an isolated episode born of the special circumstances of a covenant between the European and American manufacturers. They maintained that the industry had conducted responsible research that the government could rely on for making policy.

But confidence in the industry would be further eroded in the coming years when it was revealed that the industry's own animal studies had been so corrupted as to make them virtually useless. In 1977, the MCA learned that Industrial Bio-Test, the laboratory that had tested the toxicity of vinyl chloride on animals, was being investigated. The EPA and the FDA had swept through IBT's laboratories, finding conditions so horrendous and confused that no data coming from that lab could be considered reliable. *Chemical Week* described how "the stench of the IBT animal room, known as 'the Swamp,' was so noxious that government inspectors armed themselves with gas masks before entering it." Reporting logs were so unreliable and the control over lab conditions so deplorable that the owners were brought up on criminal charges of fraud and deception.[87]

The MCA's own investigators learned in 1979 that IBT's research on vinyl chloride's effect on rats, mice, and hamsters was so flawed that "the study by IBT is scientifically unacceptable."[88] IBT had "failed to save most tissues as specified in the protocol," had "failed to conduct histopathologic examinations of many of the tissues that were saved," and had failed "to examine sufficient organs from sacrificed animals." Specifically, "90 per cent of the brains of those animals surviving to the most critical period were never examined."[89] The MCA's consultant on the matter concluded that "the study was conducted in an extremely sloppy fashion," such that "foul play by IBT" was a definite possibility.[90]

Four years later *Chemical Week* would report that the serious problems with IBT's methods had not been a result of happenstance but that over the years IBT had "systematically falsified test data collected on scores of drugs and chemicals." One observer the journal quoted called IBT's practices the "'most massive scientific fraud' in American history."[91] How could the government continue to rely on private labs and industry research as part of its system for the development of standards, given this fact? The data that the industry had relied upon which claimed that vinyl chloride did not pose a danger were without scientific legitimacy.

But all this was as yet unknown in 1974 as the industry assured OSHA that its research could be relied on for information about potential problems. Only labor and consumer advocacy groups directly challenged this point of view. A broad coalition of unions, including the United Rubber Workers, the Oil, Chemical and Atomic Workers, and United Steelworkers (the three unions representing the vast majority of the VCM and PVC workers), joined the Industrial Union Department of the AFL-CIO and the International Association of Machinists and Aerospace Workers to argue for the "no-detectable" standard. Rubber Workers union President Peter Bommarito challenged the industry's argument that the country depended upon plastics for its progress. "This country survived for nearly 200 years without polyvinyl chloride and we can survive in the future without it," he began. "If PVC can not be made and used safely, then the proposed standard must be replaced by [a] . . . phase out [of] vinyl chloride production."[92]

Rudy Kaelin, the president of the Rubber Workers local of the Goodrich plant in Kentucky where the first cases of angiosarcoma of the liver had been discovered, said that the workers "knew for a long time that something was wrong, but did not know what, nor who to turn to." As recently as November of the previous year, when the MCA and its member companies already knew of the angiosarcomas in Maltoni's rats, the union had requested medical screenings, particularly of liver function, but had been refused by Goodrich. "We have argued for better ventilation for years with very little results."[93] The president of an OCAW local, Vern Jenson, confirmed Kaelin's opinion that the industry rarely provided workers with information about the chemicals they worked with. The workers believed that they were working with a "totally innocuous" substance. At the least, he said, "someone in our industry should have been sensitive and aware to what experimental findings were going on elsewhere in the world, and that we should have been informed in some manner that we were incurring some degree of hazard."[94]

The OCAW's Tony Mazzocchi went even further in his accusations, arguing that industry's economic arguments were a smokescreen meant to delay the implementation of a "no detectable" standard and minimize the costs of renovation and reform within the industry. "The tactic they have used is to . . . forecast economic disaster and widespread unemployment. It is our hope that OSHA will not succumb to these pressures." When one of the commissioners asked Mazzocchi whether the industry was trying to "con" OSHA, he replied that it was fine "if you wish to use the word *con*."[95] Other union spokespeople observed that "only the perverse or the exceptionally naïve or ignorant think the determination of consensus should simply be one of . . . accepting a given percentage of death and disease at a given so-called feasible limit of exposure."[96]

Other parties also weighed in on what seemed to be a labor-management confrontation over the interpretation of the OSHAct and its mandate. Andrea Hricko and Bertram Cottine, staff assistants in Sidney Wolfe's Health Research Group, made an eloquent argument for a different conception of caution than the one provided by the business community. Waiting for epidemiological proof before improving work conditions or reducing exposure to suspected carcinogens was neither practical from the scientific standpoint nor moral. "Unfortunately, [epidemiological proof] is always retrospective in nature and can only be accumulated after the harmful effects have already manifested themselves." Hricko argued that all new chemicals introduced into the human environment—whether in the workplace or through the distribution of consumer products—should be tested for their harmful effects before being put into wide use. "Had adequate animal studies to determine carcinogenic effects been conducted when vinyl chloride was first introduced as a chemical, and timely regulatory action taken on the basis of those animal studies, the subsequent human toll of disease could have been prevented."[97]

Cottine amplified Hricko's indictment of the industry's callous cost-benefit analysis, pointing out that the industry wanted to talk only about the economic costs of protecting workers and not about the social costs. By attending only to its own "short ranged financial considerations," the industry conveniently neglected the "cost of disease and death." "The pain and suffering as well as the cost to the exposed worker and his family and the social costs of insurance, hospitalization, treatment and welfare payments cannot be ignored in assessing the economics of an inadequate standard."[98]

Others argued that while the focus of public attention was presently on workers' exposure to vinyl chloride, experience with asbestos showed that "the hazard might not stop at the factory gate but that it might invade workers' homes and the neighborhoods about vinyl chloride, polyvinyl chloride facilities."[99] Hricko added that aerosol propellants were a danger "in the home as well as the occupational setting."[100]

Other union representatives asked OSHA to ensure the safety of workers in the meatpacking industry, where vinyl products were used to wrap meat. When the vinyl wrapping was heated in the packaging process, workers were exposed to vinyl chloride fumes, creating a condition known in the industry as "meat wrappers asthma."[101]

In late August, Irving Selikoff, the elder statesman of occupational medicine, told the Senate's Committee on Commerce Subcommittee on the Dangers of Vinyl Chloride of the growing uneasiness of the occupational and environmental health community with the rapid and uncontrolled growth of the plastics industry. "I believe it fair to say that in the past 20 years we have all been sort of looking out of the corners of our eyes at the petrochemical industry, and particularly the plastics industry," he began. This industry has been "growing rapidly about us and permeating every aspect of our lives." Undoubtedly, "the valuable products and their benefits were obvious." But, he said, "uneasiness existed because we knew very little concerning their biological potential, which remained largely untested and unstudied." The angiosarcoma deaths were a telling indictment of society's consumerism. "We now know that this uneasiness was justified and the lack of study . . . [was] a mistake. The discovery that one of the chemicals central to much of our plastics industry, a simple chemical, assumed to be benign, was not simple, in biological terms, and surely not benign."[102]

THE DEVELOPMENT OF THE PRECAUTIONARY PRINCIPLE

Dr. Irving Selikoff and industry representatives alike recognized that the battle over vinyl chloride was not about the dangers and carcinogenic effects of one substance. Rather, it was what the prestigious business periodical *Fortune* called "the tip of an enormous regulatory iceberg."[103] Coming shortly after the formation of the EPA, NIOSH, OSHA, and the Consumer Product Safety Commission, the storm over vinyl chloride forced regulators, industry, consumer groups, and labor to confront "all the indirect costs of running a modern economy."

Sheldon W. Samuels, the health director of the Industrial Union Department of the AFL-CIO, argued that labor saw the battle as an attempt to put an end to industry's "free ride on social costs." *Fortune* magazine, on the other hand, suggested that it was as important to prevent the death of an industry as it was to prevent workers' deaths: "If government allows workers to be exposed to the gas, some of them may die. If it eliminates all exposure a valuable industry may disappear."[104] Vinyl chloride presented a situation where "medical and economic considerations collide[d] head-on."[105]

Yet it was the language of science, rather than politics or economics, that dominated the debate about the causes of cancer, the means of prevention, and the responsibilities of the government. Consumers, labor, and public health advocates argued that there was no level at which exposure to carcinogens could be presumed effective in preventing cancers. "Advocates of the 'no-detectable level' argued for the so-called 'one-hit' theory of cancer causation," wrote Paul Weaver in *Fortune*, describing the position that there was "no such thing as a risk-free exposure to a carcinogen." The industry, on the other hand, argued that "cancers appear when the immune system breaks down." A healthy immune system had to be weakened before a cancer could develop. Industry held that "what a carcinogen does is to weaken the immune system" and that the "weakening process requires a certain level of dose." According to this interpretation, it was possible that there was "a risk-free level of exposure."[106]

This debate over whether there were safe levels of exposure to vinyl chloride forced the new regulatory agencies to formulate the principles that would guide government's role in economic, scientific, and political decisions. The argument that played out over vinyl chloride is played out today over all toxic substances.

The vinyl chloride issue brought to the fore the question first raised during the tetraethyl lead controversy a half century before: Should industry be asked to prove that a substance was safe before introducing it into the environment, or should society be forced to prove it dangerous before banning it? Since the tetraethyl lead crisis, industry had largely prevailed in this debate, but vinyl chloride represented a whole new class of chemical products of enormous importance to the chemical industry and, perhaps, society.

Writing in the *Wall Street Journal* in October 1974, Barry Kramer described the stakes. If the labor and consumer advocates' view prevailed, Kramer observed, "industry will no longer be able to assume blithely that untested chemicals . . . are safe simply because they've never demonstrated any overt harm. Like vinyl chloride, which took years to take its toll on worker health, many chemicals thought to be harmless may be equally insidious."[107] The prestigious British medical journal *The Lancet* was optimistic. "Whatever happens the vinyl chloride episode will have provided a salutary lesson," *The Lancet* wrote. "It will not be quite so easy in the future as it has been in the past for any chemical manufacturer to assume, until proved otherwise, that a chemical to which workers are exposed is carcinogenically safe."[108] Kramer quantified the seriousness of the problem, noting that there were twenty-five thousand industrial chemicals already in use and that more than five hundred chemicals were added every year, and virtually none of them had been adequately tested or followed.[109]

On October 4, 1974, OSHA published its "Standard for Exposure to Vinyl Chloride."[110] The *Federal Register* reported that the record in this proceeding was "one of the most exhaustive ever relied upon by OSHA." It had documented that three animal species—rats, mice, and hamsters—developed cancers after exposure to vinyl chloride and that "more tumors occur at higher exposure levels." The finding of cancer in animals met the criteria of the 1970 Surgeon General's Ad Hoc Committee on the Evaluation of Low Levels of Environmental Chemical Carcinogens, which held that "the finding of cancer in two or more animal species may be extrapolated to indicate a carcinogenic hazard to humans." The thirteen documented deaths among vinyl chloride workers from angiosarcoma of the liver, in addition to "evidence of tumor induction in a variety of other organs including lung, kidney, brain and skin as well as non-malignant alterations, such as fibrosis and connective tissue deterioration indicates additional oncogenic and toxicologic properties of vinyl chloride."[111]

OSHA concluded that there was "little dispute that VC is carcinogenic to man.... However, the precise level of exposure that poses a hazard and the question of whether a 'safe' exposure level exists cannot be definitively answered on the record. Nor is it clear to what extent exposures can be feasibly reduced. We cannot wait until indisputable answers to these questions are available, because lives of employees are at stake.... These judgments have required a balancing process, in which the overriding consideration has been the protection of employees, even those who may have regular exposure to VC throughout their working lives." OSHA concluded that the permissible exposure limit (PEL) had to be reduced to 1 ppm TWA, which OSHA believed could be reached through engineering controls. OSHA acknowledged industry's worry that this standard would put an especially heavy burden on manufacturers who used PVC to produce plastic products but argued that this standard should apply to every company because "at least some employees in the fabricating industry are exposed in excess of the permissible control limits."[112]

Although it was viewed at the time as a victory for labor, journalist Michael S. Brown argues that OSHA's decision to abandon the "no detectable level" for a 1 ppm standard meant that economic feasibility became "a major consideration in the determination" of other health standards.[113] Since the vinyl standard was set, OSHA has been plagued by the threat of lawsuits from industry groups demanding close attention to economic feasibility, which has resulted in lack of action on numerous substances.[114] (Even the revision of the silicosis standard which was proposed in the mid-1970s has yet to be issued, despite the fact that it has been clear for eighty years that silica dust causes silicosis and despite former Secretary of Labor Robert Reich's urging that silicosis be eliminated as a problem. Witness also that OSHA's abandonment of the recent ergonomic standard in the first months of the Bush administration, despite years of research, planning, and effort, was based on the fact that implementation of the standard would cost too much. Economic feasibility was a readily accepted factor in the consideration of danger.)

OSHA assumed that industry had the technology to enable it to implement the vinyl chloride standard immediately. The industry, however, claimed it would need to immediately reorganize its production and introduce new filtering, cleansing, and protective equipment. New plants would have to be built to replace older plants that could not easily be adapted to new processes.[115] Within a week of the publication of the new standard, the

Society of the Plastics Industries (SPI) met and decided to file a petition challenging the permanent standard in the U.S. Court of Appeals.[116]

It may be that the sense of crisis within the industry was heightened by two unrelated but parallel events. In 1973 the Arab oil embargo had substantially raised prices for crude oil, leading to a substantial rise in production costs for all vinyl chloride products. In addition, a recession in 1974–75 hit the construction industry hard, causing a severe slump in the plastics industry and particularly the producers of PVC. David Doniger writes that this was a particularly difficult time for the industry because business analysts had not predicted the slump and had, in fact, forecast virtually uninterrupted growth for the industry. Coming after an unparalleled boom in PVC consumption in the 1960s and early 1970s, the slump, combined with the challenge posed by OSHA and NIOSH, may have contributed to the intensity with which the industry resisted the government's attempt at regulation.[117] In December 1974, the various legal challenges to OSHA's vinyl chloride standard were consolidated in the Second Circuit.

Despite its public challenge to OSHA, there was little dispute within the plastics industry that vinyl chloride was a real hazard.[118] Joseph Fath, vice president of Tenneco Chemicals and acting chair of the SPI's Vinyl Chloride Monomer and Polyvinyl Chloride Producers Group, put it succinctly when he noted in an internal memo that regarding "vinyl chloride and human health[,] probably not much can be said to mitigate the fact that the two are incompatible." Fath, who had graduated from Cornell University with a B.A. in chemistry in 1944 and had since the mid-1950s been directly involved in the research and development of polyvinyl chloride, argued that the SPI had to develop a new public relations approach that addressed "itself precisely to the separation of the finished consumer good from its chemically derived raw material." He proposed "a program dealing primarily with the merits, benefits, assets and rightful place of PVC products in a modern industrial society. I believe we can easily demonstrate how PVC has benefited all of us in the supply of economical consumer goods, has aided our defense industries in preserving our political system, our communications industry in enabling us to conduct the business of our modern society and has played a key role in assuring us through the plastics industry in particular and the chemical industry in general, of a continued increase in our standard of living."[119]

This effort to convince the public that there was a world of difference between the dangers associated with VCM and the finished products made from polyvinyl chloride called for an intensive public relations campaign. In order to accomplish these objectives, relationships with the press had to be fostered, even by assisting "reporters, feature writers, etc. [in] preparing stories on vinyl chloride." The SPI's Public Affairs Committee also recommended developing strong ties with a "small body of informed, interested and effective Senators and Congressmen who can and will be ready to become an active support group for the VCM-PVC industry."[120] On December 6, the SPI and the Producers Group approved this proposal, emphasizing the objective of "the differentiation between vinyl chloride and polyvinyl chloride."[121]

The machinations of the industry as it tried to delay and limit the implementation of the OSHA standard through litigation came to a screeching halt in late January 1975 when the U.S. Court of Appeals for the Second Circuit issued its decision regarding the SPI's challenge to the OSHA standard. In a scathing review of the industry's history, Justice Tom Clark, retired from the U.S. Supreme Court, noted the long policy of delay, feigned ignorance, and irresponsibility of the chemical manufacturers. He rejected all the fundamentals of the industry's position, pointing out that while the "fatal character of VCM did not emerge until early in 1974 when the three workers in Goodrich's PVC plant at Louisville were reported, strong warning signals had appeared long before." Clark wrote, "We need not outline in detail the morbid 'Vinyl Chloride Chronology,' ... in order to illustrate the mounting evidence of VCM's carcinogenicity. Indeed, the record shows what can only be described as a course of continued procrastination on the part of the industry to protect the lives of its employees." Despite years of warnings and research, including studies dating as far back as 1949 and continuing through the acroosteolysis studies by the University of Michigan, "nothing was done." Despite Viola's early studies "the industry did nothing." Months and years went by, but "it was not until February of 1973 that a protocol was agreed upon and a research contract for animal exposure studies signed. Meanwhile, startling results from European experiments were ... kept confidential."[122]

Justice Clark identified the important regulatory principles that were being worked out around the vinyl chloride crisis. The "ultimate facts" regarding the proper standard for protecting workers were "in dispute" and "on the frontiers of scientific knowledge." Although the "factual finger" points to the need for a low permissible exposure limit, no science could definitively establish it. But "under the command of OSHA, it remains the duty of the Secretary to act to protect the workingman, and to act even in circumstances where existing methodology or research is deficient." Hence, "the Secretary [of Labor], in extrapolating the MCA study's finding from mouse to man, has chosen to reduce the permissible level to the lowest detectable one. We find no error in this respect."[123]

Despite Clark's unambiguous ruling, the SPI Vinyl Chloride Monomer and Polyvinyl Chloride Producers Group decided to proceed with a petition for a writ of certiorari at the U.S. Supreme Court. A stay was denied on March 31, 1975, however, and the 1 ppm standard went into effect on April 1, 1975.[124]

Despite all the objections by the industry, its claims of technical and economic impossibility, its legal challenges and maneuvering to stop the imposition of the standard, companies quickly and efficiently adapted to the new standard. "They offered dire warnings of plant closings, job losses, price increases and massive economic dislocation," the *New York Times* reported. But the predictions may have been nothing more than the industry crying wolf. "One year later," the *Times* noted, "not one of the doomsday predictions has proven accurate." Prices had not increased, supplies of vinyl chloride were plentiful and the industry was actually expanding, not contracting.[125] Engineering controls developed by Goodrich were fully adequate to reduce exposure, the *Times* reported. The initial costs for development, while expensive, could easily be introduced into new plants and retrofitted to older plants as well.[126] A December 2000 analysis of the costs of providing workers with a safe environment confirmed this: in the mid-1970s, OSHA estimated that it would cost industry $1 billion to comply with the standard while industry estimated it would cost up to $90 billion. The actual costs, however, in this huge and growing industry were a modest $278 million.[127]

In 1974–75 researchers documented that the dangers of vinyl chloride monomer were more far reaching than first thought. Findings indicated that vinyl chloride may be mutagenic, as well as carcinogenic.[128] Peter Infante, a young researcher with the Ohio Department of Health, found that women living in three Ohio communities with polyvinyl chloride plants "gave birth to a significantly greater number of children with malformations during the period 1970–1973" than expected.[129] In 1976, a story in the *Wall Street Journal* reported on a CDC study that indicated that vinyl chloride "apparently also causes a higher incidence than normal of miscarriages among workers' wives" as a result of "damage [to] the sperm cells of the worker-husbands." The *Journal* revealed that although the study had been presented several months earlier at a scientific meeting in Czechoslovakia, it had not been released in the United States "until

Ralph Nader's Health Research Group demanded a copy from the U.S. government under the Freedom of Information Act."[130]

The response of most companies to the possible teratogenic impact of vinyl chloride was to prohibit women of childbearing years from working in the areas of the plant where workers were exposed to chlorinated organics, lead, or mercury. H. B. Lovejoy, a company physician at a Pittsburgh Paint and Glass plant in Lake Charles, Louisiana, reported that he was "surprised and disturbed" to learn at the Health and Toxicology Committee meeting of the Chlorine Institute, a group of companies that used chlorine chemistry, that PPG was alone in "permitting women of child bearing ability" to work in those areas of the plant. Despite his conviction that PPG protected its workers from undue exposure to VCM, lead, and mercury, "the possibility of unexpected exposure remains" and that PPG should follow the example of the other companies "until such time as the courts or EEO [Equal Employment Opportunity Commission] say we must" permit them to work.[131]

In 1980, the trade press reported on more studies indicating the mutagenic effects of vinyl chloride monomer. Although *Chemical & Engineering News* quoted an evaluation by a Columbia University statistician that "the question of whether vinyl chloride is a reproductive hazard has not yet been answered,"[132] evidence mounted in the 1980s confirming various aspects of Peter Infante's observation about the deleterious effects of vinyl chloride among community residents. Joseph Wagoner, formerly of NIOSH but then working as an independent consulting epidemiologist, published a broad review of the "toxicity of vinyl chloride" in 1983. Citing a number of studies of individuals close to polyvinyl chloride plants who developed angiosarcomas of the liver, he concluded that "these study findings are supportive of the role of indirect modes of vinyl chloride exposure in the etiology of liver angiosarcoma."[133]

With the decision of the U.S. Court of Appeals in January 1975, the business community feared that its longtime domination of the industrial hygiene arena had suffered a great change. Vinyl chloride had come to symbolize "the manner in which the initiative passed out of the hands of industry," seized by what *Fortune* magazine would describe as "a loose but not uncoordinated network of regulatory agencies, government research institutes, academic medical teams, labor unions, and other groups united by a common commitment to eradicate environmental causes of disease." This network, which *Fortune* disparagingly dubbed the "regulatory-medical complex," had evolved as a result of the social movements of the 1960s and the new regulatory agencies that had arisen in their wake.[134]

Industry and OSHA each learned important lessons from the vinyl crisis about the process of regulating toxic substances. Industry learned that it needed to follow OSHA's activities ever so closely, combating the agency at every turn. OSHA's lesson was the rather dispiriting recognition that an industry could be expected to fight standards tooth and nail, to question the validity of all unfavorable scientific evidence, to mount massive public relations campaigns, and to sue OSHA whenever necessary. After 1980, rather than becoming more determined to maintain control, an intimidated OSHA tried to avoid conflict by moving slowly, usually at a snail's pace. OSHA's hope was that by careful review and compromise it might forestall industry's opposition and/or prevent the kind of exhausting process the industry had dragged OSHA through concerning the vinyl chloride standard. In the end, however, OSHA virtually retreated from its original mission of establishing a safe and healthful workplace.

OSHA's reputation as an activist agency stems almost completely from its activities in regard to a few substances and the brief period when Dr. Eula Bingham was at its head. Right after its establishment, OSHA produced standards for asbestos and thirteen carcinogens. During Dr. Eula Bingham's tenure as assistant secretary for OSHA during the Carter administration in the late 1970s, the agency added standards for acrylonitrile (another ingredient in many plastics), arsenic, cotton dust, lead, and benzene, the benzene standard ultimately suspended by the Supreme Court. But this was a tiny fraction of the number of standards recommended to OSHA by its sister agency, NIOSH.[135]

The gutting of OSHA was accomplished in part by industry's victory on the benzene standard. In the first decade of its existence, OSHA had set the lowest possible level of exposure for a chemical if it had qualitative evidence that the chemical had the potential to cause cancer. But the Supreme Court overturned the OSHA standard for benzene in *Industrial Union Department vs. American Petroleum Institute* (July 2, 1980) on the grounds that OSHA had not provided quantitative evidence that there would be a "significant risk of material health impairment" if the old standard of 10 ppm were not reduced to the agency's proposed 1 ppm. As a result OSHA and other government agencies were forced "to develop quantitative information on risks to human health before setting a standard." In the words of Justice Thurgood Marshall in his dissent in the benzene case, this placed "the burden of medical uncertainty squarely on the shoulders of the American worker."[136]

By 1981 NIOSH had recommended over two hundred fifty standards but OSHA had acted on only twenty-one of them.[137] The Reagan years saw a virtual cessation in OSHA's standard-setting and regulatory activities, as a hostile administration and a newly emboldened industrial community threatened suits and noncompliance. This pattern of inactivity based upon the fear of litigation from industry and the lack of support from Congress and the executive branch was reversed briefly during the early years of the Clinton administration. But even then OSHA focused most of its energies on preparing one major standard—for ergonomics—that Clinton approved just before he left office. Within weeks of George W. Bush's assuming residence in the White House, Congress abolished the only significant standard OSHA had established in over a decade.

EPIDEMIOLOGY OF VINYL CHLORIDE

When it became clear in 1973 that vinyl chloride was an animal carcinogen, the MCA contracted with Tabershaw-Cooper Associates to conduct epidemiological studies of the industry's workforce. While over the years there had been many problems with collecting data from member companies and other methodological problems, as early as 1974 bad news began to emerge from these studies. Tabershaw-Cooper submitted what it called its "Final Report," dated April 15, 1974, to the MCA, but the report ended up in the files of the MCA renamed "draft." On every page the words "Final Report" were crossed out and replaced by "draft."

The first results indicated "a measurable excess of digestive cancers, especially liver, respiratory cancers and other unspecified cancers in which brain cancer predominated."[138] The revised "Final Report," which was dated May 3, was substantially less pointed than the first. Despite the findings reported earlier, the report emphasized that the increased mortality and cancer rates among vinyl chloride workers were not statistically significant[139] and even below the national average for males in the appropriate age group. The "Final Report" told the industry that "overall mortality [of workers in the vinyl industry] was approximately 75 percent of what would be expected in a comparable population of U.S. males." Further, "no cause of death showed a statistically significant excess over what would be expected in a comparable U.S. male population."[140]

The *MCA News,* the trade association's newsletter, trumpeted the lack of statistical significance in a page-one headline: "Study Shows Death Rate Average for VC Workers." Its lead paragraph told readers, "The findings of a survey contracted by MCA show that vinyl chloride workers, in the aggregate, experience death rates from all causes that compare favorably with other U.S. male industrial workers." What was a warning and a matter of concern in the first "Final Report" had become a favorable finding a month later. The newsletter also reported that there appeared to be a dose-related increase in cancer rates at other sites than the liver, such as urinary organs and the brain.[141]

Epidemiologists from NIOSH who studied the report questioned its rosy conclusions. "The greatest limitation in this study," one epidemiologist observed, "is that some of the deficiencies [such as the omission of some workers with the longest exposure to VCM] tend to increase the number of expected deaths, and to decrease the number of observed deaths." This epidemiologist concluded that even "the information that they have provided is certainly not information that can reassure us on the question of carcinogencity of vinyl chloride."[142]

In August, Tabershaw-Cooper Associates reported its results in the *Journal of Occupational Medicine.* The study, which looked at 8,384 men who had worked with vinyl chloride for at least one year, "demonstrated that cancers of the digestive system (primarily angiosarcoma), respiratory system, brain, and cancers of unknown site, as well as lymphomas, occurred more often than expected in those members of the study population with the greatest estimated exposure." While the article proclaimed that "this [was] the first epidemiological study which suggests that in humans vinyl chloride may also be associated with cancer of multiple sites," the authors tried to soften the blow by reiterating claims from previous reports that "the overall mortality of the study population was approximately 75% of what would be expected in a comparable population of U.S. males" and that "no cause of death showed a statistically significant excess over what would be expected in a comparable U.S. male population."[143]

Dr. Joseph Wagoner, director of field studies and clinical investigations for NIOSH and the Centers for Disease Control, was damning in his analysis of the Tabershaw-Cooper methodology. Although 75 percent of those exposed to vinyl chloride for twenty years or longer could not be found,[144] Wagoner had identified 930 white male vinyl chloride workers who had begun their careers between 1950 and 1973. He told the U.S. Senate Committee on Commerce's Sub-Committee on the Environment that there was a "57 percent increase in deaths due to cancer, beyond what would have been expected" among vinyl chloride workers, a difference that was "highly significant." Further, he called into question the epidemiological data of the MCA-sponsored study conducted by Tabershaw-Cooper.[145] "The overall mortality risk is at variance with an earlier reported industry wide study of vinyl chloride employees which showed a deficit in total mortality," he maintained. Wagoner attributed Tabershaw-Cooper's findings to a possible flaw in its research design: the study included a "disproportionate number of recently hired employees," who presumably diluted the measurement of harm.[146] In his study, Wagoner's delimiting criterion was that the workers "had to be engaged in the polymerization for 15 or more years, since we knew indeed that we were looking for the latent effects or the effects of a carcinogen which would appear many years after a person was initially employed."[147] He had corrected for this by excluding from his analysis the "first five or 10 years after a person comes into employment."[148]

While the industry sought to focus attention on its success in attacking the problem of angiosarcoma of the liver among its workers, its own epidemiological studies confirmed the research of others, finding cancers at other sites on the body in workers exposed to vinyl chloride. The MCA's initial epidemiological study by Tabershaw-Cooper Associates had found an excess of brain cancer deaths among vinyl chloride workers, and a supplementary study commissioned by the MCA found similar results.[149] A retrospective cohort study published a year later, in 1976, by researchers at NIOSH found "an excessive number of deaths due to cancer . . . [of] the liver, lung, and the lymphatic and central nervous system."[150] In early 1979 an employee at Union Carbide's plant in Texas City, Texas, filed a complaint with OSHA based on his observation that too many of the plant's workers were developing brain tumors. Newspapers picked up the story, reporting that this plant had "an unusually high number of workers [who] . . . died of a type of brain tumor that has been linked to the cancer-causing agent, vinyl chloride."[151]

In an internal memo, Robert Wheeler of Union Carbide confided to a fellow Union Carbide physician that the company "appears to have an excess incidence of brain tumors at Texas City and at South Charleston [West Virginia]," but he doubted that it was due to vinyl chloride. Union Carbide was not as frank with its own employees, writing that it did "not yet have sufficient data to answer" the question of whether there was a "higher than normal incidence of brain tumors."[152] It appeared that of the 454 workers for whom there were death certificates on file, 110 had died of a variety of cancers, of which 11 were probably primary brain tumors.[153]

Officials of other companies acknowledged privately the legitimacy of the workers' fears.[154] Conoco's F. C. Dehn wrote privately that "several epidemiological studies ... have shown higher incidences of brain cancer when VCM is exposed. . . . There have been warnings of this type based on some animal studies, too."[155] PPG responded in much the same way it had when acroosteolysis was a problem: the company sought ways to survey workers without raising their consciousness about the cancer hazard. A suggestion that workers be sent a letter to their homes was rejected because it "would be overly inflammatory," especially in light of the "start of [labor] negotiations which will be very much concerned in part with safety and health."[156]

A two-day conference at the National Institutes of Health in the early spring of 1980 brought together thirty-five scientists who were involved in vinyl chloride research. Maltoni's continuing work on animals corroborated the fears of those who suspected that vinyl chloride was a multipotent carcinogen. Peter Infante summarized epidemiological studies that "taken together ... indicate an even greater incidence of brain cancers than liver cancers among workers exposed to vinyl chloride."[157]

In late 1980, the MCA's VCM Research Coordinators Task Group discussed a possible update of the Tabershaw-Cooper epidemiological study in order to "gain information to help in future law suits."[158] This update, done by Environmental Health Associates (EHA) for the MCA, found that "vinyl chloride workers experienced significant mortality excesses in angiosarcomas (15 deaths), cancer of the liver and biliary tract ... and cancer of the brain and other central nervous system [parts]."[159] By 1987, review articles accepted the possibility that brain cancers, even among children, could be associated with vinyl chloride exposure.[160] Even industry representatives recognized the connection. In a private memo to Conoco's legal department, W. D. Broddle, the company's director of toxicology, wrote that vinyl chloride had "some tendency to cause cancer of the brain, lung, breast and digestive tract."[161]

In 1991, Otto Wong, the chief researcher in the EHA study, went public with his findings, publishing an article based upon his research. He reasserted the "significant mortality excesses" in angiosarcomas, cancers of the liver and biliary tract, and cancer of the brain and other parts of the central nervous system.[162] The industry reacted strongly to what it perceived as Wong's violation of trust, since it had funded his research. A Goodrich manager complained to the Vinyl Institute that Wong had failed to send a draft of his paper to the MCA "for review prior to publication" and had thereby "violated their contract." He hoped that "the authors will be agreeable to add some clarifying comments in a letter to the editor."[163]

In a conference call among members of the MCA's Vinyl Chloride Panel, the MCA discussed how to respond. It appears that members did reach Wong, for in one of the most curious cases of "self-correction" Wong wrote a letter to the journal's editor, Philip Landrigan, retracting some of his most devastating findings and concluding that his own interpretation of the data rejected a connection between the excess brain cancer deaths and vinyl chloride exposure.[164] Landrigan had no idea at the time of the intense pressure that Wong was under to retract his findings. After all, Wong's "methodology was very standard," noted Landrigan in an interview with Bill Moyers. "The findings were very believable, and the retraction was really quite unexpected." Reflecting on this incident and on industry-sponsored lead research, Landrigan observed that most people "don't understand that science can be bought and paid for."[165]

By 1991 management had lost credibility among workers in the vinyl industry. Workers were no longer willing to accept the industry's assurances that it could be relied upon to protect their health, let alone that the industry should be the final arbiter of what was to be deemed safe in the workplace. Despite all the evidence to the contrary, the industry maintained a public stance that vinyl posed no risk, either to the workforce or to the broader community. Workers worried that the workplace was getting more and more dangerous and that the materials they worked with, vinyl chloride monomer and ethylene dichloride, were responsible for "high rates of employee deaths due to cancer."[166]

Workers at the Vista plant in Lake Charles, Louisiana, called the presentations by management and medical staff explaining the deaths of five employees from cancer "a snow job, bull shit." Questions from the workers were not only left unanswered but the workers also were told "to shut up and not make trouble." The workers pleaded with the company to pay attention. "We like our jobs. We like Vista; it's a good company and it pays well, but we don't want to die. We think our jobs are killing us. No one listens." In the end the workers came to feel that management just didn't care; they didn't see the workers as people. "We're just a social security number. If we die, they'll just get some other sucker to take our place. They're afraid of the liability but we just want some answers."[167]

It seems that even four years later the Vista workers were still not being heard. One company official wrote, "Study after study has confirmed there is no evidence that vinyl affects human health—not for workers in the industry, not for people living near vinyl-related manufacturing facilities, not for those who use the hundreds of vinyl consumer and industrial products."[168] The skepticism of the workforce was just one indication of the battering that had taken its toll on the chemical industry.[169]

But even as the industry came under increasing scrutiny in the early 1970s, it did manage to develop a variety of tactics to undercut OSHA and the EPA. The industry argued over what constituted good science, shifted the debate from health to economic costs, challenged all statements considered damaging to industry, and lied about what was known about the cancer-causing potential of vinyl chloride. These arguments about adverse effects of regulation on industry were all the more salient in the mid- to late 1970s, when the country entered a period of economic stagnation, high inflation, and energy shortages. At this point business began to recruit academics for scholarly justifications for its positions. Data from think tanks and academic institutes funded by industry were used to counter the champions of greater regulation. In the 1970s, for "every horror story about corporate irresponsibility that had circulated at the beginning of the decade, by its end there was a matching horror story about the shortcomings of government regulation."[170] Even the most principled and vigorous government officials were stymied. While Eula Bingham's tenure as assistant secretary of OSHA was a brief moment of regulatory activism, the vinyl crisis and the broader business onslaught instilled a long-lasting culture of fear within OSHA.

The industry had come a long way over the past decade, developing sophisticated means to influence government policies. But industry leaders still longed for the earlier era when they had much greater power. As the MCA's Government Relations Committee pointed out, in the not-so-distant past the business community was "listened to with considerable attention by those members of Congress that wore either a Republican or Southern Democrat label." But now, "business is not as influential in Washington as we would like" nor was it able to protect the varied interests of "private enterprise . . . in this country."

How did this situation come to pass? asked the committee. First and foremost the country had been fundamentally shaken and democratized by the civil rights movement, which brought the nation's attention to the plight of the powerless and to the unequal distribution of power in the corridors of Congress. In the late 1950s, Southern Democrats who controlled the chairmanships of important committees could easily promote or divert legislation of interest to the industry, recalled Don Goodall, the committee chairman. "But that day went out with the one-man, one-vote drive that took place more than a decade ago, and for a variety of other reasons."[171] By the late 1960s and early 1970s, in addition to the gains brought by the civil rights movement, labor was better organized. Television informed the public about environmental and industrial issues in ways not previously available. In addition, "the wide exposure TV gives to candidates tends to open up the selection process," leading to greater discussion of political issues. Finally, the committee pointed out, public interest groups used the media to gain the public's attention to a degree never attained before. These changes left business grappling with how to regain the initiative in setting policy.[172]

Toward this end, business began to look for the next generation of chief executive officers in their legal and public relations departments—executives who spoke the language of lobbyists and politicians and who were prepared to shape the regulatory climate. One survey of CEOs revealed that the amount of time they devoted to "public issues" had doubled between 1976 and 1978. Irving Shapiro, chosen as CEO of DuPont in 1974 because of his skills in government relations, was the first head of DuPont with no background in engineering, science, or finance. He was the epitome of the "modern business leader," with "one foot in the boardroom and the other in Washington."[173]

In fact, the CEOs of the two hundred largest U.S. corporations got together in 1972 to form the Business Roundtable, which, according to *Fortune*, "was the biggest and baddest lobbying group in Washington." Called the "Green Berets of business influence," the Roundtable "helped defeat a slew of pro-labor laws" and government regulatory actions in the 1970s.[174] In view of the new political environment, it was difficult for environmental, consumer, and labor advocates to fashion an effective opposition to industry's closed ranks. Each new federal action became the focus of intense, acrimonious, and divisive discourse as conservative and business groups framed every issue as a battle over America's future. Advocacy groups were faced by a wall of intense resistance and were forced to decide between competing strategies of political reform. Should they be content with occasional small victories in legislative arenas, particularly in light of the rolling back of earlier legislation and regulation? Or should consumer groups set their sights on grand goals of the sort that bear fruit only over time?

Future battles over regulation of the chemical industry would come from newer, less institutionally predictable community groups that could not as easily be manipulated by industry's lobbyists, lawyers, and political action committee money. In the 1980s and 1990s the struggle would be waged between the chemical industry and the drastically refigured and politically empowered constituencies of the labor and civil rights movements, environmentalists, and a core of professionals who came of age in the activist 1960s and were trained in the post-NIOSH, post-OSHA era.

Ol' Man River or Cancer Alley?

While labor unions and consumer advocates were battling the chemical industry in the 1970s, communities around the country began protesting against the industries whose pollution of their air and water was endangering their health. Many of these struggles took place in the South, where a large portion of the chemical industry had found the political and economic environment more friendly to their interests than in the industrialized corridors of the Northeast and Midwest. Also in the 1970s Louisiana emerged as one of the nation's leading centers of vinyl chloride and polyvinyl chloride production. Louisiana was rich in natural resources and offered a low-cost labor force and a state government eager to provide lower taxes and lax environmental regulations.

What industry did not anticipate was the powerful resistance of residents who organized their communities; demonstrated against plants; allied themselves with union activists, who provided support and inside information about company malfeasance; joined with national environmental groups with access to national media; and linked up with public interest lawyers, who challenged the alliance between the industry and the state.

THE POWER OF THE MONEY OF THIS CORPORATION

Even in the early twentieth century, Louisiana had an intertwined relationship with the petroleum industry, which had been drawn to Louisiana by its abundant natural resources. The state's first oil wells were drilled in 1901 on the west side of the Mississippi River near White Castle, a town just south of the capital, Baton Rouge.[1] By 1920, large-scale drilling had begun in most of the state's sixty-four parishes, which are similar to

234

counties. By the end of the decade, following the election of Huey Long as governor (1928), the oil and gas industry had become a mainstay of the state's economy. Standard Oil constructed its first refinery in Baton Rouge in 1909, and the extraction of oil in the state skyrocketed from 548,000 barrels in 1902 to 92,000,000 barrels in 1939 to 214,000,000 barrels in 1952.[2]

In the years around World War I, the Standard Oil Company revolutionized the production of organic compounds by isolating hydrocarbon chains (the basis for many synthetic fibers) from petroleum refinery production rather than coal tar. This has been considered the "petrochemical industry's starting point,"[3] enabling the industry to move beyond the production of fuel alone and establishing a vast synthetics industry that later included vinyl chloride and polyvinyl chloride. In a half century, petrochemicals became a staple of the new American economy, finding their way into virtually every type of consumer and industrial product: plastic bags, automobiles, water pipes, computer chips, paints, medicines, carpets, clothes, shoes, luggage, furniture, heat shields for rockets, and diapers.[4]

An epic battle between the petroleum industry and the people of Louisiana can be traced back to the populist crusade of Governor Huey Long to rein in Standard Oil. (Long was governor from 1928 through 1931, and though he was elected to the U.S. Senate that year he continued to run the state until his assassination in 1935.) In 1928 Long, recognizing that Standard Oil and other major oil producers needed Louisiana's oil and natural gas to expand their industry, proposed an increase in the tax on natural resources (called the severance tax) and a change in the way the tax was applied. He recommended that the tax be based upon the quantity of oil and gas removed from the ground rather than on the market value of the resource when it was extracted. This effectively placed "a heavier burden on the oil and gas industries," which set the stage for a conflict that would burst into the open the following year.[5]

In 1929 Long sought to further increase the tax revenues from industry through an "occupational license tax"—specifically, a tax on the refining of oil—to provide more funds for education. Standard Oil responded by funding an intensive lobbying campaign (some would say the company paid off legislators) and defeated the bill in the state legislature. T. Harry Williams, Long's biographer, relates the sordid and heavy-handed politics that went into the defeat of the tax bill. The president of Standard Oil's Louisiana division, Daniel R. Weller, recruited a well-known political figure whom Williams refers to as "Jim." The company reserved an entire floor of Baton Rouge's chief hotel, the Heidelberg, near the Statehouse.

To his floor of the hotel [Jim's] associate brought legislators and people from all over the state who could exert pressure on the legislators. Jim used whatever methods of persuasion he had to: they were usually blunt. The associate summarized them: "By the time Jim got through paying 'em off things were pretty hot." Surviving members of the legislature remember Jim's activities. "The money he spent was terrific," said one. "You could pick up $15,000 or $20,000 any evening then."[6]

Yet the extraordinarily popular Huey Long had resources of his own and in the end exerted enough pressure to force the bill through. Seeking revenge, Standard Oil organized a campaign to impeach Long. In what historian Alan Brinkley describes as "a tumultuous meeting of the House" involving "a jammed voting machine, hysterical shouting and swearing, flying fists, thrown inkwells, and the bloodying of a Long opponent by a Long ally,"[7] Long was accused of attempting to bribe members of the legislature, misappropriating government funds and state property, carrying concealed weapons, and even disposing of and destroying furniture and fixtures from the Governor's Mansion. Ultimately, he was impeached but not convicted. Long counterattacked, distributing circulars statewide announcing that the real issue was his populist opposition to greedy Standard Oil: "I had rather go down to a thousand impeachments than to admit that I am governor of the state that does not dare to call the Standard Oil Company to account so that we can educate our children and care for the destitute, sick, and afflicted. If this State is still to be ruled by the power of the money of this corporation, I am too weak for its governor."[8]

Nevertheless, despite almost revolutionary rhetoric, it was a fact that Long's state was extremely dependent on taxes from the oil and gas companies. And with these tax revenues, Louisiana was able to build an infrastructure of roads and bridges that rivaled the more industrial states of the northeast. At the beginning of Long's administration, the "state highway system comprised fewer than 300 miles of paved roads and only three bridges; by 1935, there were 3,754 miles of paved highway, forty bridges, and almost 4,000 miles of new gravel farm road."[9] The state also established one of the most extensive free public hospital systems in the nation, largely based on the taxes provided by the oil and natural gas industries.[10] Louisiana began programs aimed at increasing adult literacy; increasing elementary and high school attendance rates; providing night-school classes and free textbooks for public, private and parochial schools.[11] As Brinkley points out, Long's reforms put into place an infrastructure that was essential for the future industrial development of the state.[12]

In the 1940s petroleum reserves were discovered off the Gulf of Mexico coast, and by 1947 offshore drilling began in earnest. By 1955 there were more than 700 proven oil and gas fields throughout the state with more than 21,000 wells, making Louisiana one of the leading oil-producing states in the nation. From the 1930s through the 1950s, the oil and gas boom provided Louisiana with its richest source of revenue. By 1954–55, 23 percent of the state's income came from mineral leases and royalties, and another 12 percent came from taxes on other natural resources.

Even though by 1949 Louisiana ranked first in per capita aggregate state taxes, meaning that the state received huge revenues, the real burden on the state's citizenry was actually quite low. The state was still largely poor and rural, ranking thirty-ninth in the nation in per capita average income, yet it ranked third in terms of money spent per citizen for government operations. In 1957–58 Louisiana's per capita expenditure for education was $64.68, compared with a national average of just over $39. Louisiana provided an average of $46.50 per citizen in welfare expenditures, while the national average was $16.64. Similarly, the state provided its health and hospital system with an average of $14.19 per citizen while the national average was $11.46. (Neighboring Texas, which also had tremendous oil and gas reserves, spent $41.61 on education, $16.83 on welfare, and $6.02 on health and hospitals.) Such broad social spending led conservative critics, by 1960, to charge that "Louisiana has become a 'welfare state' and that it performs too many services for the individual members of its citizenry." One critic suggested that "responsible individualism, and the dignity of man may again become the militant faith of our people so that they will successfully challenge the advocates of collectivism and the irresponsibility of the 'welfare state.'"[13]

The petrochemical and refining industries seemed to be the one area of manufacturing to thrive in Louisiana, which eventually became one of the nation's leading chemical and refining centers. The Mississippi River corridor between the ports of Baton Rouge and New Orleans was extremely rich in natural resources: oil, gas, brine, sulfur, fresh water drawn from aquifers, and huge salt domes that could store vast oil surpluses.[14] More than 600 salt domes lay beneath the surface along the Gulf Coast, some "as large as a mile wide and six miles deep," providing extraordinarily cheap storage for hundreds of millions of barrels of oil and other materials essential for the petrochemical and chemical industries.[15]

Between 1937 and 1959 the number of sugarcane farms in Louisiana decreased from 10,260 to 2,686, and the average acreage of the remaining—and largely consolidated—plantations increased from 28 to 101 acres.[16]

Over the course of the twentieth century, the large plantations that had dominated the antebellum and postbellum eras gave way to ever larger corporate farms, turning sugarcane production into a big business. Mechanization fundamentally altered the work process, forcing thousands of former field hands into increasing poverty and dependence.

Although the plantation system dissolved, most of the state's poor remained rooted in the land and the social relationships that had dominated the plantation communities.[17] Many still remember the near-slavery conditions under which they grew up. Amos Favorite, who later became involved in a major environmental rebellion in the Mississippi River corridor, recalls his youth on the Waterloo sugarcane plantation in Geismar during the 1930s: "It was educated slavery. Us colored children were only allowed to go to school three months a year until seventh grade. It cost too much to go see the doctor in Gonzalez [Louisiana]. The plantation vet would look at us when he came to check the animals." Favorite abandoned his schooling completely at the age of nine when his mother died and he was forced to cut cane for twenty cents a ton.[18]

One account of this system written in the 1950s captured the nature of the exploitation. The plantation master was still the "rock" upon which the whole society rested. He fought to preserve the "paternalism, racial advantage, family prestige and cultural rank" that had characterized the sugar regime. At the same time he adopted "machines, science, financial finesse and administrative competence" to bring rationality and modernity to the plantation system. The new boss played a dominant role in the community—often controlling the movie theaters, drugstores, and even the banks. The plantation workers remained as dependent as ever, subject to dismissal and blacklisting if they objected in any way to the place given them in the unspoken social contract of rural sugar society. "A hired man is always in danger of becoming a fired man, dismissed not only from his plantation but from the entire cane belt, where the blackball rolls with the speed of a telephone call."[19]

Between 1940 and 1955 most sugarcane fields were mechanized, as fifty or more men could be replaced by a single harvester "requiring the services of an operator and two helpers."[20] But the workers who remained on the larger, mechanized sugar farms did not benefit from the wealth produced by mechanization. Little or nothing was done to fix their dilapidated houses. It was not unusual for African American families to live in a one-room house constructed of boards between which daylight could be seen. Located on narrow dirt roads that marked the borders between the old plantations, many of these structures lacked indoor plumbing and electric-ity. In 1950, the average annual income in St. James Parish, home of the town of Convent, where environmental justice struggles would later occur, was $713 per year, one-fifth of the amount that government identified as the poverty level in the New Orleans area. And this was not even the poorest county in the sugar region; neighboring St. John's Parish recorded an average income of $663. These communities were often run like company towns. The local stores, owned by the plantation, forced workers into perpetual debt by selling to them on credit with high interest rates, thereby tying them to the low-paying jobs that predominated in the area.[21]

Despite the fact that Louisiana was still responsible for three-quarters of the nation's domestic sugar production, the state's identity had changed from one dotted with sugar plantations to one dotted with the factories, oil derricks, and cracking towers of a growing petrochemical industry. A 1958 article in *National Geographic* remarked that "an astonishing complex [of large industrial plants] has sprung up, involving some two billion dollars in new or expanded operations. Chemicals, manufacturing, and processing establishments occupy mile after mile of Mississippi frontage. Steel towers rise and derricks dot the levy edge, until the region from New Orleans to Baton Rouge seems one great chemical-industrial plant."[22] By the mid-1950s, chemicals and chemical products ranked first in the value of manufactured products in Louisiana.[23] In 1956 the Ethyl Corporation began construction of a vinyl chloride monomer plant and W. R. Grace Company built a polyethylene plant in Baton Rouge.[24]

The industry's movement into this area was not driven by merely economic considerations. Industry counted on the political powerlessness of the mostly poor, African American population, virtually all of whom were deprived of the right to vote. By concentrating their refineries and other factories in these communities, industry gained access to cheap land without worrying about political opposition. This would change as the Civil Rights movement of the 1960s set the stage for a long process of political empowerment that would eventually disrupt the South's age-old arrangements between industry and the state.

DOW IS THE PLANTATION NOW

Part of industry's decision to move to Louisiana's Mississippi River corridor had to do with the fate that had befallen the plants it established along the Gulf Coast, particularly in Texas, during the 1940s and 1950s. When Dow initiated a program of expansion in Texas, planning to make it the center of the company's growing empire, it had not expected to be faced by one of the strongest labor-organizing drives in the south. From Beaumont to Freeport to Corpus Christi, twenty-three unions, including the Oil, Chemical and Atomic Workers Union (OCAW), the Longshoremen, and the Oilfield, Gas Well and Refinery Workers, set about organizing the thousands of black and white chemical workers hired to run the plants.[25] According to Dow's official historian, "at any given moment at least one of the locals and more often several were threatening a strike."[26] In 1955 and 1956, strikes largely closed down Dow's operations in Freeport.

Frustrated by this labor unrest, Dow decided to extend its southern operations to Louisiana's Mississippi River industrial corridor. In 1956, Dow purchased the old Union Plantation, which was located in Plaquemine, ten miles south of Baton Rouge. This 1,700-acre sugar plantation, owned by the descendants of Andrew H. Gay, who had purchased the site at a tax sale during the Civil War, employed more than six hundred men and women in the early twentieth century.[27] The plans for the plant in the community of eight thousand people quickly grew from an initial investment of $20 million to $75 million, "the biggest single expansion the company had attempted since 1940." The plant, comprising seven major projects and thirty-five minor ones, became the largest petrochemical complex in Louisiana (and one of the largest in the world), quickly gobbling up land from several other plantations, including Reliance, New Hope, Mayflower, and Homestead.[28] The site, extending westward inland from the Mississippi River, was twenty-three miles north of a Dow property that contained the Napoleonville salt dome, a source of brine necessary for the production of chlorine. Chlorine, in turn, was used in the production of ethylene dichloride, a feedstock for vinyl chloride monomer and other plastics.[29]

Dow was counting on the fact that Louisiana remained a segregated state, populated in part by poor blacks so desperate for work and feeling so powerless that they could be counted on not to cause the kind of labor unrest Dow had experienced in Texas. But just as the new Dow plant opened, the Civil Rights struggle intensified in Louisiana and changed a situation that had seemed so propitious for Dow.

The Congress of Racial Equality (CORE) began major organizing drives to register voters and to desegregate stores, public buildings, and the workforce. In May 1958, New Orleans, one hundred miles downriver from Baton Rouge, had desegregated its bus and trolley lines after several years of demonstrations and court cases. But change was not going to come easily in Louisiana. Outside of New Orleans, the Ku Klux Klan and other white supremacist groups continued to instill terror in rural African

American communities. "Between 1957 and 1960 the NAACP struggled to stay alive outside of New Orleans," observes Adam Fairclough in *Race and Democracy*. Presidents of local branches of the National Association for the Advancement of Colored People [NAACP] refused to hold meetings for fear of retribution. In fact, "the NAACP had no functioning branch in Louisiana's capital city between 1956 and 1962."[30] As a result, CORE brought in a group of "young volunteers who assembled in Plaquemine in July 1963 [and] inaugurated a new phase of the civil rights struggle in Louisiana."[31]

Much as the Student Nonviolent Coordinating Committee [SNCC] had done in Mississippi, CORE flooded the state with volunteers who challenged segregation and thereby threatened the power of planters, industrial leaders, and state and local officials whose rigid discriminatory practices were at the heart of segregationist policies. In Iberville Parish, in which Plaquemine and the new Dow plant were located, no African Americans had been allowed to register to vote since 1960. In Plaquemine itself, northern volunteers were "appalled by the poverty and squalid housing conditions" in the black communities. "In an unincorporated area of Plaquemine—one of two black neighborhoods deliberately gerrymandered out of the town's boundaries—people had to draw their water from pumps and relieve themselves in outhouses or in the woods."[32] Although the number of African American registered voters rose 800 percent during World War II to 7,561 people in 1946, blacks still accounted for only 1 percent of Louisiana's registered voters at a time when they constituted about a third of the state's total population. Not until the massive voter registration drives and passage of the federal Voting Rights Act of 1965 would there be at least one black registrant in every parish of the state.[33]

In June 1963 the civil rights activists in Plaquemine demanded a wide range of reforms, including an end to segregation of public facilities and employment discrimination and "the annexation of two black neighborhoods that currently received no municipal services." Although demonstrations continued until mid-August, the mayor, Charles Schnebelen, refused to negotiate and insisted that the protesters "submit their demands to the City council in the usual manner." The local black leadership recruited James Farmer, CORE's national director, to come to Plaquemine to lead what would become the city's largest civil rights demonstration to date. On August 19 one thousand people marched on City Hall. More than two hundred people were arrested, including Farmer, who was jailed and as a consequence was unable to deliver his scheduled speech at the famous March on Washington. After Farmer was released, however, he was still in jeopardy, for the police had deputized white citizens and vigilantes who undertook a violent repression of the demonstrations. Farmer got out of town by hiding in a casket that was carried by hearse to New Orleans.[34] He later claimed that he had "never seen such police treatment in Mississippi or Alabama. . . . Police did not just break up the demonstrators, but pursued them into churches, homes, and any other shelter they sought."[35]

Imagine the situation in Louisiana. The chemical industry had built massive chemical plants across the state and was planning for the development of more plants. A huge civil rights struggle was playing itself out, and the consciousness of local citizens was being raised. Citizens were becoming more attuned to the environmental impact of the petrochemical industry and more vigilant about the damage it was doing. Then in the 1980s and 1990s, two communities in the Plaquemine area discovered that a growing number of their water wells were polluted with chemicals used in the production of vinyl chloride. Morrisonville, a largely black community situated on the river bordering a Dow plant, had been founded in the 1870s by slaves freed from the Australia Plantation, just north of Plaquemine.[36]

Fearing potential lawsuits for damages resulting from explosions, pollution of water tables, or diseases resulting from air pollution, Dow tested a new strategy to deal with the local consequences of environmental pollution; the company would simply buy the town and all the homes in it.[37] Just as damaging federal data were about to be released in 1989, Dow let it be known to the residents of Morrisonville that it was the only buyer in town, and if they didn't sell to Dow, their property would later be worthless.[38] One of the last to leave, G. Jack Martin, a deacon at the Nazarene Baptist Church, the historic heart of Morrisonville, summarized his experience: "Dow didn't exactly ask for our input. They just came in and told us what they were going to do. I guess Dow is the plantation now."[39] The town's "big mistake," according to Martin, was that it "sold Dow some land in 1959." Before that, there had been a greenbelt between the town and the plant, but the company "built on it right out to the fence until they were on top of us."[40]

While most of the residents accepted Dow's offer to buy out their home and land, about twenty Morrisonville families refused. "Dow doesn't pay for attachment to land, for the inheritance that is in this community," said Rosa Martin, Jack's wife and the town's informal historian, who owned a house so close to the plant's property that the plant's loudspeakers could be heard inside her brick home.[41] In the end Morrisonville was abandoned. (In 2001 the Louisiana Department of Health and Hospitals "discovered high levels of vinyl chloride" in the drinking water of a community in

Plaquemine, leading to lawsuits and continuing controversies over chemical plants in the area.)[42]

A similar drama played out in the town of Reveilletown, just south of Plaquemine. Residents of this primarily African American community had complained about the fumes and emissions from the plant and argued that "the entire community was poisoned by vinyl chloride emissions loosed from Georgia Gulf's manufacture of plastics." One of the residents of Reveilletown, Janice Dickerson, became active in the environmental justice movement and helped organize a candlelight vigil in 1989 "in which black and white environmentalists mourned the death" of the community.[43] The Georgia Gulf Corporation, realizing that the protest might result in lawsuits brought by the residents, razed the town and constructed homes for residents elsewhere.[44]

The companies considered the buyout an effective way to protect residents from possible harm from dangerous explosions and toxins released into the air. "It makes sense in putting a [buyout] program together instead of waiting for an accident," remarked Michael Lythcott, a consultant who helped design similar efforts for other companies.[45] Environmental activists saw the issue differently. Mary Lee Orr, the executive director of the Louisiana Environmental Action Network (LEAN), stated that "companies are reducing their problems by moving people instead of reducing accidents and pollution."[46] Nor was this approach specific to Dow or Louisiana. As the *New York Times* noted, "Prodded by lawsuits over pollution and damage claims from a number of explosions, several of the nation's largest oil and chemical companies are spending millions of dollars to create safety zones by buying up the homes around their plants."[47] All that is left to mark the sites of Morrisonville and Reveilletown today are a signpost and a fence in the shadow of giant chemical plants, the graveyard of Morrisonville's Nazarene Baptist Church, and an open-sided wooden prayer site, built by Dow, for family members visiting the graves.

WELCOME TO CANCER ALLEY

Before the buyouts of the 1980s, older communities found their environments threatened by effluents belching from cracking towers and smokestacks, leaking from pipelines, and streaming from salt domes used for oil storage. In Texas and Louisiana, leaks from these salt domes were a major problem for communities.[48] The Mississippi River itself was used by chemical manufacturers as an open sewer for industrial wastes and by-products. By the early 1970s, the Mississippi River had become a threat to the population living along its shores. One longtime resident remembers that in the 1950s and early 1960s, she would go to the top of the flood levees that kept the river from destroying the surrounding sugar country to swim, draw water, and wash clothes. She remembers being baptized in the river and recalled community and church events along its shores.[49]

By the early 1970s, these activities were nearly impossible. Oil and chemical companies virtually shut off access to the river for much of the area's population by building docks and storage areas for the huge barges that took refined products to New Orleans or up the Mississippi to Baton Rouge, Memphis, St. Louis, and other cities.

By the late 1970s, chemical pollution was becoming the focus of concern not only for workers in the vinyl plants but for the general population as well. In 1978, as New York's Love Canal dominated headlines across the nation, researchers at the National Cancer Institute began mapping cancer hotspots, where cancer incidence rates were growing most rapidly. "Cancers that in the past have been related to industrial exposure [in the plant] have continued to increase even after the effects of . . . cigarette smoking have been removed," Marvin Schneiderman of the National Cancer Institute told the National Conference on the Environment and Health Care Costs in 1978. Showing a map of the United States with high incidence areas darkened, he illustrated that Louisiana was virtually blotted out. "It would be nonsense for me to assert that all this increase was due to industrial [pollution] exposure," he noted. But, "It would be equivalent nonsense and possibly criminal to assert that none of it was."[50] The beautiful state of Louisiana, once widely known for its pelicans and bayous, had become "a blotted out" area on a map showing areas of industrial pollution.

But the severity of the pollution did not keep industry from seeking to expand; nor did it keep the state from encouraging that expansion. During the 1970s, the Mississippi River corridor was viewed as ripe for investment by foreign companies. German and Japanese corporations, looking for new outlets for their capital, turned to the American South as an appropriate place for many of their most polluting industries. As historian David R. Goldfield explains in his survey of the South in the post–World War II era, "much of this influx [of capital] resulted from the export of polluting firms from Germany and Japan." He quotes the Japanese consul general in Atlanta, who explained that "older industries . . . are being phased out in Japan and exported to other countries. . . . We will put these high pollution industries where there is space and water enough to handle them . . . like here in the South."[51] (One local newspaper recalls that by the 1960s and 1970s, industrial plants were so dense along the river that "some began calling the region 'America's Ruhr Valley.'"[52]) Japan's reputation in vinyl chloride production had been sullied because of a tragedy that occurred in Minamata Bay, Japan, in the early 1960s. Forty-three people died and an unknown number of others were blinded and brain damaged after a vinyl chloride factory dumped into the bay huge quantities of mercury salts, which are used in the vinyl chloride production process. Between 1953 and 1960, 111 people were poisoned by eating contaminated fish and 19 "congenitally brain-damaged children were born."[53] Since that time, many others have died or been damaged by the long-term effects of the poisons.[54] Since at least the 1960s Japan has tended to export its environmentally destructive industries while maintaining a relatively strong environmental record at home.[55]

The conflict between industry and the environment escalated. Industry grew tremendously, and so environmental pollution became worse and worse. In the early 1970s, the Environmental Defense Fund issued what it called "the first evidence in this country . . . that carcinogens in drinking water are in sufficiently high concentrations to endanger human health." The study focused on the Mississippi River in Louisiana because some communities used only river water and others used only groundwater for drinking and household uses. Although the evidence was "fragmentary," the findings suggested a link between pollutants and cancer. The study found that "nine parishes in [Louisiana] are among the forty-five cities and counties in the United States that have the highest reported cancer death rates for white males."[56] By the early 1980s, Louisiana displaced New Jersey and its chemical industry along the turnpike as the nation's most polluted state.[57]

In 1982, Louisiana faced an industrial disaster that demonstrated that the toxins inside the factory endangered not only workers but also people at large. A train that included numerous chemical tanker cars derailed in Livingston, a town between the chemical centers of Geismar and Baton Rouge. Forty-three cars filled with petroleum, vinyl chloride, tetraethyl lead, phosphoric acid, methyl chloride, styrene, toluene diisocynate, or ethylene glycol derailed, shattering windows and setting off "a series of explosions . . . at the derailment site in the middle of town."[58] Fumes, fires, and spills over several days led to the evacuation of 2,700 people who were "kept from their homes for two weeks."[59] Clean-up workers "built a network of earthen ditches and pools to collect vinyl chloride as it seeped from the cars" in order to "quicken the burnoff of the vinyl chloride, allowing the clean-up to continue." Although no one could predict exactly how the fumes would affect people in the surrounding area,[60] Livingston became a metaphor for the acute danger that the chemical industry posed as it expanded through the 1980s. When Formosa Plastics announced plans to build a polyvinyl chloride plant in north Baton Rouge close to its source of vinyl chloride monomer and other plastic feedstocks, it did so in part "to insure that it never has another Livingston."[61]

Between 1984 and 1989, one of the nation's longest management lock-outs took place at the BASF chemical plant in Geismar. Geismar, the site of large chemical plants owned by BASF, Shell, and other manufacturers, was long known for its filthy plants and lax environmental controls. BASF, the world's second largest chemical company, had built the largest of its more than eighty U.S. chemical facilities in Geismar in the late 1950s. In February 1970, the president of the OCAW local gave a vivid account of the dumping of chemical waste in Geismar: "We have three chlorine units. The company used to put the tail ends off in a sump and pump it into the Mississippi River, but they've come up with a cheaper idea where they dump it right into the plant ditches and chlorine disposal towers. . . . We are constantly smelling this chlorine, according to which way the wind blows, and one of the plants has a ditch around it on three sides, so we constantly smell this chlorine all day, twenty-four hours a day, depending on what job you're working at."[62]

The lockout at Geismar was part of a broader attempt to undercut the union movement in BASF's American plants. It took place during the hey-day of President Reagan's anti-union activities. The company had proposed a contract that included a wage freeze for a year, cuts in health care provisions, and the right of the company to contract out certain jobs to nonunion companies.[63] When the union rejected these provisions, the company "escorted 370 of the workers outside the plant, locked the gates, and vowed not to let the workers—or the union—return."[64]

Not only was the lockout a sign of BASF's disdain for workers, but it was also the occasion of a new alliance between the labor movement and the residents of the region, who were becoming attuned to pollution. Richard Miller, a New Yorker who had worked with Tony Mazzocchi, legislative director at the OCAW, traveled down to rural Geismar, planning to stay a short time. According to Mazzocchi, Miller became deeply involved with the BASF workers and eventually became a chief organizer for the union. Looking around for allies in the fight against BASF, he found many workers and their families and neighbors who were deeply preoccupied by the issues of health and safety. Workers told stories about the irresponsible ways of BASF. People pointed to the dramatic impact of the chemical plant on the environment: pecan and other trees died or no longer bore nuts or fruit; cars were covered with a white powder that corroded their finish. By focusing on environmental issues, the union was able to forge strong ties with workers and other local people.[65]

With its long history of attention to occupational and environmental health, the OCAW was the perfect union to begin a campaign against BASF for polluting the region's air, ground, and water. Using billboards, print advertisements, radio broadcasts, and demonstrations, the OCAW sought simultaneously to build support for the locked-out workers and to indict BASF for its unsafe and environmentally dangerous practices. By providing information to local environmental organizations, the OCAW helped challenge BASF's toxic dumping practices, claiming credit for stopping the construction of a $50 million petrochemical plant. The union also helped establish environmental groups, including the predominantly African American Ascension Parish Residents Against Toxic Pollution, Louisiana Workers Against Toxic Chemical Hazards (LA Watch), the Geismar-based Clean Air and Water Group, and the Louisiana Coalition for Tax Justice.[66] In return, the local people provided the OCAW with information and showed a willingness to join the campaign against BASF.

The union was relentless in its attempt to reveal BASF as the despoiler of the Mississippi River, even establishing contact with the Green Party in Germany and pointing out BASF's history as a company that prospered during the Nazi era. By demonstrating BASF's role in the environmental destruction of the Rhine River in Germany, the union began to forge a public consciousness about BASF's role in the despoiling of the Mississippi River as well. *Chemical Week* credited locked-out BASF workers with creating the term "Cancer Alley" to identify the lower Mississippi River in the mid-1980s: "It was BASF workers whose 'Welcome to Cancer Alley' billboards publicized the moniker that still stigmatizes the area."[67] Other banners and billboards dubbed the area "Bhopal on the Bayou."[68] Although the workers finally ratified an unsatisfactory contract in December 1989, after a sixty-six-month lockout, the union had survived and the workers had profoundly influenced the community by raising consciousness about environmental toxins. According to the Louisiana Environmental Action Network, "many workers and citizens in Louisiana will never again look at the state's huge petrochemical industry through the same eyes." After the strike, the union and the National Toxics Campaign combined to hire a full-time organizer who could continue to foster ties between labor and the environmental movement.[69]

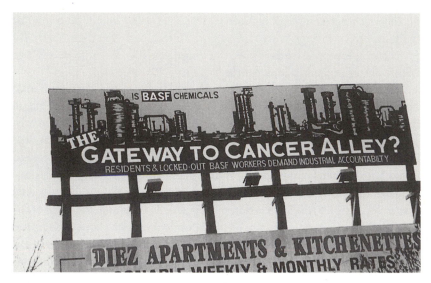

17. The Gateway to Cancer Alley? Gonzalez, Louisiana. The OCAW strike against BASF united labor and environmentalists against the chemical industry along the Mississippi River. This and other billboards popularized the link between the chemical industry and environmentally induced cancers. Source: Willie A. Fontenot.

A NATIONAL SACRIFICE ZONE

Three industrial catastrophes in the late 1970s and early 1980s firmly implanted in the public mind the image of the chemical plant as a dangerous monster. At Love Canal in Niagara Falls, New York, the irresponsible dumping of chemicals forced residents to move out of their homes. In Times Beach, Missouri, dioxin-tainted oil sprayed on the town's unpaved roads to keep down the dust ultimately polluted the town, which had to be abandoned and destroyed. (Dioxin is a term used to describe a number of toxic byproducts of the burning of chlorinated wastes. It is easily absorbed into human and animal tissues.) But the tragedy that befell Bhopal, India, in 1984 was beyond imagining. A methyl isocyanate leak at a Union Carbide plant killed 3,800 people and sickened 200,000. (Methyl isocyanate is an intermediate compound used in the production of insecticides and herbicides.) "Witnesses said that a densely populated area of about 15 square miles was turned into 'one vast gas chamber.'"[70] The following year a leak at another Union Carbide plant in Institute, West Virginia, served as a warning that Bhopal could happen anywhere.[71] It was becoming clear that industry could no longer be trusted to protect the general population.

Soon after these tragic events, Congress mandated that the EPA produce a Toxic Release Inventory (TRI) of 328 toxic chemicals, specifying where in the United States each of these substances was used or produced. This would make it possible for individuals and their consultants in a community to know with some degree of reliability the specific chemicals and other toxins that were being released into the air, water, and land around the factories. The EPA made copies of the Toxic Release Inventory available to the public through the Government Printing Office, local officials, and public libraries in 1989.[72] Based on information supplied to it by industry, the TRI became, in the words of *USA Today,* "A First Peek 'Behind the Plant Gates'" and a basic tool in community organizing efforts, providing activists with critical information in their struggles to identify the grossest polluters.[73] According to *Chemical Week,* the TRI effectively "branded Louisiana as the most polluted state in the U.S.—because of its chemical plants."[74] Agrico-Chemical on the Uncle Sam Plantation in Convent was identified as the "leading water polluter" in the nation.[75] Larry Adcock, plant manager of Dow Chemical in Plaquemine, acknowledged that "the TRI numbers were so big that they just scared the hell out of everybody."[76] And the entire nation would soon hear from Oprah Winfrey that the lower Mississippi was "a national sacrifice zone . . . [where] lives are being forsaken."[77]

Two kinds of environmental groups operated in Louisiana. Long-established organizations like the National Wildlife Federation, the Sierra Club, the Audubon Society, and the Nature Conservancy had active state chapters that addressed issues like the maintenance of the natural ecology and even of historic sites like old plantation homes. Newer groups like LEAN and Greenpeace had active chapters in Lake Charles (in western Louisiana), Baton Rouge, St. James Parish, and other river communities. The newer groups formed alliances with African American and Cajun organizations to address the ill effects of industrial plants on their communities. These activists were angry that the factories offered neither economic revival nor sensitivity to the sanctity of their neighborhoods, homes, and lives; the factories promised only to reap great profits for big industry. These newer activist groups were willing to engage in tactics foreign to the more conservative environmental groups. In 1988, Greenpeace activists challenging the Georgia Gulf Corporation in Plaquemine "partially plugged a wastewater pipe in the Mississippi River . . . to protest chemical waste dumping"[78] and in the 1990s unfurled giant banners on the dome of the state capitol in Baton Rouge denouncing the collaboration of state officials with industrial polluters.

Also in 1988 a group of both radical and more traditional environmental groups, including LEAN, Greenpeace, and the Sierra Club, joined labor unions like the OCAW to form the Louisiana Toxics Project. This coalition staged "The Great Louisiana Toxics March"—from Baton Rouge to New Orleans—"to protest the destruction of the southern Mississippi region . . . an industrial wasteland of enormous chemical factories spewing filth on a massive scale."[79]

The Great Louisiana Toxics March began on November 11, 1988, in Devil's Swamp, just north of Baton Rouge. Once a pristine area famous for its abundant wildlife, Devil's Swamp had been designated a Superfund cleanup site as a result of its pollution by a chemical plant. Several hundred people assembled there—workers from chemical plants, their family members, and union and environmental activists. They walked south through towns along the Mississippi River and past nearly 130 chemical plants, spreading their message in placards and in song.[80] Organizers promised that thousands of people would walk for at least some part of the route, enjoying "red beans and rice, jambalaya, gumbo; rhythm and of blues, gospel, jazz, and zydeco; rallies, meetings, reports, forums, and workshops."[81]

It was an incredible scene as the sounds of Louisiana mingled with the rhetoric of environmental organizers. In Baton Rouge the marchers were addressed by Martin Luther King III. The march encountered opposition along the way, first in Paulina, a small town along the river, where four marchers were "warned off" of the ITO plant property for trying to talk to company officials, and then in Jefferson Parish, where the sheriff "demanded several hundred dollars for official escort services from the marchers." In Orleans Parish, where marchers had paid $200 for a parade permit, local officials demanded more money as payment for an escort through the town. After nine days, the marchers finally arrived in New Orleans, having garnered enthusiastic support from people along the way. Most significantly, the march was a huge step toward building the sort of environmental coalition necessary to take on Louisiana's chemical establishment in the coming decade.[82]

In 1988 Louisiana elected for governor a congressman named Charles E. (Buddy) Roemer, a Harvard-educated reformer who voters hoped would take on industry.[83] He replaced Edwin Edwards, who had been indicted by the federal government on charges of graft and other misdeeds. Roemer refused to take any industry money during his campaign, accepting only

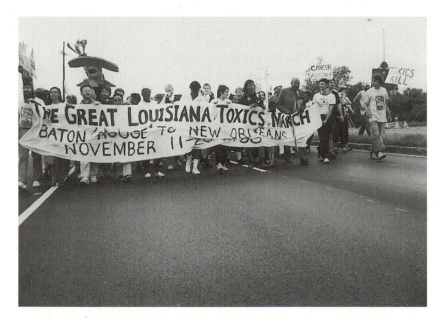

18. The Great Louisiana Toxics March. In late 1988, a coalition of labor and environmental groups marched 100 miles from Devil's Swamp, north of Baton Rouge, to New Orleans. The march gathered the support of national civil rights figures such as Jesse Jackson and Martin Luther King III. Source: Willie A. Fontenot.

political action committee contributions. Calling his election a "revolution," Roemer brought into his government people with no ties to Louisiana's long-standing political machine or to petrochemical money.[84] He broke with Edwards's policy of "selling" commissionerships as part of his political patronage system; instead, he put an ad in the *Wall Street Journal* for the Department of Environmental Quality (DEQ) commissioner's position and received two hundred resumes, many from people associated with the chemical industry. Rather than hiring from the established networks of lawyers and industry people within the state, Roemer chose Paul Templet to be DEQ commissioner. As the head of Louisiana's first Coastal Management Program, Templet had taken on Chalin Perez, one of the most powerful political figures in Plaquemines Parish, over the issue of coastal wetlands management. (Perez's father, Leander Perez, had played a major role in the parish during the Civil Rights movement when he vowed to put any Freedom Rider who "invaded" his turf into the swamps of Plaquemines Parish, "where they would be eaten alive by mosquitoes."[85]) Templet left Louisiana in 1979 and continued his work on wetlands management in

American Samoa. He returned to the state to teach at Louisiana State University, where he was tapped by Roemer.[86]

In hiring Templet, Roemer threatened the Faustian bargain the state had made with the chemical industry—that the state would sacrifice its environment in exchange for the tax revenues and jobs the chemical companies would provide. Roemer increased funding to the Department of Environmental Quality, raising its budget from $25 million to $68 million by 1991 and more than doubling the number of its personnel, particularly those involved in the enforcement of environmental regulations.[87]

Under Templet's direction, the DEQ "required the state's top 36 polluters to produce new waste reduction plans within 60 days."[88] The DEQ had been in existence for only five years and, according to Templet, "had been a very quiescent agency."[89] While he headed the DEQ, the Louisiana legislature passed more than twenty new environmental laws and the department established eighty-one sets of regulations, far more than had been in existence up to that time.[90] He also introduced an "environmental scorecard" that tracked each company's air, water, and land pollution emissions. Companies that failed to improve their environmental record over time were stripped of state-granted tax exemptions. The scorecard signaled to chemical manufacturers that Louisiana could no longer be counted on for lax regulations of environmental pollution and for tax breaks with no strings attached.[91] In an attempt to "embarrass them into action," Templet spoke very publicly about the dangers that industrial pollution presented to Louisiana's citizens.[92]

Eight years after he left office, Templet recalled his "amazement" at the power wielded in Louisiana's state political establishment by the chemical and oil interests. He remembered that he literally feared for his safety when he challenged industry. But rather than seek refuge in obscurity, he decided he would become "very visible," in the hope that visibility would better ensure his safety. He started riding a motorcycle "because it was easier to see any tampering than with a car." Templet estimated that in the end he forced industry to spend an extra billion dollars for environmental controls[93] and that during the Roemer administration industrial emissions dropped 50 percent.[94] When Roemer's term was over, Templet returned to LSU only to find that his salary had been cut by $10,000 because, he believes, of pressure from industry which had begun to fund faculty members involved in environmental research.[95]

The chemical industry, wary of Roemer's "efforts to dispel Louisiana's image as lax on environmental enforcement,"[96] instituted programs to control environmental pollution in an effort to forestall intervention by the state.[97] A program called Responsible Care was set up by the Louisiana Chemical Association in 1988 to clean up the worst of its polluters and to dispel its own image as "environmental pirates," according to Bob Haun of the BASF plant in Geismar.[98] Just as often, the industry chose not to clean up its pollution but simply to buy out and remove an entire community, as it did with Morrisonville and Reveilletown. The buyouts were an implicit acknowledgment by industry that these towns were being polluted or would be polluted in the future.

The chemical industry saw Roemer's reforms as temporary roadblocks to its plans for further expansion in Louisiana. The industry knew that a state traditionally dependent on the chemical industry for tax revenues and jobs would be unwilling to block development of potential sites. Impoverished St. James Parish, which straddled the Mississippi thirty miles south of Baton Rouge, was one of many sites that were already zoned industrial and still had substantial tracts of plantation land available for development. In 1991 the state, clearly still eager to welcome more industry, planned to designate St. James Parish an "attainment zone," making it ripe for development by a chemical company.[99] Despite the rumblings by Roemer, the industry retained its long-standing influence in the legislature and could count on continued large tax breaks. As Randall Helmick, an industry representative, pointed out, Louisiana had a "tax equalization policy" that allowed the state to match or surpass the incentive programs of any other state, even those of neighboring Texas.[100] In other words, the Statehouse was bent on keeping Louisiana as attractive to industry as ever.

Even Roemer's reforms, which were essentially populist, were part of a move to open Louisiana to what Roemer considered "cleaner" chemical productions, particularly plastics. Roemer had sought to get ICI America, a Delaware firm, to build a plant in St. Gabriel Parish, promoting it as a clean project. He encouraged other plastics manufacturers to use locally produced feedstocks to produce polyvinyl chloride and other polymers, and he plowed resources into LSU to develop centers for polymer science and to train plastics engineers. A Taiwanese firm, Formosa Plastics, opened a plant at Point Coupee along the Mississippi to produce polyvinyl chloride pipe, using resins from a new Baton Rouge production unit. Roemer encouraged other international companies to consider Louisiana their American home. Louisiana increased its overseas marketing budget to promote foreign investment in the state, particularly investment by Japanese firms.[101] Roemer was clearly not intent on destroying the chemical industry, even if the industry was correct in believing that chemicals had "certainly lost its most-favored-industry status."[102]

Eventually Roemer alienated every political constituency in the state. After a quick start in which he passed an educational reform package, including pay raises for teachers, promoted environmental awareness, and reduced the state's dependence on the petrochemical industry, his administration initiated few more reforms.[103] By 1991, Roemer's popularity had so plummeted that he faced credible challenges from even such disreputable characters as David Duke, the former grand wizard of the Louisiana Ku Klux Klan, and former three-term governor Edwin Edwards, a man twice indicted for corruption—and recently convicted.[104]

Edwards won reelection, and his return to politics reinforced industry's long-standing prominence in the state government. Throughout the 1970s and 1980s, Edwards was as forceful a political figure as Huey Long had once been. In many ways he symbolized the corruption at the heart of Louisiana politics that made it only too easy for the industry to wield its power.[105] Despite Edwards's campaign pledges that he would not undo Roemer's efforts to improve Louisiana's environmental record, among his first acts as governor was to appoint Kai Midboe, an industry consultant, as the secretary of the state's Department of Environmental Quality. As a lawyer in Baton Rouge, Midboe had represented the oil and gas companies; his appointment was viewed by labor and environmental activists as an indicator of bad policies to come. The Oil, Chemical and Atomic Workers characterized Midboe (and some of Edwards's other appointees) as having "a track record of hostility to environmental concerns" and connections to the Louisiana Chemical Association.[106]

It didn't take long for Edwards to confirm the worst fears of environmentalists. "Louisiana grew up with the chemical industry," Edwards declared, and it was clear he was not one to try to challenge it.[107] The *Engineering News-Record* noted that it "took only two days in office [for Edwards] to scuttle an environmental tax abatement program it took his predecessor, Buddy Roemer, three years to set up." Roemer and Templet had set up a property tax exemption system that had linked tax breaks to compliance with "state and federal rules on emission control and pollution prevention."[108] Edwards, however, maintained that any linkage between corporate investment and environmental protection would necessarily discourage investment. The chemical industry cheered Edwards's action.[109] Kai Midboe also suspended the environmental scorecard, saying it was "a draconian burden on industry." Kevin Reilly, the new secretary of the Department of Economic Development, announced that Edwards was preparing to "rescind the scorecard altogether" because it put Reilly in an impossible position, making him "both a policeman and a salesman. The scorecard just hampered my efforts and I resented it."[110]

It was clear to industry that the state, from the governor on down, would "rather do things with industry than do things to industry," reported *Chemical Week,* which also noted that "the investment and regulatory climates in the state have improved."[111] The industry also sought to shift more of the tax burden away from the chemical companies and back to individual citizens. As *Chemical Week* observed: "In most of the U.S., about 40% of state revenues come from corporate taxes and 60% from income and other individual taxes; in Texas and Louisiana, the proportions are reversed."[112]

The companies and the state increasingly envisioned an international role for themselves, hoping to find foreign markets to deal with the overcapacity of the industry in the early 1990s. One industry executive pleaded with industry colleagues to "understand how bad over-expansion can be," stressing that the development of foreign markets was central to any successful business strategy.[113] By 1995, the head of the Louisiana Chemical Association (LCA) was trumpeting the industry's continued modernization program and expansion into foreign markets, becoming the second largest exporter of chemicals in the country: "One-quarter of Louisiana's chemical production is shipped internationally, so it's essential that plants here invest the capital necessary to retain world-class status."[114]

By undoing Roemer's reforms Edwards intended to reassure an industry increasingly attacked by established environmental groups and angry grass-roots organizations. "From parish to parish," *Chemical Week* remarked shortly after Edwards took office, "the local environmental movement may be the strongest of that in any industrial state."[115] Louisiana citizens would no longer accept that foul smells, polluted water, and chemical waste dumps were a necessary byproduct of economic progress. While Louisiana had only eleven designated Superfund sites (primarily because the state had not done the work necessary for the federal government to list all of them as such),[116] as many as one thousand areas were contaminated by chemicals. Some of these were in historic, well-heeled communities, and many others were in poor people's neighborhoods.[117] It is no wonder local opposition grew.

GOOD SCIENCE?

Given that state government in Louisiana showed little propensity for controlling industry, the task fell to environmental activists, who had long depended on local residents to report suspected toxins to them. These activists would forward residents' reports to professionals for confirmation. For example, residents of St. Gabriel, located in the heart of Cancer Alley, had long worried that the Ciba-Geigy, Pioneer, and ICI plants, which produced chlorine, benzene, and a variety of herbicides, were harming the health of local residents.

Kay Gaudet, who owned a pharmacy in St. Gabriel, concluded from her daily conversations that many residents were being poisoned by toxins from these plants. She conducted an informal survey of the town of 2,100 people and discovered that 63 women suffered 75 miscarriages between 1985 and 1988, a seemingly large number in such a small community.[118] Gaudet, unaware of Peter Infante's studies of stillbirths and miscarriages in Ohio but armed with her own data, traveled to Washington to testify before a congressional committee on the environment. Her testimony generated an enormous amount of publicity because it came in the midst of the 1987 gubernatorial race.[119] Buddy Roemer, then a congressman, learned of Gaudet's work and called the Louisiana attorney general's office to suggest that it conduct an investigation of miscarriages in the area.[120] Soon local reporters flocked to the town, and with them came public health experts from Tulane.[121]

In short order, the Tulane School of Public Health and the CDC's Agency for Toxic Substances and Disease Registry joined forces to conduct a two-year epidemiological study of "midterm and late term miscarriages of women with documented pregnancies between the ages of 18 and 50 who lived in St. Gabriel, Carville, and Sunshine between 1982 and 1987."[122] Jim Gentry, an environmental activist and the community representative on the panel that reviewed the design of the study, "wanted the questionnaire to ask women who have suffered miscarriages how close they lived to chemical plants and to describe pollution in their neighborhoods." Tulane and the CDC rejected these and similar suggestions as too subjective and not quantifiable, causing Gentry to conclude: "I think the study will be good science, but I'm not sure it will be complete science."[123]

In 1989 the experts found the miscarriage rates statistically "were no higher than the state average," provoking an angry response from Gaudet and other local activists who were convinced of the validity of their informal finding.[124] Gaudet believed that the betrayal of her community was the result of a less than vigorous scientific study, designed by experts specifically to explain away what she had observed. She criticized the methodology of the epidemiological study: it covered too large an area; it included only documented pregnancies and miscarriages; and it did not include an appropriate control group. She also criticized researchers for conducting interviews over the phone rather than going "door to door," thereby excluding poor residents who did not have phones and others unwilling to share personal information over the phone. She came to see this use of science as virtually useless as a community resource. "It's going to be this thing around your neck, having to deal with scientific papers that say there isn't a problem," she said. "Federal and state governments are not ready to take responsibility and admit what they've done to us."[125]

Looking back ten years later, Gaudet noted her own naïveté in thinking that science could ever fully satisfy communities affected by industrial pollution. She had come to fear that even the best science could not prove danger. "I would be very shocked," she observed, "if there ever was a study that was conclusive." The apparent rigor of the methodology itself actually served to hide the effects of toxic chemicals on the community: if such a "thorough" study failed to prove the relationship between chemical exposure and miscarriages, then, it was assumed at an official level that there must be no relationship. Scientists' inability to uncover the obvious in St. Gabriel led Gaudet to a deep skepticism about the science itself: "I would never encourage a community now to do a study."[126] Community activists in other parts of the state were having similar experiences. Even Florence Robinson, a biology professor from Southern University who lived in Alsen, the site of Devil's Swamp, believed that the state's insistence on statistical proof was little more than an attempt to avoid the issue and to shirk the responsibility for proving danger: "The burden of proof is on us [the residents]. That's not how it should be. . . . Can [local resident] Mrs. Pate prove that her rash comes from any particular chemical company?"[127]

Marise Gottlieb, an epidemiologist at Tulane University, studied lung cancer death rates in twenty southern Louisiana parishes in the early 1980s and concluded that those living within a mile of a chemical plant or refinery had a four times greater chance of dying of lung cancer than those living two to four miles away. She concluded that lifestyle factors could not possibly account for such dramatic differences. Critics from industry and elsewhere pounced on her conclusions, claiming that many other factors such as differentials in smoking rates might account for the differences. Gottlieb agreed that further studies were necessary to establish a causative relationship, but she could never get any further funding from industry: "We were making a lot of progress. You have to ask why it stopped." She assumed that she "was doing the 'wrong' kind of work" and surmised that "had I said there was no relation, everyone would have been happy." Instead of funding Gottlieb's work, the governor, Edwin Edwards, appointed a task force to look at cancer research. It concluded in March 1984 that "the available data suggest no single cause for the high incidence of cancer in Louisiana."[128]

THE TUMOR REGISTRY

In the late 1980s Greenpeace brought in independent experts to break the impasse between local activists (and their few academic allies) and state officials. Using government data, Greenpeace published two studies indicating that harm to the Mississippi and to the health of those living near the river increased as the river flowed south to the Gulf of Mexico. The study showed that cancer rates were low in Minnesota, where the river originated, but increased dramatically by the time the river reached Louisiana and the gulf. Greenpeace concluded: "The increases along the river are stark, and cannot reasonably be attributed to chance."[129] While most critics, as usual, suggested a host of other factors that could explain these mortality patterns, one respected environmental newsletter, *Rachel's Hazardous Waste News,* asked: Does the epidemiological data gathered by sympathetic investigators "prove industrial pollution causes cancer? It does not. Does it make you think twice about moving into a high chemical neighborhood or neighborhood with lots of dumps? It does us."[130]

The dramatic gulf that had developed between community activists and conservative scientists and their business allies can be seen in a struggle in the 1980s over The Louisiana's Tumor Registry. The registry was established in the late 1970s by the Louisiana legislature. In 1983 it published its first volume, *Cancer in Louisiana,* which presented mortality data from cancer from the 1930s through the 1980s. Like more informal surveys before it, the registry indicated a high cancer death rate among Louisiana residents. By 1988, the Tumor Registry included data on cancer incidence as well as cancer death rates throughout the state; by the mid-1990s the registry comprised no fewer than eight volumes of data.[131]

In response, the Louisiana Chemical Association contracted with an epidemiologist, Otto Wong, who was consulting for the Chemical Manufacturers Association to evaluate the epidemiological evidence on carcinogenicity of vinyl chloride. Wong concluded that the Louisiana environmental data could not prove that cancer was caused by emissions but must be the result of the residents' lifestyles. "South Louisiana people tend to smoke more, eat low amounts of fresh fruits and vegetables, and work in high-risk industries associated with lung cancer." In addition to the dubious step of including "high risk industries" under the heading of "lifestyle," he refused to accept that those industries had any effect on cancer rates among nearby residents. Wong called for "more quality research" to establish any link between environmental exposure to chemicals and cancer.[132] (See chapter 7 for more about Wong.)

About the same time, Vivien Chen and her colleagues at the LSU Medical Center in New Orleans began publishing annual reviews of the Tumor Registry's data in an attempt to explain the high mortality rates in southern Louisiana by comparing them with cancer incidence rates. They found that, with two exceptions, incidence rates in the parishes in the Cancer Corridor were similar to cancer rates for other populations throughout the nation, raising questions about the commonly held belief that there was a link between industrial pollution and disease. She recommended closer long-term studies and concluded that attention had to be turned to issues of elective personal behavior, not industrial clean-up. "Any effective cancer control programs in Louisiana," she maintained, "must emphasize and be directed towards prevention and cessation of tobacco use." She restated this conclusion in her annual reviews of the data from the Tumor Registry throughout the 1990s.[133]

The chemical industry used these studies to resist any claim by communities that pollution from chemical factories was dangerous. Trade association journals trumpeted the studies as "an opportunity to get at the truth about Louisiana and its reputation as cancer alley."[134] The Louisiana Chemical Association announced that Chen had proved to their satisfaction that the major problem in Louisiana had not to do with pollution but the "lack of early detection and limited access to needed health care." The industry even went so far as to suggest that environmental justice activists, by continuing to harp on toxic pollution, were in essence further delaying "efforts to initiate new programming to address those factors— tobacco, diet, access to care—that could significantly reduce cancer death rates."[135] Scholars from conservative think tanks also eagerly echoed Chen's conclusions. In a Cato Institute article titled "Does Environmentalism Kill?" the writer detailed Chen's data and then concluded that environmentalists themselves were responsible for the high mortality rates by opposing industry attempts to bring new jobs and resources to the region.[136]

Many local activists and even some elected government officials reacted in a dramatically different way. They saw Chen's studies as seriously flawed in both design and methodology. Robert Kuehn, the head of the

Tulane Environmental Law Clinic, complained that close study of her data did not "readily allow identification of childhood cancers" and that she obscured specific local cancer rates by failing to present "cancer data by the Parish of occurrence but instead grouping Parishes by broad...regions." He also summarized criticism by others that the registry failed to report on "the numerous tumors by residents of Louisiana that are detected by out-of-state hospitals."[137]

Richard Ieyoub, writing both "as a parent, and as Attorney General of the State of Louisiana," likewise complained that the "childhood cancer data is not presented in Volume 8(1) in a way that would readily allow identification of those rare childhood cancers and the parish of occurrence of such cancers which have, apparently, appeared in some locations in Louisiana in unusual numbers." The attorney general, elected in 1995, was concerned about the issue of "'clusters' of rare childhood cancers [that] have been detected in specific locations in Louisiana." He objected to the fact that the broad parameters by which the registry categorized cancer deaths hid specific children's cancers and failed to identify small clusters. The fact that the registries reported cancer by region (which combined a number of parishes), when in fact the Toxic Release Inventory was organized by parish, made it impossible to link pollution to the clusters in particular communities. "Such grouping of parishes and presentation of cancer incidence data by 'region' may obscure differences in cancer incidence which may exist between industrial and agricultural parishes—and... may obscure other important intraregional differences."[138]

James Cox, a state senator from Calcasieu Parish, where Lake Charles, the other major center for the petrochemical industry is located, extended the complaints of Kuehn and Ieyoub in a letter to Chen. Cox complained that the Louisiana Tumor Registry was incomplete because "numerous cases of cancer in citizens in my district are not diagnosed here in Louisiana." Many of his constituents traveled to Texas, he held, and many other Louisiana children went to St. Jude Children's Hospital in Memphis, Tennessee. "I have been informed...that you admitted that there were no current reciprocities for data exchange with out-of-state hospitals frequently used by Louisiana residents," he observed. Cox objected to the differences between Chen's public and professional presentation of the very same data, observing that the limitations of her study, though reported in professional journals, were absent in her public statements about the relationship between childhood cancer and the chemical exposures. "One certainly cannot make any general statements that there is no increased incidence of

Cancer in Louisiana, if all of the data has not been compiled."[139] Paul Templet, the former Department of Environmental Quality administrator and now a professor of environmental science at LSU, also criticized Chen's epidemiology for not finding a method for associating distance from chemical plants to birth defects and other illnesses.[140]

It became distressingly clear that communities could not depend on outside scientific experts to corroborate their anecdotal evidence of a link between chemicals and disease. In fact, the net effect of hiring experts tended to be to weaken the authority of communities by making those experts the sole arbiters of truth. In community after community in the Louisiana toxic corridor, residents performed surveys that uncovered significant health problems, only to discover that what was so obvious to them was not confirmed by the professional epidemiologists. While residents looked to a broad array of indicators to show that pollution was hazardous, the state's epidemiologists usually focused on one particular bodily insult—usually cancer—as representative of community health status.

The story of the development of vinyl chloride plants in Louisiana is one of collusion between industry and state government. Louisiana appealed to industry for a number of reasons: it had a rich supply of natural resources, a state government eager for the jobs and tax revenue industry could bring, and the remnants of a plantation system that left African Americans poor, in need of work and, until relatively recently, too disenfranchised to pose much of a threat to industry. The petrochemical industry moved right in, leaked and pumped its chemicals into the environment, and ignored any indications of the toxic nature of its product. Where some saw an attempt to exploit and develop the state's natural resources—oil, gas, salt, and port facilities—for the benefit of the people of Louisiana, others saw a confirmation of the state's commitment to industries which would blithely exploit the land and the people for the benefit of their shareholders.

Sociologist Robert Bullard sums up the situation in America's chemical heartland: "By default, the region has become a . . . sump for the rest of the nation's toxic waste. A colonial mentality exists in the South, where local government and big business take advantage of people who are politically and economically powerless. Many of these attitudes emerged from the region's marriage to slavery and the plantation system, which exploited both humans and the land."[141]

What was occurring in Louisiana was an extreme example of a problem that was facing environmentalists and consumer advocates across the country. A recalcitrant industry, joined by a conservative political establishment, was threatening to undo years of environmental legislation and reform. Through corporate contributions to political leaders and the establishment of numerous political action committees, business was testing the very boundaries of democracy.

A Hazy Mixture

Science, Civil Rights, Pollution, and Politics

Driving south from Baton Rouge on Interstate 10, one passes through suburbs and strip malls and comes to Louisiana Route 44, which winds south to the east bank of the Mississippi River. Route 44 continues past old plantations, monuments to slave rebellions, and an African American history museum housed in an old plantation where gowned ladies give guided tours. Soon the landscape of pastoral towns gives way to giant industrial complexes spread out along what now becomes the River Road. To the west, a huge levee hides the Mississippi River from sight and blocks river access from the desperately poor communities interspersed among the industrial plants.

Cracking towers and brightly burning gas plumes dominate the landscape. Giant pipes straddle the road, crossing overhead to join refineries and granaries on the left to the river ports and docks on the right. Signs identify old plantations that are now home to sprawling chemical and grain storage facilities. Metal pipes—some glistening silver, some red with the dust of bauxite, used to make aluminum—run along the road.

As one drives past the old Uncle Sam Plantation, site of IMC Agrico's Uncle Sam Plant, one enters the town of Convent, which was named for the Convent of the Sacred Heart established in 1825 on that site by French missionaries.[1] Convent appears to be little more than a string of houses, trailers, and plants. The town center is composed of a parish office building, the Catholic church, and a post office. A gas station with a small general store serves as the central market. The northern part of town, called "Freetown" (for the former slaves who settled there in the 1860s), is where Shintech, a Japanese-owned plastics company, proposed to build a giant plastics manufacturing facility in 1996. The residents, mostly African Americans, live in dilapidated wooden houses reminiscent of old slave quarters

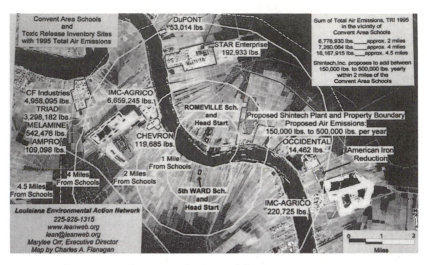

19. Map of Convent and vicinity. This map of the Convent, Louisiana, region shows the siting of chemical plants in relation to schools. It also indicates the proposed site of the operation that Shintech later abandoned. Source: Louisiana Environmental Action Network (LEAN).

situated on dirt roads that meander away from the river to dead-end in fields abutting huge mountains of industrial waste. One such dirt road, "so narrow that the postman won't drive down it," borders the huge sugarcane fields of the former St. Rose, Helvetia, and Wilton plantations.[2] It is here that the community mounted a protest that resulted, for the first time, in the federal government's pre-empting the authority of state officials and industry over the issue of environmental justice and environmental racism.[3]

The three-mile by one-hundred-mile stretch of land between Baton Rouge and New Orleans, where Convent is located, is the very heart of "Cancer Alley." Behind the levee, more than one hundred firms manufacture sulfuric acid, ethylene, fertilizers, petrochemicals, and vinyl chloride. In 1995 these companies poured more than thirty-eight million pounds of toxins into the air, soil, and water. The EPA now requires these companies to report toxic releases to the federal government, so it is a matter of record that the alley contains approximately 40 percent of Louisiana's plants that "contribute 53% of the total TRI air releases in the State."[4] These industries largely account for Louisiana's ranking as one of the most heavily polluted states in the country in the 1990s.[5] According to the EPA, "Louisiana industries had the largest total toxic releases from 1989 to

Table 9.1. Toxic Air Pollutant Releases (Averaged) per
Person per Year (1995)

United States (12.1%)*	7 lbs/person
Louisiana (30.8%)	21 lbs/person
Corridor parishes (36.8%)	27 lbs/person
St. James Parish (49.6%)	360 lbs/person
Convent area (83.7%)	2,277 lbs/person

*Percentage of the population that is African American.
SOURCE: "From Plantations to Plants: Report of the Emergency
National Commission on Environmental and Economic Justice in
St. James Parish, Louisiana" (September 15, 1998). Data were drawn
from the 1995 federal Toxic Release Inventory, TELC.

1993," second only to Texas in the years 1994 to 1997.[6] Twenty-four percent of the state's population and 34 percent of its African American population live there.[7] While on average, 7 pounds of toxic materials were
released nationwide into the air for every person living in the United
States as a whole, 2,277 pounds of pollutants were released into the air for
every person living near Convent (Table 9.1).[8]

The effect of these chemical emissions on the health of the population
appears quite significant. According to the Deep South Center for Environmental Justice, rates of leukemias and lyphosarcomas, breast cancers
and colon cancers are much higher here than would be statistically predictable.[9] The population living here felt powerless to oppose industry. But
all this would change.

In October 1996 the Shintech Corporation, one of the world's largest
producers of polyvinyl chloride plastic, announced plans to build a massive
integrated vinyl chloride plant on a 3,700-acre sugarcane field in Convent.
Shintech hoped that by 2005 the facility, which would cost $700 million to
build, would be manufacturing up to 1,000,000 tons of polyvinyl chloride
a year, with a projected 11 percent increase in air pollution.[10] Given the
industry's history of unbridled expansion, Shintech could not have imagined that the small community of Convent would ultimately see to the
demise of its plans.

The state of Louisiana, Republican governor Murphy J. (Mike) Foster,
and the administrators of the Louisiana Department of Environmental Quality (DEQ) all eagerly committed themselves to supporting Shintech, which
promised to create about 165 jobs. In anticipation of bountiful revenues,
the state promised to award Shintech a ten-year industrial property tax

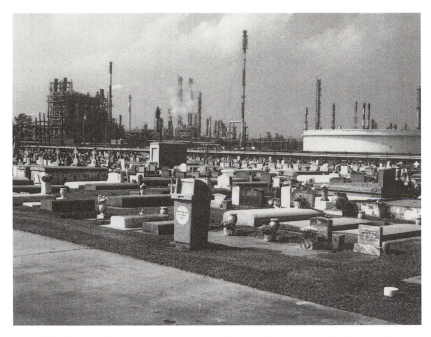

20. Holy Rosary Cemetery, surrounded by the Union Carbide chemical plant. This graveyard, in the midst of a huge chemical plant, was once just outside the now-vanished Mississippi River town of Taft, Louisiana. Source: David Rosner and Gerald Markowitz.

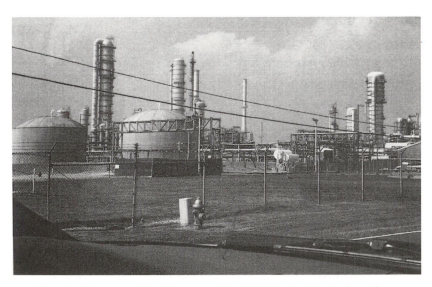

21. Chemical plant, north of Convent. The IMC-Agrico Uncle Sam Plant is one of the many chemical complexes that dot the Mississippi River banks between Baton Rouge and New Orleans. Source: Gerald Markowitz and David Rosner.

exemption of $94.5 million, or approximately $787,000 as a subsidy for each permanent job created.[11] In May 1997 the DEQ issued four air quality permits to Shintech, clearing the way for construction to begin.[12]

Convent residents immediately organized protests against the building of the plant, appealing to the Environmental Protection Agency to overrule the hasty decision by the DEQ. The EPA, for the first time in its history, responded by holding up air and water permits until certain technical aspects of the plant's impact on water and air quality were cleared up and questions of environmental justice were investigated. In the end, Carol Browner, administrator of the EPA, did not have to decide on the permits because Shintech chose to withdraw its proposal.

ENVIRONMENTAL RACISM— ENVIRONMENTAL JUSTICE

Back in February 1982, when President Reagan appointed Anne Gorsuch administrator of the EPA, it was clear that he meant to dismantle the agency in fact if not in name. In the first year or so of the Reagan administration, "no new enforcement cases were filed by the EPA against hazardous waste sites," although there were "more than eighteen thousand sites around the country [that] were known to EPA to qualify for clean up under the legal definition of Superfund."[13] It became clear to the public that "unlike its predecessors, the Reagan administration could not be trusted to protect the environment."[14]

A reinvigorated and much more confrontational environmental movement rose up in response. Many people "joined environmental organizations for the first time, producing sizable membership gains for many of the national organizations in the 1980s."[15] Mainstream environmentalism had its roots in conservationist and preservationist values, however, and was seen by many African Americans as a decidedly white, middle-class movement often oblivious to issues of economic and racial justice. For Whitney Young, head of the Urban League, "the war on pollution... should be waged after the war on poverty is won." He saw the environmental movement as diversionary, "ignoring the most dangerous and most pressing of our problems."[16] Furthermore, traditional environmentalism had at times been associated with some of the more reactionary social movements of the twentieth century, such as the often racist eugenics crusade, further undercutting African American support for the movement.[17]

Two particular cases pointed to the role of racism in decisions to site sources of pollution in poor neighborhoods. In the late 1970s an African American community group in Houston, Texas, sued the city for placing a landfill in its neighborhood. The residents ultimately lost the case, but the suit was of value in that it documented that the city had sited incinerators, landfills, and other waste sites in poor black and Hispanic neighborhoods.[18] In 1982 in Warren County, North Carolina, five hundred people were arrested for protesting the county's plans to build a hazardous waste facility in their community. Benjamin Chavis Jr., then of the United Church of Christ and later the executive director of the National Association for the Advancement of Colored People (NAACP), coined the phrase "environmental racism" to denote the "mounting evidence of discrimination" in environmental decisions.[19] In 1987 Chavis and the United Church of Christ published *Toxic Wastes and Race in the United States,* the first systematic analysis of the placing of toxic waste sites in poor communities.[20] In 1990 Robert Bullard published *Dumping in Dixie.*[21] The same year, a group of academics and environmentalists gathered at the University of Michigan for the Conference on Race and the Incidence of Environmental Hazards. Afterward its leaders met with the first Bush administration's EPA administrator, William Reilly, to request that the EPA investigate the use of race as a determinant of environmental policy. Reilly acknowledged the legitimacy of their concerns by establishing the Environmental Equity Work Group.[22] The following year, more than six hundred people attended the First National People of Color Environmental Leadership Summit, organized by Chavis, Bullard, and others in Washington, DC.[23]

By the 1990s organizations in Louisiana and around the country were documenting the fact that a disproportionate number of chemical plants were being placed in minority communities. Greenpeace found that the percentage of vinyl chloride monomer and ethylene dichloride plants situated in minority communities in Louisiana was "237 percent greater than the national average."[24] Beverly Wright, Pat Bryant, and Robert Bullard documented the efforts of communities up and down the Mississippi River to stop the establishment of plants and reduce toxic releases of "more than two billion pounds between 1987 and 1989." These toxins were being released into many working-class river communites, for example, Alsen, where more than 77 percent of the residents (98.9 percent of whom were African American) owned their own homes.[25] Eleven lead smelting and plastics plants, a hazardous waste incinerator, and two Superfund sites had made the area almost unlivable for residents. (The Superfund, the popular name for the Comprehensive Emergency Response, Compensation, and Liability Act of 1980 (CERCLA), established a priorities list of polluted sites and identified polluters who were to be held responsible for funding a reclamation effort.[26]) The Devil's Swamp area in Alsen had once been "something like out of a Walt Disney movie" with "beautiful lakes and the cypress trees and white cranes and the blue herons," according to E. W. Pate, a local resident.[27]

But by the late 1960s nearby chemical plants had dumped so much noxious waste there that fires began to erupt. In 1969, the levee broke and "hundreds of thousands of contaminants [were] spilled . . . into the Mississippi River."[28] The trees died, the birds disappeared, and the fish developed tumors. Residents started complaining to the state about their own physical ailments; some could barely work in the soil of their own backyards because toxic chemicals burned their eyes and skin. Others experienced chronic headaches, bloody noses, and skin rashes. While state officials acknowledged residents' exposure to various chemical pollutants, in the absence of "hard evidence" from the community they would not accept that these chemicals caused the health problems residents were experiencing. "They have to come up with a little bit more information than that for me to start delegating or redirecting my resources," remarked Kai Midboe, Governor Edwin Edwards's head of the Louisiana Department of Environmental Quality in 1993.[29] Midboe excused his inaction by explaining, "I cannot address concerns [of] people that—you know, when people say 'I feel' or 'I'm concerned' or whatever." Rather than attribute it to pollution, state officials agreed with the Louisiana Chemical Association that the "higher than normal death rate from cancer" in Louisiana was due to "lack of early detection, [and] lack of proper health care."[30] (See chapter 8, page 259, endnote 135.)

The obligation of the federal government to respond to environmental justice issues derives from Title VI of the 1964 Civil Rights Act, which prohibited discrimination by any program or agency that received federal funds. The EPA established an "elaborate administrative procedure" for citizens to follow to file civil rights complaints against any recipient of EPA financial assistance, including the Louisiana DEQ.[31] Even more attention was paid to environmental racism during the Bush administration. In February 1992 the EPA's Equity Workgroup issued a report titled *Environmental Equity: Reducing Risk for All Communities*, which noted the dearth of reliable information regarding the relationship between environmental hazards, class and race. The March issue of the *EPA Journal* focused on questions of equity and environmental pollution. All of this activity generated tremendous media attention and later in 1992, the EPA established the Office of Environmental Justice to monitor the effects of industrial pollution on minority and poor communities.[32]

Nonetheless, the EPA failed to take action in numerous cases where industries had placed polluting plants in minority communities like those in the Mississippi River corridor. "The illegal discrimination in siting unwanted facilities became so rampant and so obvious," one scholar asserted, that in February 1994, President Bill Clinton issued Executive Order 12898,[33] which directed all federal agencies to "analyze the environmental effects, including human health, economic and social effects, of federal actions, including effects on minority communities and low income communities" and to "make achieving environmental justice part of [federal agencies'] mission."[34]

This order was taken by industry as a dangerous sig-nal that the federal government was prepared to intervene on behalf of aggrieved citizens. As the *Oil & Gas Journal* stated, it was "economic and racial poison loft[ed] on wings of pretty-feeling words."[35] In Louisiana the chemical industry feared that "Louisiana is a real test-bed [of the environmental justice movement] because we have so many plants in rural areas."[36] Daniel Borne, president of the Louisiana Chemical Association, maintained that the decisions to place so many factories in poor and African American communities along the Mississippi was based not on race or class but on economics: here was cheap land and good access to the river. Industries were also looking for communities that historically had offered little political opposition.[37]

LOUISIANA—THE STATE RUN BY A BUSINESSMAN

The real battle between the chemical industry and local community groups, the state and the federal government would erupt in 1995 when Mike Foster, a wealthy, well-connected Republican, was elected governor of Louisiana. (Foster had strategically switched from the Democratic to the Republican Party before the primary, thereby overcoming a splintered field of opponents that local reporters referred to as "Noah's Ark" because it contained "two white female Democrats, two black Democratic congressmen, and two former Republican governors.")[38]

Foster, who had made his fortune in sugar farming and oil, quickly formed alliances with some of the most reactionary and racist public officials in Louisiana and the nation. He was the only governor to support Pat Buchanan in the 1996 Republican presidential race. The Louisiana branch of the National Association for the Advancement of White People gave him its vote of confidence.[39] Several years later a grand jury investigated a revelation that Foster had had secret dealings with David Duke's campaign organization during the campaign, paying Duke $152,000 for a mailing list of 80,000 Duke supporters.[40] A month after taking office, Foster "announced an end to state affirmative-action programs and declared that racial discrimination no longer existed."[41] Foster's environmental policy clearly consisted of making the state friendly to the chemical industry; he wanted a "DEQ chief who 'works with industry on a non-adversary basis.'"[42]

By 1996, the state's dependence on the chemical industry had reached its zenith. Of the $2.44 billion in new investment in Louisiana in 1996, fully $1.23 billion, or 50 percent, came from the chemical and allied products industry. The "next closest sector was petroleum refining, with $341 million."[43] By 1997, in an article titled "Gulf Coast Fishing: Luring Firms with State Incentives," *Chemical Week* enthused that "chemical projects accounted for almost 60%—more than $2.2 billion—of Louisiana's total industrial investment of $3.8 billion in 1997, and the chemical industry's share of 1998 projects announced so far is outpacing last year."[44] As Kevin P. Reilly Sr., the secretary of the state's Department of Economic Development, said, "The Louisiana chemical industry is a driving force in the state economy and a major component of the U.S. chemical sector," accounting for one quarter of the nation's petrochemical production.[45] Lawrence C. Scott, an economist at Louisiana State University (LSU), predicted in 1996 that the chemical industry would add at least six hundred jobs over the next two years.[46]

But not everyone was so pleased about this growth. Some political leaders believed that Louisiana was "relying too much on the oil, gas and petrochemical industry." Even though the economy was booming in the mid-1990s, some feared that the state was being lulled into a complacency that would inhibit creative planning for the future. "The urgency for diversification has disappeared," declared Jerry Luke LeBlanc, the chair of the Louisiana House Appropriations Committee.[47]

In 1996 Foster's administration was quite open about its willingness to cater to industry. His office ran an ad in the *Wall Street Journal* bearing the heading, "Louisiana—The State Run by a Businessman." The ad depicted a government official bending over backward, asking, "What has Louisiana done for business lately?" while the copy below pointed out that during a time when lawsuits plagued industry, Louisiana could offer limits on corporate liability, a prohibition against punitive damages, and the requirement that plaintiffs prove negligence.[48] By 1997 Foster's Department of Environmental Quality had not only backed away from any confrontations with the industry, but also had reduced penalties and fines on industrial polluters by nearly 90 percent from Roemer's 1989 levels; in 1997 industry's total penalty assessment was $736,000, down from more than $8 million in 1989. Robert Kuehn, head of Tulane's Environmental Law Clinic, pointed out that the "signal the State is sending from a profit standpoint is that you might be better off breaking the law and taking your chances." The Louisiana Chemical Association praised the DEQ's program for promoting voluntary compliance, noting that "you don't make progress by harassing people to get compliance."[49]

Foster went even further than Edwards in removing environmental impediments to industrial development.[50] Toxic releases "in Louisiana increased by 8 million pounds, or 4.5 per cent from 1995 to 1996"[51] and by another 3 million pounds the following year.[52] Although Texas ranked number one in toxic emissions, Louisiana surpassed Texas in the amount of toxins emitted per person by nearly three to one.[53] In 1998, Paul Templet, the former head of Governor Buddy Roemer's DEQ, remarked that as a result of the pro-business policies of Foster and Edwards, "Louisiana's chemical industry releases are still four times the national average, and they appear to be rising again."[54]

This pro-business atmosphere was precisely what the chemical companies wanted. But some saw it as blatant collusion between industry and the state government. It was shortly after Mike Foster took office in 1996 that Shintech, the U.S. subsidiary of Japan's multinational plastics manufacturer Shin-Etsu, announced that Louisiana was one of three states under consideration for a giant plant. Shintech was planning a "manufacturing complex that would include chlor-alkali, ethylene dichloride, vinyl chloride monomer (VCM), and polyvinyl chloride (PVC) production." Shintech already had a plant producing 2.8 billion pounds of PVC in Freeport, Texas, but that plant depended upon Dow Chemical for its feedstock of VCM and Shintech wanted to be free from such dependence. The new plant would be huge by any standard; it would cost as much as $700 million to build and would produce the feedstock and plastic in one integrated process; its annual capacity would be 495,000 tons of chlorine, 550,000 tons of caustic soda, 1.1 billion pounds of VCM and 880 million pounds of PVC.[55]

The Louisiana DEQ's Kevin Reilly laid out for Shintech the lengths to which the state would go to encourage the company to locate in Convent: the Industrial Tax Exemption program exempted "new and expanding manufacturing facilities from local and parish *ad valorem* (property taxes) for a period of five years with a provision for an additional five years." The Louisiana Enterprise Zone Program authorized the state to provide "a one-time tax credit of $2,500 for each new permanent job added to the payroll at startup or during the next five years." In addition, the Industrial Revenue Bond program, the Inventory Tax Credit Program, the Freeport Laws, and the establishment of Foreign Trade Zones all sweetened the pot for Shintech.[56] (The Louisiana Coalition for Tax Justice estimated that a ten-year property tax exemption would total more than $94 million over ten years, including over $27 million in exempted school taxes. In addition, they estimated that as an enterprise zone, Shintech would receive an additional $412,500 in tax credits, plus tax rebates of $25 million.[57])

Nine months after Foster's inauguration, Shintech chose about six square miles on a former sugar plantation in Convent in St. James Parish.[58] St. James Parish, which straddled the Mississippi River forty miles north of New Orleans, had approximately 21,000 residents and more than a dozen industrial plants, "including two petrochemical plants about two miles from the proposed Shintech site."[59] In July 1997, the Louisiana Department of Environmental Quality issued Shintech three separate construction and operating permits for plants to produce chlor-alkali, vinyl chloride mono-mer, and polyvinyl chloride, maintaining that "adverse environmental impacts had been minimized or avoided to the maximum extent possible."[60] Although the plant would emit methanol, vinyl chloride, ethylene dichloride, chloroform, carbon tetrachloride, hydrochloric acid, chlorine, and ammonia[61] and might have deleterious health effects, the Louisiana DEQ concluded that the "social and economic benefits of the proposed Facility will greatly outweigh its adverse environmental impacts. Notably, the Louisiana constitution requires balancing, not protection, of the environment as an exclusive goal."[62]

In 1998 *Time* magazine featured Louisiana in a special report ("Louisiana No. 1 in Terms of Subsidies per Capita") that linked tax breaks for large companies and the state's heavy industrial pollution and extreme poverty. During the 1990s, the article reported, Louisiana "wiped off the books $3.1 billion in property taxes alone," claiming this was necessary to attract jobs to the state. *Time*'s analysis noted, however, that Louisiana paid huge amounts in lost revenues for the few jobs created. For the nine jobs created by Dow Chemical in Plaquemine from 1988 to 1997 the state paid a total cost of $96 million in tax breaks and other incentives, or $10.7 million per job. Georgia Pacific, also in Plaquemine, cost the state $46 million for 200 jobs, or $230,000 per job.[63] Paul Templet noted that "as these subsidies rise, the income disparity between the rich and the poor rises."[64] In June 2000 the *New York Times* reported that Louisiana had the "second highest poverty rate of any state . . . and the gap between its wealthiest and poorest residents is the nation's widest and is growing."[65]

The loss in state taxes mostly affected public works projects, road and bridge maintenance, schools, and medical clinics. Since industries were generally located along the river in economically distressed and politically disenfranchised black communities, those communities bore the brunt of the lost revenues.[66] "In some Louisiana parishes...20% or more of the industrial property taxes goes to education. So every tax break granted to a company translates into less money for schools," noted *Time*.[67] Templet believed poor services, a weak educational base, and especially pollution would undermine the long-term financial health of the state. He wrote that "a clean environment not only is good for business, but is probably a necessary condition for a healthy economy over the long term."[68]

The loss of tax revenues for education left Louisiana with a profound dilemma. The state sought to attract high-tech companies that would pay higher wages, but by undermining the schools state officials made it impossible to provide a skilled workforce for these new industries. Still, the state clung to the chemical industry as its best hope for economic improvement. Loren Scott, an LSU economist, argued that it was self-defeating to deny the right to construct in these communities: "It's a tricky issue because if you deny these plants the ability to come into those areas, those people are almost assured of remaining low-income. You can bring in furniture production, textiles, food processing, but they are low paying industries. It means you work and still wind up poor." On the other hand, Scott pointed out, it was unrealistic to expect that the state would attract Silicon Valley industries "when you're next to last in [standardized test] scores and either last or next-to-last in high school graduation rates."[69]

The chemical industry would provide *some* opportunity. Robert Kuehn agreed that the lack of an educated workforce imperiled the state's economic prospects. But his analysis diverged dramatically from Scott's, as he observed that although the state's tax exemption policies might provide a few high-tech jobs for white professionals from outside St. James Parish or even from outside the state, it was an illusion to think that these industries would benefit the poor and poorly trained residents of these river communities.[70]

The residents of Convent knew that the residents of nearby Wallace had prevented the building of a chemical plant in their midst. When the Formosa Plastics Corporation, a Taiwanese-held company, wanted to build a rayon plant on the site of the 1,800-acre Whitney Plantation on the west bank of the Mississippi,[71] the company made the case that the plant would bring jobs and income. Wallace residents retorted that the chemical industry thus far had done little for the unskilled, largely African American, residents of their small community, but instead had hired skilled, generally white workers for all but the most menial positions. The proposed factories would require high-tech skills, which the local black residents did not have.[72] One survey in St. Gabriel, in Iberville Parish not far from Plaquemine, found that local residents held 164 out of 1,878 permanent jobs, or

8.7 percent.[73] Wilford Green, who had lived in Wallace his entire life, expected that the only jobs available for African Americans in Formosa Plastics' proposed plant would be "the same kind of job that my father had —cleaning the yard, cutting the grass, cleaning the toilets. Are we going to have administrative jobs? Nobody's saying that to us, no!"[74]

Furthermore, many residents feared that industry would bring more air pollution and disease to their community. Many of the companies receiving the greatest subsidies were the filthiest and most damaging to the river region's sensitive ecology. For example, IMC-Agrico, which received $15 million in property tax relief between 1988 and 1997, was a major polluter in Louisiana, releasing 12.8 million pounds of toxic chemicals in the manufacture of fertilizers and other chemical products; Rubicon, Inc., a chemical company in Geismar, released 8.4 million pounds of chemicals and was exempted from $9 million in property taxes; Monsanto released 7.7 million pounds of toxic chemicals but Louisiana "excused Monsanto from payment of $45 million in property taxes over the past decade."[75]

Just as industry feared, the Clinton executive order provided some legal and political clout for the residents of St. James Parish wishing to protest. Emelda West, a seventy-one-year-old African American woman who was one of the prime movers of the group called St. James Citizens for Jobs and the Environment, which opposed Shintech's plans, said of Clinton: "I don't guess he knew I existed. But he did have people like me in mind."[76] West is a widow whose college-educated children had been forced to leave the state because of the lack of opportunities. Being a charismatic speaker of extraordinary energies, she proved to be an extremely effective organizer. She knew and talked to everyone in town about Shintech's plan, distributed leaflets, and took visitors on tours of the back roads near the industrial plants.[77] Once made aware of the possibility of another huge chemical plant in their area, residents began to act. St. James Parish already had nine chemical plants, and residents were not willing to watch Shintech erect another factory "within five miles of 11 other industrial facilities (nine of which were major sources on Louisiana's emission inventory system for toxic releases)."[78]

Some wrote to their newspapers. One woman complained that she didn't "want an additional 600,000 pounds of toxic air contaminants in my already-overburdened area."[79] Other women like Pat Melancon and Gloria Roberts joined Emelda West in protesting Shintech's plan to build in their backyard. Roberts, a retired schoolteacher, did much of the research documenting the demographics of the area around the proposed plant. Although most of her neighbors had been bought out she refused to move from her split-level house surrounded by property owned by Conoco. Melancon, who was white and a retired teacher, was a major speaker on behalf of the parish's black, white, and Cajun residents. Together these women went door to door to warn neighbors of Shintech's plans and to galvanize opposition. They held meetings in churches, assembled petitions, wrote to state and national officials, and began to develop alliances with local and national environmental groups. They made contact with the Louisiana Environmental Action Network (LEAN) and Greenpeace, both of which had been carrying on statewide campaigns against the chemical industry.

Residents knew from their own experience with the existing plants in St. James Parish that in addition to the usual pollution, emergencies and chemical accidents were common occurrences. Residents were often awakened by sirens or alarmed by radio alerts warning them not to leave their homes or workplaces. The smell of solvents continually wafted through the air, making it hard for residents to believe the companies' assurances that nothing was amiss. Residents were particularly anxious because, in the event of a major accident or explosion that might release massive amounts of toxic chemicals into the air, evacuation would be nearly impossible. They feared they would be trapped by dead-end streets, the narrow River Road, and railroad tracks that crisscrossed the area. Furthermore, chemical releases into the air could travel a mile in less than a minute, especially when hurricanes and other storms swept in from the Gulf of Mexico, whereas it might take even a responsible company as long as twenty minutes to detect releases and warn nearby residents.[80]

In nearby Ascension Parish, a 500,000-gallon storage tank at the Borden Chemicals and Plastics plant had exploded in 1997, its "detonation heard for miles around, forcing the closing of Louisiana Route 1 and the voluntary evacuation of some neighbors." The same plant had released eight thousand pounds of "hazardous materials," including vinyl chloride mono-mer.[81] In Lake Charles, to the west, the other major site of chemical and plastics production in the state, a jury found the Condea Vista Chemical Company liable for "wanton and reckless disregard of public safety" for dumping between nineteen million and forty-seven million pounds of ethylene dichloride, a feedstock for vinyl chloride monomer, into the lake itself. At the time, the company had admitted leaking only thousands of pounds of the suspected carcinogen and, had it not been for the lawsuit, the true extent of the spill would never have been revealed.[82]

Soon after beginning public protests against Shintech in the spring of 1997, residents met with lawyers at Tulane University's Environmental

Law Clinic in New Orleans.[83] For years the Tulane Environmental Law Clinic, a training ground for third-year students interested in environmental law, had played a significant role in a number of important challenges against industry in Louisiana. It represented residents of Ascension Parish in getting the state to enforce regulations for the underground storage of hazardous waste. It also represented the St. John's Citizens for Environmental Justice, the Congo Square Foundation, a Vietnamese immigrant association, and the local Audubon Society chapter in successful challenges in numerous environmental issues.[84] Together with community groups, the students quickly developed a legal and public policy strategy to force the EPA to intervene under a variety of federal statutes and regulations. They argued that the disproportionate impact of environmental pollution from the proposed plant on the poor, African American community of Convent would violate Title VI of the Civil Rights Act of 1964. The clinic further argued that the proposed plant's effluent would also violate Title V of the Clean Air Act.[85]

The threat of pollution from chemical plants was not unknown to the federal Environmental Protection Agency. Twenty years earlier[86] the EPA, while trying to reassure the public that vinyl chloride emissions didn't "pose an imminent hazard to people living near the plants," had to acknowledge "that some hazard does exist and that our population deserves the protection afforded by regulatory action."[87] The EPA estimated that VCM and PVC plants probably discharged two hundred million pounds of VCM and fifty million pounds of PVC each year into the nation's air, water, and soil.[88] It also "estimated that approximately 4.6 million people [who] lived within five miles" of the plastics plants were potentially exposed to levels of vinyl chloride monomer that could cause up to twenty extra angiosarcoma deaths nationwide.[89]

AND THEY'RE NOT IN IT FOR THE MONEY

The intervention of Tulane, the state's most prestigious university and premier law school, helped turn what was a local "not in my backyard" (NIMBY) movement into a statewide initiative that gained national attention from both the chemical industry and the U.S. government. The industry was aware of the public relations disaster it faced if the construction of a plant were stopped because the industry was found guilty of environmental racism. Until then no group had kept a company out because of environmental racism, although nineteen other environmental justice complaints were under consideration, three in Louisiana and six in Texas.[90]

As *Chemical Week* noted, the Shintech protests were much more danger-ous and potentially precedent setting than protests in the past.[91] A victory in Convent would mean real trouble for industry in the future.

When local residents, in conjunction with Greenpeace and the Tulane Environmental Law Clinic, filed a complaint with the EPA, they challenged the traditional hegemony of the petrochemical industry in the state. The industry understood, as did Emelda West and other local residents, that the stakes had been raised. *Chemical Week* declared that the EPA's decision as to the validity of the residents' complaint would "offer the first insight on the EPA's interpretation of President Clinton's 1994 Executive Order requiring federal agencies to address the health and environmental effects of their policies on minority and low-income communities."[92] The publi-cation agreed with opponents of the plant that "this is a test case with national significance that will demonstrate whether EPA is committed to carrying out the environmental justice [provisions of Clinton's executive order]."[93] In August 1997 the Office of Civil Rights of the EPA decided to accept "for investigation a complaint alleging that Louisiana Department of Environmental Quality (LDEQ) has violated Title VI of the Civil Rights Act of 1964."[94] The Tulane law clinic supplemented its complaint by docu-menting that the Shintech plant would be an even worse polluter than pre-viously revealed. They asserted that the Shintech facility would produce up to 550,000 pounds of volatile organic chemicals like vinyl chloride monomer and 138,000 pounds of other toxic chemicals such as chlorine that would add to the 7.2 million pounds of toxins that were already emit-ted into the air in Convent.[95]

The reaction to the EPA's action was not uniformly positive. The Baton Rouge *Advocate* declared that the federal agency "hardly could have picked a worse place to try out this hazy mixture of science, civil rights, pollution, and politics."[96] But it was Governor Foster and the Louisiana Department of Economic Development that led the fight to save Shintech's plant. Given the state's long-term view that "chemicals drive the Louisiana economy," it is not surprising that they would portray the residents' protest as an attempt by "outsiders" to deprive a poor community of jobs.[97] Foster saw the staff of the law clinic as the chief culprits, calling them "a bunch of vig-ilantes out there to make their own law," and he claimed that Tulane's and Kuehn's actions were hampering the state's economic growth.[98] The state secretary of economic development, Kevin Reilly, accused the clinic of leav-ing "the university open to the charge of being irresponsible at best and pursuing elitist social engineering goals at worst."[99] Foster went so far as to threaten Tulane by calling for a re-examination of the tax breaks that

Tulane received from the state; he urged Louisiana businesses to stop donating to Tulane.[100] Robert Kuehn was bemused by all the fire directed at him personally and at the clinic. As he put it, "This group of citizens is up against the entire state government, not to mention Shintech's team of lawyers. Here we are a few student attorneys and a supervising lawyer. I'm not sure why they're all shook up."[101]

Kuehn certainly knew why the state was going after him and the Environmental Law Clinic. Established in 1989 in response to the environmental crises across the state, the clinic defended poor communities throughout the state from the actions of the chemical industry and the inaction of the state itself. In addition to responding to requests from local groups concerned about pollution issues, the clinic hired a community outreach coordinator to ensure that local communities were aware of the help the clinic could provide.[102] The Louisiana Environmental Action Network, which had been founded in 1987 and had helped organize the Great Toxics March, enthusiastically welcomed the clinic's students and their mission. LEAN's newsletter noted, "Louisiana's environment has a new lawyer, a whole office full of them—and they're NOT in it for the money."[103]

Edward Sherman, the dean of the Law School, and Eamon Kelly, the university's president, both refused to buckle under the governor's threats, arguing that the mission of law clinics is to defend those too poor to hire private lawyers, that the university had the right to academic freedom, and that under the law it was the obligation of the university to protect the citizens of Louisiana. Sherman reminded everyone that Tulane University, as the largest private employer in New Orleans, supported economic development, but "in representing the [Convent] neighborhood group the clinic is simply invoking the proper legal channels to enforce the environmental laws."[104] He praised the clinic, asserting that it had "been attacked so frequently, in part, because it has been effective. Its impact has been stricter enforcement of environmental laws."[105]

The threats against Tulane's Environmental Law Clinic were more than mere words. Opponents turned to the state Supreme Court in their efforts to stop the clinic from opposing Shintech's plant. The Chamber of Commerce of New Orleans and the River Region petitioned the court to re-evaluate the rules under which university law clinics operated in Louisiana. Robert Gayle, the president and chief executive officer of the chamber, wrote to Chief Justice Pascal Calogero accusing the clinic of trying to "push and impose the social views of the faculty and students in the courts of the state of Louisiana.... We respectfully request that proper amendments be made to discontinue the use of Supreme Court rules to foster social positions left solely to the unregulated judgment of a faculty member capable of influencing and directing students to file suits [as] qualified members of the Bar."[106] In October the Louisiana Association of Business and Industry joined the chamber to object to Tulane's "obstructionist practices and [its] fostering social positions that conflict with the business community." The association "asked the court to amend rules that allow students to practice as attorneys."[107]

This was not the first time that a governor and the petrochemical industry had asked the court to "clip the wings" of the Tulane clinic. According to the New Orleans *Times-Picayune*, in 1993 the head of the Louisiana DEQ, Kai Midboe, at the urging of then Governor Edwin Edwards, "wanted the clinic muzzled so that he could get on with the job of making nice to the petrochemical industry."[108] Edwards himself had threatened to stop state funding for a new downtown basketball arena to be used by Tulane and to cut tuition assistance to Louisiana residents who attended the school.[109] To the surprise of many, the Louisiana Supreme Court summarily dismissed the state's requests to redefine the role of law clinics in defending the poor. The clinic was allowed to continue its work.

Having lost in the Supreme Court, the Louisiana chemical industry mobilized to try to take control of the Supreme Court itself by funding campaigns to defeat the liberal justices who had acted against their interests. Of the $577,256 donated to candidate Chet Traylor in his 1996 successful bid to defeat liberal Justice Joe Bleich, almost half came directly from oil and gas industry executives, their lawyers, and Louisiana business and industry.[110] When Chief Justice Calogero and two other judges faced reelection in 1998, there was reason to fear that the chemical industry would go after them.[111] The *Times-Picayune* attributed the upset in the court to political maneuvering, stating, "The Supreme Court is all of a dither.... It seems unlikely that the justices have suddenly discovered complexities in an issue summarily decided less than five years ago. Changes in the political landscape would seem to be responsible."[112]

In June 1998, the court ruled that the Tulane Clinic and all other law clinics in Louisiana could represent only individuals with incomes below the guidelines established by Congress for the Legal Services Corporation. In so doing the court delivered to industry the verdict it had paid for. The verdict meant that the clinics could represent only organizations where 51 percent of its members had incomes below these stringent guidelines and in cases where the group had no affiliation with any national organization. Because these qualifications were nearly impossible to meet, the ruling made it "more difficult for the poor and working poor to get representation in complicated, expensive lawsuits, such as those involving environmental issues."[113] Harold Green, a community organizer for the Southern Christian Leadership Conference, the venerable organization founded by Martin Luther King Jr., declared that "for all intents and purposes, it pulled the rug from beneath our feet."[114]

Eamon Kelly, Tulane's outgoing president, was direct in his disgust over the narrowness of the court and its willingness to disempower the poor, African American communities of Louisiana. Kelly echoed the cry of the Civil Rights era in proclaiming that it was "almost impossible for the working poor, who in our state are disproportionately African Americans, to have access to equal representation before the law." "This is power politics, pure and simple. This is the Governor, business community and the courts combining to deprive the working poor of their right to counsel.... In a course I teach on the developing world, I describe some Third World countries where the poor and minorities do not have access to legal representation. It is sad to be able now to include Louisiana as a case study in my course."[115] Of course, Governor Foster saw it differently. "The court is finally tightening up on that bunch of outlaws trying to shut everything down."[116]

While the state had a long tradition of political corruption, usually it was a local affair; now Louisiana was under scrutiny from the rest of the country. As the New Orleans *Times-Picayune* described it, the "High Court [had become the] Target of Disgust." While the state Supreme Court had sometimes made "itself a state-wide laughingstock...this time the whole country is in stitches." Members of the American Association of Law Schools called for a boycott of New Orleans as a convention site because the court's decision was "a travesty" and "beyond the pale."[117] Robert F. Kennedy Jr., in an address to students at Tulane, denounced the governor and the Supreme Court ruling as shortsighted and antidemocratic. "If we want to do what Governor Foster wants us to do, treat the planet as a business in liquidation, we'll see a few years of economic prosperity. But our children... will inherit a denuded landscape, poor health, and lost resources." Kennedy identified Tulane and the law clinic as "the front line" of democracy, providing a progressive vision for the future.[118] In contrast to Foster's narrow vision for bringing Louisiana into the industrial twentieth century, Kennedy and others argued that Louisiana had an opportunity to advance to the twenty-first century. Louisiana, with its access to national markets through the Mississippi River and international markets through the port of New Orleans, was too crucial to the country's long-term development to allow local politics, a culture of political corruption, and the narrow interests of the petrochemical industry to supersede the nation's needs.

Under pressure of intense national scrutiny, the court loosened its ruling in March 1999, allowing clinics to serve people with incomes up to twice the federal poverty level. Still, as Robert Kuehn, director of the Tulane Environmental Law Clinic, pointed out, Louisiana remained the only state "with an explicit financial limit on representation." He felt the ruling forced "the group to ask its members how much money they earn as a condition of membership and that creates a chilling effect on belonging to a group or seeking the help of a clinic."[119]

THE BIGGEST COINCIDENCE OF THE YEAR

Industry officials probably never imagined that Tulane, LSU, and other universities in the state would ever be so ungrateful as to try to resist them, given that these universities received more support from industry than from any other entity in the state. The chemical, gas, and petrochemical industries, after all, "accounted for $28 billion of the state's $110 billion gross state product," and the industry had contributed mightily to the state's universities. Freeport McMoRan, one of the world's largest manufacturers of chemical fertilizers, contributed $2.5 million to LSU to start the Institute for Recyclable Materials, $1 million to LSU's cancer center and $1.6 million to the University of New Orleans for its Center for Environmental Modeling. C. B. Pennington, a leading oil man, gave LSU $125 million to construct the Pennington Biomedical Research Center and, when he died in 1997, his $250 million estate was distributed among the Pennington Research Center, the Pennington Foundation, and his grandchildren. Texaco donated "a twenty-year free lease for a building that houses [Tulane's] Public Health School facility." Freeport McMoRan contributed $1 million to Tulane's Bio-Environmental Research Center and Shell and Exxon contributed $2 million to Tulane's Environmental and Waste Management Program. Ethyl, Texaco, and Claiborne Gasoline all endowed an LSU chair, while Freeport McMoRan endowed a Tulane chair and two LSU chairs and Pennington endowed two chairs at Tulane.[120] As Barbara Koppel observed in *The Nation*, this was probably only the tip of the iceberg. "Efforts by journalists and others to get the universities to reveal their funding sources (apart from data about endowed chairs) have been stonewalled: Tulane's status as a private institution allows it to remain silent and although LSU is a public university, it created a private foundation through which it funnels its grants."[121]

Soon after the confrontation between Tulane and the governor, the Environmental Law Clinic's lawyers discovered that Kevin Reilly, the head of Louisiana's Department of Economic Development, had joined with Shintech's public relations firm to compile files on and to investigate several groups that had opposed Shintech, among them the clinic and Greenpeace. Reilly had used state funds to compile an "enemies list," reported the *Times-Picayune*. When accused of using state funds to identify the tax status of one group that opposed the Shintech project, Reilly exclaimed, "You're darned right I looked up their records. . . . I'm going to use every legitimate method at my command to defeat them."[122]

Foster also worked to split the African American community by forging an alliance with the NAACP's state and local branches to persuade them to support Shintech. In August, Ernest Johnson, the head of the state NAACP, went to Convent with the governor to talk to residents about the proposed plant. The next month, Johnson announced that the state branch would remain "neutral" in the dispute, explaining that "the local chapter had endorsed the plant" because in an area with substantial unemployment, the plant promised jobs.[123]

More outrageous was what the Baton Rouge *Advocate* called the "biggest coincidence of the year."[124] It was revealed that the Louisiana Economic Development Corporation had approved a $2.5 million loan for minority businesses to a group headed by Johnson on the very day that he had announced the NAACP's neutrality. Although Governor Foster said that any suggestion of "linkage is really ugly and unpleasant and I'm offended by it," a *Times-Picayune* investigation reported that the state agency had "rejected staff recommendations and waived procedures to approve" the grant.[125]

This seedy attempt by the governor and state officials to promote the chemical industry's interests at any cost and to undermine local opposition to a polluter erupted into a national firestorm in September 1997 following the EPA's decision to deny Shintech air quality permits. Despite dozens of previous petitions from communities around the country, this was "the first time the [Environmental Protection] Agency has granted a citizens' petition for review under Title V of the Clean Air Act." The EPA thus temporarily overruled the state agency[126] by agreeing to consider the charges that Shintech's choice of the largely African American Convent site amounted to environmental racism. Thus the EPA established a precedent for arguing environmental racism as a reason for denying an industry the right to expand. The EPA had previously made clear that environmental justice complaints were to be decided not on the basis of intent to discriminate but on the impact of actions, irrespective of intent. These EPA decisions had flown in the face of a number of Supreme Court decisions from the previous ten years that placed the burden of proof on plaintiffs to show the intention of employers, industries, and others to discriminate.[127]

Industry representatives understood the radical implications of the EPA's action. Shortly after this decision, the *Oil & Gas Journal* stated the industry position quite clearly, complaining in an editorial that "the notion of environmental justice has escaped its jar in the Clinton Administration and flitted into the real world of people and money." It warned that "before an outright infestation develops, someone should find an effective pesticide."[128] Another chemical trade publication argued that the "EPA's approach to weighing environmental justice petitions" amounted to an intrusion on state's rights.[129] Robert Bullard, perhaps the nation's leading scholar of environmental justice, saw the EPA's consideration of the Shintech case as a *Brown vs. Board of Education* for environmentalists.[130] Just as that 1954 Supreme Court decision had laid the ground for desegregation, so this decision by the Carol Browner's EPA made it reasonable for poor, minority communities to expect that they could challenge industry over the issue of environmental racism.

Galvanized by the EPA's decision, the residents of Convent mounted an astounding national campaign to demonstrate to Washington that the country was watching. In addition the campaign further energized the environmental movement. Civil rights leaders like Jesse Jackson and entertainers Bonnie Raitt, Dave Mathews, Michelle Shocked, and Wynton and Branford Marsalis (themselves natives of New Orleans) weighed in on behalf of the community.

As residents awaited the EPA's final ruling, they continued to challenge the state and the governor through public hearings and public protests. In Convent a parade of local, state, and federal officials attended public hearings to demonstrate to the EPA that they were sensitive to the potential impact a new Shintech plant would have on the community's well-being. Members of Congress, including Democratic Senators Paul Wellstone of Minnesota and Carol Mosely-Braun of Illinois and Democratic Representative John Conyers of Michigan, urged the EPA to decide in favor of the community.[131] In Baton Rouge, Greenpeace joined with LEAN to educate residents of the state and urged them to support the Convent struggle. They held demonstrations and unfurled banners from the Capitol.

The combination of protests, legal actions by Tulane's law clinic and community groups, ongoing negative publicity, and the threat of a precedent-making federal action finally caused Shintech in September 1998 to withdraw its plan to build the plant at the Convent site. As a result of Shintech's decision, federal EPA administrators were spared the responsibility of making a potentially explosive decision, the state of Louisiana was spared the opprobrium of the press, and the chemical industry was spared having the EPA intervene to control the activities of one of their industries, which would have meant a significant shift of power from the corporations to the communities.

Convent and the Tulane Law Clinic had won, but it was largely a bittersweet victory. In the end, Shintech simply built a smaller plant across and up the river in Plaquemine, next to a Dow plant that could supply Shintech with materials. Shintech attempted to portray its new plant site as proof that it didn't practice environmental racism. Plaquemine, according to Shintech spokesperson Dick Mason, "has a smaller minority population, lower poverty levels and higher relative income levels than the St. James Parish area."[132] In the words of the *New York Times* headline, Shintech "Evades 'Environmental Racism' Test."[133] But Tulane legal clinic director Robert Kuehn pointed out that the demographic evidence Shintech was offering could "be traced to 1991 when Dow bought out and relocated the predominantly black community of Morrisonville."[134] In other words, the predominantly African American community in question had already been moved out by Dow.

Greenpeace quickly announced that "the battle against Shintech is now shifting to Plaquemine, Louisiana."[135] Within months of the announcement that Plaquemine would be the site of the new plant, residents formed a group called People Reaching Out to Eliminate Shintech's Toxins (PROTEST).[136] Dow had in 1997 released 3.7 percent more air pollutants than it had in 1996[137] and its Plaquemine plant had been the scene of several explosions and major leaks during the 1980s and 1990s. In October 1994 fires at the plant resulted in the release of seven thousand to eight thousand pounds of chlorine into the air, prompting the town to initiate the practice of what they call "Shelter in Place."[138]

This program, used throughout the Louisiana chemical corridor and Lake Charles, ostensibly protects community residents when chemicals are accidentally released from a plant. The program is simple and generally quite ineffective. When sirens from a plant ring and announcements on the radio warn that a release of toxic materials has occurred, residents are supposed to seek shelter indoors and turn off their ventilation systems, if they have them. In Plaquemine, for example, sirens awakened residents in more than four hundred homes at 3:40 AM on October 3, 1994. The Community Alert Network, a telephone alert system, and radio stations warned residents to remain indoors and to close their windows. The River Road, Louisiana 1, was closed for the rest of the day as drifting fumes and the toxic smell of chlorine covered the area.[139] (For many of the poor, whose homes were often little more than shacks, Shelter in Place must have seemed a cruel joke, for their homes were rarely airtight.)

This time, unlike in Convent, the governor sought to head off trouble by meeting with Plaquemine residents.[140] Officials from Shintech also listened to residents' concerns in an effort to appear to be sympathetic and responsive.[141] Still, local protests continued, attracting to Plaquemine activists like Lois Gibbs, who had emerged as a national leader after organizing community residents to protest against Hooker Chemical's dumping of chemicals at Love Canal in Niagara Falls, New York.[142] But the protests at Plaquemine were much diminished by Shintech's success in convincing residents that the company would be a good corporate neighbor. In addition, permits to construct the plant were granted much more quickly than they had been at Convent. Construction began early in 2000.

The case of Shintech raises the question of how a poor, politically powerless African American community managed to triumph over a giant chemical company during an era when appeals to justice had often fallen on deaf ears. In the 1960s civil rights groups and even the federal government were quick to act when blatant racial discrimination was demonstrated. But more recently, citizens who charge discrimination by state governments and industries receive little help from a federal government whose policy is decidedly pro-corporate—encouraging oil exploration, opening up federal lands for mining and logging, and relaxing federal air pollution standards. Yet there is resistance, and the linking of health issues with traditional environmental and labor concerns may be a potent force in stimulating a new, grass-roots opposition to corporate power. What seems to account for the success in Convent, Louisiana, was that the protests of residents were heard and joined by traditional and activist environmental groups, labor activists, lawyers, and some in the federal bureaucracy committed to social justice. This committed coalition exerted its collective power and defeated an incredibly powerful corporation.

SCIENCE AND PRUDENT
PUBLIC POLICY

Environmentalists who might disagree on many issues have been united in their common distrust of chemicals, factories, and new technologies that they believe are radically altering the ecological balance that is the basis for life on this planet. Although such issues rose to new prominence with the debate over global warming, as early as the 1960s and 1970s some of the nation's leading scientists saw in the new chemicals the potential for ecological catastrophe if they were not controlled.[1] These researchers outlined the many ways chemical pollution was wreaking havoc on our environment: fish were being killed off in the Great Lakes and the Hudson River; birds and other animal life were being destroyed; asthma rates were soaring as a result of pollution and urban smog; and cancer and other diseases were proliferating. While these researchers called for a concerted effort to develop better data on the relationship between industrial pollution and disease, they also argued that, in the absence of final proof, the government must step in to protect a fragile environment from a host of man-made insults. In essence, these scientists were calling for a different approach to evaluating environmental danger. As the signers of the Wingspread Statement on the Precautionary Principle put it in January 1998, the principle of precaution should be the overriding policy in environmental matters. Rather than await definitive proof that may never come, society must require a certain degree of confidence in a material's safety before allowing it into the human environment.

Others maintained that there must be convincing scientific proof of danger before policy makers had the right to intrude on the private reserve of industry in America. Conservative intellectuals, in particular, challenged environmentalists' assumptions that there was a causal connection between chemical exposures and the rising epidemic of cancers. For example, Edith

Efron, whose research was funded by the Olin and Pepsico foundations, wrote in her 1984 book, *The Apocalyptics: Cancer and the Big Lie,* that elite scientists had perpetuated a tremendous hoax by claiming that cancer was a product of industrial production. She claimed that science itself had demonstrated exactly the opposite, that there was little or no scientific proof of a link between cancer and exposure to a variety of chemicals. Ideologically driven radical scientists from elite universities had intimidated other scientists, she wrote, and kept them from proclaiming this truth. Conservative intellectuals even argued that there was no reason for government to act because technological innovation combined with a resilient earth would easily absorb any man-made insult.[2]

Another author, Elizabeth Whelan, the president of the American Council on Science and Health, an organization founded in 1978, made virtually the same argument in *Toxic Terror,* published in 1985 and again in 1993. Whelan found "an astounding gap between the consensus in the scientific and medical community on environmental issues versus what was being presented in popular publications, on television and radio and in books" for the layman. She argued that the "extreme environmentalist movement" had needlessly terrorized the public into believing that chemicals were unduly hazardous and called for "Americans to recognize the severity of the gap between science and popular public thought, and the dramatically unpleasant side effects that a continued embracing of environmental alarmism will have for our country." Why, she asked, "are the media so gullible when it comes to swallowing whole the utterances of the doomsayers?" and "why haven't the vast majority of American scientists and physicians come forward publicly in defense of the truth?"[3]

The American Council on Science and Health (ACSH), distinguishing itself from "so-called consumer-advocacy organizations that misrepresent science and distort health priorities," claims to represent "mainstream science, defending the achievements and benefits of responsible technology within America's free-enterprise system."[4] Many understood the organization, which receives financial support from major chemical industries and conservative foundations, to be a front for industry.[5] In "The ACSH: Forefront of Science, or Just a Front?" *Consumer Reports* noted in 1994 that the ACSH received "40 percent of its money from industry, particularly manufacturers in the food processing, beverage, chemical, and pharmaceutical industries, and much of the remainder from industry-sponsored foundations." Major contributors included American Cyanamid, Dow, Exxon, Union Carbide, Monsanto, and Uniroyal Chemical Company, the very companies that had fought against the vinyl chloride standard.

Consumer Reports argued that "sometimes, the council appears more interested in fighting regulation than in promoting good science or health."[6] As Sheldon Rampton and John Stauber noted, with the exception of its opposition to the tobacco industry, the ACSH has denied the relationship between asbestos, Agent Orange, DDT, lead, and chemical food additives and environmental disease.[7]

Some argue that the government should not concentrate on the elusive, ambiguous relationship between chronic illness and long-term exposures to environmental pollution, but should devote its attention and resources to widely accepted links between disease and tobacco, alcohol, poor diet and personal behavior, not industrial activities or policies. They also maintain that it is facile to minimize the question of economic development. In his 1998 book *The Promise and Peril of Environmental Justice*, Christopher Foreman faults environmental activists for failing "to confront the inevitable tradeoffs between economic opportunity and environmental risks." In Foreman's view, "these risks are, in the grand scheme of things, mostly relatively low and manageable." In the case of Convent, Louisiana, Foreman's view is that many of the residents "anxiously awaited construction of a proposed plastics plants, only to see the EPA delay approval as a result of lobbying by an activist coalition that was probably unrepresentative of community sentiment." The most important issue should be economic development, which, if halted by calls for environmental justice, will only "produce its own victimization of minorities."[8]

Citing studies that call into question the validity of the fear of cancer among residents of these river communities, journalist Henry Payne writes that "the idea that a PVC plant is somehow less healthy than other factories illustrates radical environmentalists' exploitation of the regulatory process to oppose industrial development" rather than a statement of scientific validity.[9] Along with conservative and business groups, Payne argues that "people with below average incomes generally live closest to pollution sources"[10] because they chose to take advantage of low rents.

Stephen B. Huebner, the Jeanne and Arthur Ansel Fellow in Environmental Policy at the Center for the Study of American Business at Washington University, for example, tried to explain the close connection between factory sitings, hazardous waste dumps, and poor people's communities by arguing that the poor themselves were at work in creating this concordance: "Economic forces play a role in shaping the racial and economic characteristics of neighborhoods surrounding undesirable facilities. When an industrial facility is sited, property values in the surrounding areas may fall. Over time, relatively wealthy residents may leave the neighborhood, while the relatively poor, for whom it is more costly to leave, may remain. In addition, the increased affordability in housing may create an inflow of new, less affluent residents." Huebner believed that "economic disparities induce minorities to 'move to the nuisance.'" For Huebner, the problem was not that industries choose predominantly poor and black communities to place toxic waste dumps and polluting industries but that the poor themselves make a rational economic decision to seek out these communities because they want to benefit from the low property values there (and, presumably, the unhealthy quality of life).[11] If the federal government intervened and prevented industrial polluters from siting in poor communities, "that outcome could be detrimental to communities seeking the economic benefits [low property values, jobs, and low cost of living] associated with hosting industrial activity, and would hardly be 'just' for the affected residents."[12]

The business community stated the issue even more brazenly, arguing that "poverty makes its sufferers share with cost-conscious industrial developers an affinity for cheap real estate. To elitists, that economic verity comes across as cruel injustice; most poor people probably call it the chance to have work and a place to live."[13]

Not all conservative arguments are as crass as these. Aaron Wildavsky, Julian Morris, and others have argued that there is a danger in being too cautious. While certain technologies that have "serious negative effects and few beneficial effects (the plague and nuclear war are examples), imposing a general prohibition on the use of new technologies until solutions have been found to all their potential harmful side-effects is a recipe for stasis."[14] For many of these authors the recent concerns of environmentalists about the potential impact of new chemicals and new technologies on the environment are exaggerated and have the potential for undermining American industry's long-standing commitment to innovation and progress.

DIFFICULT TO QUANTIFY, EASY TO SMELL

Environmentalists base their arguments on the belief that people's health is more important than the uncertain and uneven impact of economic development. The problem for environmentalists has been that although certain chemicals are toxic, it has often been difficult to show to the satisfaction of government regulators a direct correlation between particular chemicals from smokestacks and sewer pipes and the specific illnesses in clusters of people in particular communities. In situations where low-level exposures are suspected of causing harm among small populations, the small sample size makes it impossible to demonstrate statistical significance. Furthermore, without appropriate controls, specific characteristics such as age, socioeconomic condition, or other personal or community factors can lead to false conclusions if they cannot be measured or are not controlled for. While the suspicions may or may not be correct, any conclusion regarding cause and effect is open to serious criticism.

Common sense and observation leave the public convinced of the link between chemicals and their watering eyes, burning skin, and labored breathing. Francis Adeola, of the University of New Orleans, states, "Unequivocally, a disproportionate exposure of the people of color to hazardous wastes and environmental illnesses in the state of Louisiana constitutes a serious environmental injustice." However, he laments, "the available statistics [data gathered] on the causes of death do not provide enough breakdown to allow a systematic examination of deaths due to toxic wastes and other environmental hazards."[15] In the end the inability of epidemiology, toxicology, and statistics to demonstrate very small effects have been used by conservative critics who fashion the lack of statistical significance into the argument that such effects do not exist.

In her book *Uncertain Hazards,* Sylvia Tesh explains that the central shortcoming of epidemiological studies is their need to focus on an identifiable and measurable entity; for example, researchers can look at cancer incidence but cannot accurately look at the variety of outcomes, such as neurological disorders or reproductive problems, suffered by many of the populations at risk. In the absence of extraordinarily sophisticated and extremely expensive longitudinal studies, there is little chance that any but the most unambiguous and obvious problems will be uncovered.[16] As one physician who studies disease in industrial settings puts it, "I'm usually the last to know when there's an environmental problem. Even then I can only find anything of significance when virtually everyone in a community or a factory already knows the problem exists."[17]

Environmental epidemiologists who work outside the laboratory attempt to study a complex world in which contamination and exposure to toxins can come from a variety of sources, including air, water, or land. Because of the many dynamic relationships between populations and their environments, it is virtually impossible to control the huge number of factors that can account for different lengths (and intensities) of exposure, specific chemicals or chemical mixes, or routes of exposure. "Normal science worries more about false positive errors," explains Peter Van Doren, a political scientist at the University of North Carolina, and this bias "has the inevitable side effect of increasing" the risk of missing real disease. By requiring a 95 percent confidence level of statistical probability of the proof of danger, an inordinate number of studies inaccurately report no danger when in fact danger does exist. "False negatives," he argues, are a real problem for community studies because the conservative nature of statistical analysis decrees such a high threshold of proof that much meaningful evidence is often rejected in favor of the "null hypothesis" of no causal relationship.[18] Traditionally, statisticians would "rather falsely claim no association between variables when there is one than claim an association where it does not exist."[19]

Tesh gives the example of a small city of 100,000 people and the risk of cancer. Since cancer is a fairly common disease and accounts for 20 percent of all deaths nationwide, one might expect that of the average of 872 deaths in the community annually, 175 would be from cancer. If a certain plant spewed an airborne carcinogen that caused 10 extra deaths from cancer, these people would not cause a statistically significant rise in the mortality rate of the city as a whole because "10 extra cancer deaths in that city could not be distinguished from the expected variation. And it would not be statistically significant at the 95 percent confidence level."[20] Tesh's analysis confirms the astuteness of the reaction of the pharmacist in St. Gabriel, Louisiana, Kay Gaudet: "Risk assessment will probably fail to support the claim by members of grass roots environmental groups that their health is endangered by exposure to pollution."[21]

In large measure, conservative analysts have used epidemiological studies to raise doubts about environmentalists' and community residents' fear of industrial pollution. In part, this is because of a difference in the understanding of what constitutes proof of danger. In essence, the conservative arguments rely on a view of science, and of epidemiology in particular, that is overwhelmingly reductionist. It sees the world in mechanistic terms that cannot account for the complexity of interactions and social relationships that determine outcomes in complex systems.[22] But mainstream epidemiology increasingly rejects this reductionist assumption. Scientists such as Kenneth Rothman, Mervyn Susser, Ezra Susser, David Ozonoff, Steve Wing, and Samuel Shapiro are much more sophisticated in their analysis of the role of epidemiology in the uncovering of environmental diseases. They point to the fact that no single study (epidemiological or in any other discipline) is definitive and that no discipline alone can complete the process of proving causality. Rather, it is the accumulation of evidence and the direction of that evidence that shows causality. Even tobacco's relationship to lung cancer was not "proven" by a single study, epidemiological or otherwise. Rather, it was the accretion of epidemiological evidence that leaves few, if anyone, in doubt of the reality of this causal link.

In Louisiana, the inability of Vivien Chen's studies to find harm, even when everyone—professionals and lay people alike—knew there was a problem, undermined public faith in her methodology. Jim Gentry had worked as an environmental lab technician at Dow Chemical in Plaquemine for nineteen years and had sat on the state panel that reviewed the epidemiological design of the miscarriage study conducted in St. Gabriel. He became frustrated by the discrepancy between the results of specific studies, which showed at best a weak association between chemicals and miscarriage, and the seemingly legitimate conclusion drawn from simple observation that there was a link. He asked if the fact that the state study could not statistically demonstrate harm meant that danger did not exist: "When you walk out of the house and the smell almost knocks you down, when your neighbors call and ask you to step outside and see if you can figure out what's in the air, when birds die in the backyard, when you get headaches from the fumes, how do you tell people that there's nothing wrong?"[23]

Much of the pressure on the EPA comes from the fact that the number of Title VI Civil Rights complaints have grown and the EPA knows its tools for establishing harm to minority residents are problematic. It is necessary for the EPA to find "tools that could be used repeatedly with some ease" when communities make claims of environmental racism.[24] When the Office of Civil Rights (OCR) of the EPA receives a complaint based on issues of environmental justice, it has to "determine whether the complaint states a valid claim." If, after review the office accepts the complaint, it investigates to determine "whether the permit at issue will create a disparate impact, or add to the existing disparate impact on a racial or ethnic population."[25] If the EPA finds that the permit creates a disparate impact the state agency that issues the original permit has "the opportunity to rebut the findings, to propose a plan for mitigating a disparate impact, or to justify the impact." If no voluntary solution is found, the OCR can "start procedures to deny, suspend, or terminate funding of the agency."[26]

The problem with this procedure is that the Office of Civil Rights needs "a method of measuring or estimating the difference in the impact [of polluting facilities on] population subgroups."[27] The OCR needs to know if there are substantial differences in the impact of pollution on different groups and whether these differences can be considered harmful to specific populations. Since the determination of such a differential impact greatly affects policy decisions, it has to be based on sound methodology and science that can be subjected to peer review. The case of Convent, Louisiana, is illustrative: the EPA's Scientific Advisory Board set out to evaluate the available methodologies for assessing risk. The first stage used by the EPA in the Shintech case, the Relative Burden Analyses, sought to analyze the average burden per person of toxic emissions released from the smokestacks of factories located in their midst, using the Toxic Release Inventory data gathered during the previous decade. The second methodology, Cumulative Outdoor Toxics Concentration and Exposure Methodology (COATCEM), follows the dispersion of specific toxins and carcinogens from their source to the communities affected and estimates "cumulative cancer risks and non-cancer health effects of the chemicals."[28]

But there are major problems with both methodologies. While the first was seen as "simple, transparent, easy to use and understand," it had fundamental weaknesses that "significantly limit[ed] its utility." The most significant weakness was that all data were collapsed into one pseudo-chemical; no distinction was made between the various chemicals released into the air by a plant in an area. The Science Advisory Board determined that, although the second methodology, COATCEM, had "potential for future use" because it differentiated between chemicals and their relative toxicity, it too had significant weaknesses. It was more expensive and required a greater degree of scientific expertise, making it difficult for community groups and the EPA to use it. While both methodologies were developed to evaluate the threat of air pollution, neither could evaluate the threat to human health posed by polluted drinking water, soil, underground injection sites, or spills. Nor could these methodologies identify the effect of acute, short-term exposures whose health effects could be "significantly higher than the calculated steady state levels." And neither could take into account that "some emitted chemicals are stable while others are reactive" or that some chemicals are released as vapors and some as particles.

Of special concern to the EPA's Science Advisory Board was the fact that both methodologies depended upon the TRI data given to the government by specific companies. "These data are useful but have certain limitations, since they are self-reported by facilities and are often based upon estimates rather than upon monitored emissions." Not all facilities are required to report TRI data to the government nor are all chemicals "emitted from a facility required to be reported." Because even these incomplete and uncorroborated data are averaged over the course of a year, and because toxic releases occur periodically, using annual data could significantly misrepresent exposure levels.[29] In recognition of the weaknesses in the methodologies, the committee made certain recommendations to improve the methodologies—changes in data gathering, reporting, and specificity. But overall the committee was not particularly hopeful about the possibilities for better accuracy.[30]

But new studies of workers exposed to very low levels of vinyl chloride monomer (VCM) provide hope that other branches of science may have something to add to the environmental debates. Dr. Paul Brandt-Rauf of Columbia University and his colleagues reported in 2001 that workers exposed to levels of VCM below the current permissible exposure limits develop "specific mutations in the *ras* oncogene and the p53 tumor suppressor gene." While the impact of this subtle biological change may appear obscure to us today, the authors suggest that biomarkers may prove extremely useful "for monitoring human exposures to occupational and environmental carcinogens." The use of such biomarkers may mean that we may not have to wait for epidemiological proof of the effects of chemicals in terms of human disease, but rather "biomarkers can provide intermediary evidence for potential hazardous (or protective) exposure levels that can enhance risk assessment for occupational and environmental exposures and better inform regulatory decisions."[31] Today our body burden of potentially dangerous endocrine disrupters is haunting a new generation of scientists worried about a host of new subtle mutagenic and teratogenic effects on generations yet unborn.[32]

The issue of evaluating environmental causes of disease becomes even more complex when we ponder the implications of a 2001 Centers for Disease Control (CDC) report that indicates that a host of synthetic materials are now constituents of our bodies whether we live in a polluted region or not. As Clair Patterson demonstrated in the case of lead nearly forty years ago, now the entire earth is covered with synthetic materials that have insinuated themselves into everyone's bodies. While lead was one of few pollutants present in our bodies a half century ago, now phthalates, pesticides, organochlorines, and heavy metals are present as well. The CDC study is expanding and will undoubedly document more and more synthetics in our body tissue. The implications of the presence of these chemicals in our bodies are virtually impossible to fathom, and they make studies looking for health effects even more problematic.

Theo Coburn's *Our Stolen Future* and Joe Thornton's *Pandora's Poison: Chlorine, Health, and a New Environmental Strategy* raise important questions about where we are heading and what we can do to avoid unknown and inestimable problems. They maintain that older paradigms of danger from industrial products centered on the immediate impact and/or the cancer-producing potential of toxins. The synthetic compounds in use today, especially the chlorinated hydrocarbons (of which vinyl is one of the most prevalent) pose a new kind of danger. Although cancer is still of concern, these synthetic chemicals may be causing new classes of disease and damage to the body that are too subtle to even measure. Specific concerns have been raised about the possibility of endocrine disruptions and genetic mutations—leading to neurological and physiological changes that will affect generations to come. Thornton, a research fellow at Columbia University's Center for Environmental Research and Conservation, argues that the organochlorines, like polychlorinated biphenyls (PCBs), can "reduce sperm counts, disrupt female reproductive cycles, cause endometriosis, induce spontaneous abortion, alter sexual behavior, cause birth defects, impair the development and function of the brain, reduce cognitive ability, interfere with the controlled development and growth of body tissues, cause cancer, and compromise immunity."[33]

If this is true, and certainly Thornton makes a powerful argument to support his contention, then the complexity of the problem that scientists and policy makers face is greater than ever. The only prudent course is to adopt a strategy used for pharmaceutical regulation for decades: test materials for safety before they are widely distributed through the environment and avoid mass exposures that may create problems taking decades of suffering to correct. This is certainly the lesson of lead's history. In 1991 the National Research Council's Committee on Environmental Epidemiology acknowledged the dilemma of environmental epidemiology, especially with regard to environmental exposures and the public's health. They found that "insufficient data [were] available for evaluating the impact on public health of exposure to [toxic] substances."[34] The commission opted for caution: "Although the effect on large populations of very low levels of toxic pollutants is unknown, action must be taken now to protect public health in the future."[35]

Such caution is even more important in light of the unfulfilled mission of regulatory agencies such as the EPA to evaluate what can and should be known about the dangers of chemicals in the environment. If the problem were simply that it is impossible to find out the dangers associated with various chemicals, a case might be made for privileging "progress" over precaution. But the EPA is so underfinanced and understaffed that even the most basic evaluations of most new chemicals are not done. According to the EPA, in 1998 only 43 percent of 2,800 chemicals produced in volumes of one million pounds a year or more had basic toxicity data and only 7 percent had a complete set of basic screening level toxicity data.[36]

In March 2001, the CDC's National Center for Environmental Health, under the direction of Richard Jackson, released a study indicating that there has been a remarkable decline in levels of lead in people's blood over the last two decades, since the phasing out of leaded gasoline and the elimination of lead in household paints. The case of lead is an indication of the importance of the precautionary principle in practice. The lead industry assured workers and consumers for decades that lead was safe and was essential to the success of modern industrial America. Yet, Americans have managed to live with dramatic decreases in the use of lead in a variety of products and have seen the benefits of its elimination. Similarly, the chemical industry worked hard to convince people that plastics equaled prosperity and that plastics were safe. It has become clear that lead and plastics have their place in modern culture, but many people argue that the materials do not deserve a special privilege as untouchable and unregulated substances. Several European countries have taken the position that polluting industries should be subject to special taxes, a financial burden that could trigger technological innovation and possibly allow societies to lower taxes in other areas.[37]

Until the late 1990s the critiques of environmentalism focused mostly on local or national disputes. But recently the arguments have taken on international dimensions, especially during and after the debates over the Kyoto Protocol on Global Warming. The international discussions have significantly raised the stakes in what was once a relatively limited debate about how to respond to particular crises like Love Canal or Convent, Louisiana, or specific threats like lead and vinyl. Issues that were once of concern to particular companies and communities are now of concern to multinational corporations and the world.

The Business Roundtable, founded in 1972 as an association representing two hundred of the nation's largest corporations to counter the government's growing regulatory role, has taken an active role in debates concerning environmental pollution. In recent years, the Roundtable has actively opposed the Kyoto Protocol. Its members argue that to delay implementation for developing countries would put the United States at special disadvantage economically, that voluntary efforts to stem the release of greenhouse gases should prevail over mandatory requirements, that the development of new technologies rather than conservation and energy efficiency should be the focus of U.S. efforts. This influential body has argued that there is no imminent crisis and that the long-term nature of global environmental change gives us the opportunity to study the science of global change more closely to be able to arrive at conclusive judgments. "Because climate change is a complex issue which will evolve over many decades," the Business Roundtable asserted in 1996, "no policy commitments should be made until the environmental benefits and economic consequences of global climate change proposals are thoroughly analyzed and reviewed."[38]

Does this mean that policy making should remain paralyzed as we seek to develop more and more information? Or, in George W. Bush's words regarding global warming, do "we need more studies"? Perhaps we need a different approach, one that takes science's uncertainty not as a sign that there is no danger but as a sign that serious danger might well exist. If this approach were taken, we would have a very good policy model, one that emphasizes restraint and caution, rather than unchecked technological advancement, as the principle by which policy should be developed. Such an approach might become ever more important as we contemplate the newer health issues that the chlorine industry presents to us. Perhaps we should consider the admonition of the National Research Council in 1991: "Until better evidence is developed prudent public policy demands that a margin of safety be provided regarding potential health risks. . . . We do no less in designing bridges and buildings. We do no less in establishing criteria for scientific credibility. We must surely do no less when the health and quality of life of Americans are at stake."[39]

CONCLUSION

Over the course of the twentieth century the tension over industry's responsibility for ensuring the safety of workers and the general population has only increased. When Mrs. Emmers wrote to President Roosevelt in 1933 asking for help with her child who was disabled from lead poisoning, she did so with little hope that either industry or the government would respond. In fact, she was informed that the government could do nothing except recommend her to charity.

How different things look today. For one thing, a Mrs. Emmers would not be alone. She would talk to her neighbors, and if they noted a pattern in the health problems of their children they might very well organize themselves to take action. Her husband's union would most likely be attentive to the occurrence of medical problems and would either raise the issue with management or go directly to the Occupational Safety and Health Administration (OSHA) for redress. Mrs. Emmers or the union might enlist help from a local Committee on Occupational Safety and Health (COSH) or from environmental groups, which might in turn lobby for regulations to control the industry responsible for harming her husband and daughter.

A modern-day Mrs. Emmers would probably not be so polite, nor would she assume that industry was on her side. Like Mrs. West, Mrs. Melancon, and Mrs. Roberts of Convent, Louisiana, she would know from the history of the last century that industry could not be trusted with her family's health and safety. She would have read or heard news about the activities of the asbestos and tobacco industries and the Ford and Firestone companies, which, in pursuing their own financial interests were negligent about the health and safety of workers and consumers. Knowing about Love Canal, Three Mile Island, and Bhopal, she and her neighbors who were poor and (more likely than not) African American or Hispanic would be suspicious of any large industry moving next door and wonder why the company had chosen their community. As a citizen and voter, she would be familiar with terms like "global warming," "environmental impact" and "toxic wastes" and would be aware of protests by environmental groups worried about industry's effect on the environment or even the globe.

The history of the lead and vinyl industries gives us a window into why the relationship between industry and the public is so strained today. These industries responded to potent evidence of the danger of their products by hiding information, controlling research, continuing to market their products as safe when they were known to be dangerous, enlisting industrywide groups to participate in denying that there was a problem, and attempting to influence the political process in order to avoid regulation. There are those who find the actions of the lead and vinyl industries so egregious as to constitute a subversion of democracy. They believe that by promoting secrecy, interfering with scientific research and thereby inhibiting the free exchange of ideas, by buying the loyalty of elected officials with donations to political action committees and with soft money contributions, by threatening economic abandonment and unemployment if communities insist upon safety and health regulations, these industries posed a serious threat to political democracy in the United States.

The question is this: How representative are lead and vinyl of general corporate behavior? Some would argue these are rogue industries, atypical of the general business culture. But this itself would be an article of faith, not fact, since neither the public nor the academic community has the opportunity to review the internal histories of most other American corporations. At the present time industries are not required to make internal corporate or trade association documents available to the public. These documents, which help the public understand what information industry possessed on particular toxins and what actions industry took in regard to those toxins, generally enter the public record by way of lawsuits. In the case of lead, lawsuits by lead-poisoned children, states, and municipalities against the lead industry have made such documents available. In the case of vinyl, lawsuits by poisoned workers against some of the largest chemical and petrochemical companies in the world have led to the discovery of documents that show lying, manipulation of government officials, and secrecy as tools used by industry to protect its product. What emerges is a history of deceit that is strikingly similar to that of the asbestos and tobacco industries. As with asbestos and tobacco, the lead and vinyl industries knew of dangers from their products but chose to ignore or conceal them. In fact, they actively deceived the public about the safety of their products. While we may not yet know the actions of all industries with regard to industrial toxins, by now we do know that at least four or more major industries engaged in very similar activities to keep information from the public and to prevent regulation of products that they knew to be dangerous.

Society is now holding corporations to new standards of ethical behavior. The National Consumers League first began putting its consumer safety label on products and *Good Housekeeping* magazine began using its "Seal of Approval" back in the Progressive era. The dramatic expansion of a consumer economy and the simultaneous creation of consumer groups brought to the fore the obligations of industries to the public. National legislation, as well as local ordinances, sought to protect consumers from adulterated food, impure drugs, and the like as early as 1906. In the 1910s and the 1920s, legislators argued over the need to protect consumers from industries that acted negligently or irresponsibly.

There is no question but that industry has had a moral and ethical obligation to protect consumers for at least a century. Similarly, industry has had an obligation to its workforce. The massive industrialization that transformed the cities of the nation created a heightened awareness of the dangers of the new society that was increasingly seen as threatening and dangerous. By the early decades of the century, industry itself acknowledged this transformation by organizing its own National Safety Council, whose "Safety First" motto became synonymous with good corporate citizenship by the 1920s. Warnings about danger in the industrial setting and the reorganization of work and the introduction of safety equipment all spoke to this radical reorientation that shifted responsibility for accidents from the worker to the employer. Simultaneously, state after state passed workers' compensation statutes that also acknowledged the obligations of industries to protect their workforce. In this light, no one today can argue that the actions of the tobacco industry and the asbestos manufacturers decades ago in hiding dangers of their product from the public were moral.

Whatever the ethical history of industry may have been, the fact remains that the general public, given what they have learned of industrial disasters and harm to workers and populations resulting from industry inaction, feel suspicious of industry and more hesitant than ever to allow industry total responsibility for their health. All over the world the struggle between industry and the public over responsibility for the public's health is being played out. In Hudson, New York, a cement company's proposal to build a plant on the Hudson River—where General Electric dumped PCBs a generation ago—has met serious opposition from the community, which is concerned about the health and environmental effects of such a plant. In the working-class neighborhood of Mossville in Lake Charles, Louisiana, African American residents have organized to challenge the assurances of the plastics and petrochemical companies that the chemicals used in their plants will cause no harm. In San Diego, California, and Tijuana, Mexico, Anglo and Hispanic environmental activists have joined forces across the border to stop the dumping of toxic materials in Mexico.

As we have seen in the history of lead and vinyl, residents who were worried about harm from industrial toxins generally began by taking their grievances to the company. When they felt that an industry was neither providing them with sufficient information nor addressing the conditions that were harming workers and community residents, they often began to push for regulation of the industry. It was at this point, sensing the possibility of government regulation, that the industry generally got behind voluntary compliance as the best way to "regulate" industry.

The first government responses to grievances in regard to industrial pollution occurred on the local and state levels. In these instances the government acted less like a policeman and more like a partner interested in working cooperatively with industry through organizations like the National Safety Council and the American Conference of Governmental Industrial Hygienists. But as it became clear that state, local, and voluntary efforts were inadequate to cope with the massive environmental and occupational health problems that emerged after World War II and as the movement for government regulation heated up, federal agencies like the Occupational Safety and Health Administration (OSHA), the National Institute for Occupational Safety and Health (NIOSH), the Environmental Protection Agency (EPA), and the Consumer Product Safety Commission (CPSC) were established. These agencies were significant not only for what they actually did to protect the public and the workforce, but even more for the fact that they lent legitimacy to the work of researchers outside industry, establishing the principle that industry must not be solely responsible for sponsoring the research and considering the data. They provided a generation of students in medical and public health schools with employment outside industry, and they began investigating issues once considered the preserve of the laboratories of the chemical, auto, and lead industries.

In the mid-1970s, confronted by increased regulation and greater opposition from activist communities, industry formulated new strategies to regain the upper hand and to prevent further regulation of its activities. Through trade associations, political lobbying, and contributions to political action committees, industry sought to influence legislators and rein in federal agency administrators. The most powerful CEOs established industrywide organizations like the Business Roundtable, while smaller businesses relocated their trade associations to Washington to represent industry's position at the highest levels of government. At the same time, they contributed large sums of money to defeat the political candidates who were most dangerous to them. As a result, the business community from the late 1970s through the 1990s was very successful in neutralizing the demands of the national organizations of consumers, environmentalists, and labor that had proven so troublesome in the 1960s and 1970s.

Such actions by the business community convinced many people that regulation is susceptible to pressure from politicians. No longer was the task of activists to push for legislation; the issue became one of who controls the legislators. There is no more telling example of industry's power to affect the legislative process than the election of George W. Bush. Immediately upon taking office in 2001, Bush, known to be a friend to industry, appointed Gale Norton to head the Department of the Interior. Norton, a former lobbyist for NL Industries, the modern incarnation of National Lead, was quick to claim that the lead industry had first learned of the dangers of its product to children in the 1940s and had acted immediately to remove lead from paint, when in fact industry documents indicate that they had known more than twenty years earlier that their product was killing children. Bush quickly reversed President Bill Clinton's adoption of the OSHA ergonomic standard, suspended the reduction of the arsenic standard for drinking water, and promoted oil exploration in a part of Alaska's protected wilderness. Bush also announced that the United States would not sign the Kyoto Protocol on Global Warming, claiming that "more research" needed to be done. Even in the wake of the September 11 attacks, the Bush administration acted to restrict public access to information about polluting industries and restricted journalists' and historians' access to government documents previously available through the Freedom of Information Act.

Americans, who are generally not of one mind when it comes to the question of regulation, nevertheless express widespread support for protection of the environment, that is, people's health and the nation's ecology. But as recent events regarding Enron have shown, an American public interested in regulation may be governed by an administration very much in alliance with industry and therefore not interested in regulation.

For this reason many people are concluding that they cannot count on government for protection and are turning to the courts as the arena through which to seek redress of their grievances.

National policy is increasingly worked out through liability suits, class action suits, and civil actions brought by individuals, groups of injured persons, and state attorneys general. In addition, the enormous victories of the asbestos plaintiffs in the 1980s suits against Johns Manville and the joint action brought by state attorneys general against the tobacco industry began to shift the balance of power. In the past, plaintiffs in liability lawsuits were at a distinct disadvantage in civil court because they had so little money compared to the huge corporations, which hired giant law firms, engaged an army of expert witnesses, and invested in legal and other research. Since the victories of plaintiffs in the asbestos litigation and the recent tobacco settlements, plaintiffs' law firms are, for the first time in history, as big as, and in many cases even bigger than, industry defense firms and can therefore devote the resources to do the research, and to mobilize the army of lawyers and experts necessary to prepare cases adequately. Recently, cities like New York, Chicago, Milwaukee, St. Louis, and San Francisco have engaged major firms to sue the lead industry for the injury to individual clients, while states have sued to recover the costs of special education programs, hospital costs, costs for detoxifying children's housing, and the like. The state of Rhode Island recently won a major victory when a judge ruled that a conspiracy case it had brought against the lead industry could go forward.

The issues that emerged in the lead and vinyl story continue to be important as we debate the future of the nation and of the planet. How should we deal with the industries' secrecy about the harmful effects of their products? Will legislation that requires industries to reveal their products' danger be sufficient to protect consumers? Like drug manufacturers, should industries regularly warn us of their products' potential harm? Should industries be allowed to simply export their poisonous manufacturing processes to less developed countries with few environmental regulations?

The international, even global, aspects of pollution have forced a reevaluation of the methods that Americans have used to control pollution. In the past, the "exportation" of polluting production plants to Mexico, Thailand, and other countries was largely overlooked by a complacent population enjoying low-cost clothing made from synthetic fibers manufactured overseas. Similarly, exporting dangerous materials banned at home, like DDT and tetraethyl lead, to other countries has outgrown its former status as an ethical dilemma. With today's new awareness of the global impact of pollutants, whether in the United States or in Southeast Asia, exporting pollution has begun to transcend job loss or morality. The stakes have been raised, both for society and individual corporations. At the turn of the twenty-first century, Italian magistrates have brought criminal charges against twenty-seven managers of Italian chemical companies for ignoring and hiding information that led to the deaths of vinyl chloride workers and the discharge of dangerous toxins that led to pollution of the Venice lagoon and possible endangerment of the health of surrounding communities.

What can we learn from this history? Perhaps most importantly, we can recognize that it is absolutely essential to have as much openness and free access to information as possible. Without such information Americans are dependent upon the limited and sometimes inaccurate information given to them by companies. And it is ever foolish to forget that industry's first obligation is to its shareholders, and that all too often industry values secrecy over openness if only out of jealous protection of its competitive position. But when it comes to public health, the society has a right to insist that the community's interests come before the shareholders' profits. It is not enough for industry to tout the benefits of its products; it must also inform people of their potential dangers.

This is not a radical proposal. This is already common practice in the advertisements of pharmaceuticals and many household cleansers. But the requirement that companies include warning labels or inserts on products that contain dangerous materials is not sufficient. Far too little money is spent by industry, itself or by independent scientists, to evaluate the seventy thousand chemicals that are currently in wide commercial use. Further, we must remember the warnings of Drs. Linda Rosenstock (former head of NIOSH) and Marcia Angell (editor of the *New England Journal of Medicine*), who bring our attention to the insidious ways that industry affects the institutions that are meant to independently evaluate the toxicity of new products.

The issues of global warming and the subtle impact of numerous chemicals on our bodies force us to confront the limitations of our traditional tools for evaluating danger. Preventing endocrine disruption and subtle neurological change demands a level of precaution as sophisticated as that required to make sure that our milk is untainted, our meat uncontaminated with bacteria, and our grains not covered with deadly pesticides. As history has proven, science is often unable to give us the knowledge we need. Some have called for better science before judging a chemical

hazardous. But as Dr. Philip Landrigan has observed, what "often constitutes lovely science...frequently constitutes very poor public health
because it delays for many years the enactment of good health protective
regulations."[1]

We may never know the true extent of the damage lead, vinyl, and
countless other chemicals have done to our society, not to mention the
damage that trade associations have done to our democratic institutions.
Nor will it ever be possible to evaluate the lost potential of individuals
whose intelligence has been slightly lowered, whose behavior has become
a bit more erratic, whose personalities have been altered in ways impercep-
tible to scientific measurement. We will never know the social, economic,
and personal costs to society from the lost potential of our citizens.

NOTES

INTRODUCTION

1. Emmers is a pseudonym. See: A. W. M. to President Roosevelt (November 8, 1933), National Archives Record Group (NARG) 102, Records of the Children's Bureau, Central File, 1933–36, File: Diseases Due to Metallic, 4–5–17.

2. Marcia Angell, "Is Academic Medicine for Sale?" *New England Journal of Medicine* 342 (May 18, 2000), 1517.

3. Linda Rosenstock, "Global Threats to Science: Policy, Politics, and Special Interests," in A. Grieco, S. Iavicoli, and G. Berlinguer, eds., *Contributions to the History of Occupational and Environmental Prevention* (London: Elsevier Science, B.V., 1999), 113. See also Linda Rosenstock and Lore Jackson Lee, "Attack on Science: The Risks to Evidence-Based Policy," *American Journal of Public Health* 92 (January 2002), 14–18.

4. Ibid., 112.

5. Ibid., 111, 113.

6. "Talks Agree on Global Ban on 12 Very Toxic Chemicals," *New York Times* (December 11, 2000), Section A, 16.

CHAPTER 1. THE HOUSE OF THE BUTTERFLIES

1. David Rosner and Gerald Markowitz, "The Early Movement for Occupational Safety and Health, 1900–1917," in Judith Walzer Leavitt and Ronald Numbers, eds., *Sickness and Health in America: Readings in the History of Medicine and Public Health* (Madison: University of Wisconsin Press, 1985), 507–21.

2. Arthur B. Reeve, "The Death Roll of Industry," *Charities and the Commons* 17 (February 1907), 791.

3. Alice Hamilton, M.D., "Industrial Diseases, with Special Reference to the Trade in Which Women Are Employed," *Charities and the Commons* 20 (September 5, 1908), 655, 658.

4. See Allison L. Hepler, *Women in Labor: Mothers, Medicine and Occupational Health in the United States, 1890–1980* (Columbus: Ohio State University Press, 2000), 36–37.

5. Thomas Oliver, "Lead Poisoning and the Race," *British Medical Journal* 2 (October 28, 1911), 1096–98.

6. Thomas M. Legge and Kenneth W. Goadby, *Lead Poisoning and Absorption* (New York: Longman's, Green and Co., 1912), 35.

7. Alice Hamilton, "Lead Poisoning in Illinois," in American Association for Labor Legislation, *First National Conference on Industrial Diseases,* Chicago, June 10, 1910 (New York: AALL, 1910), 29, 33. See also Alice Hamilton, "The White-Lead Industry in the United States," U.S. Bureau of Labor, *Bulletin No. 23* (Washington: GPO, 1911), 189–223 for discussion of the widespread prevalence of lead poisoning among workers in the white lead industry.

8. Alice Hamilton, "Lead-Poisoning in Illinois," *Journal of the American Medical Association* (hereafter *JAMA*) 56 (April 29, 1911), 1240–44.

9. Alice Hamilton, "Hygiene of Lead Industry," Address to Meeting of Superintendents, National Lead Company, Chicago (December 7, 1910), 10, Alice Hamilton Papers, A-22, no. 29, Schlesinger Library, Radcliffe College.

10. Alice Hamilton, "The White-Lead Industry in the United States, with an Appendix on the Lead-Oxide Industry," in U.S. Bureau of Labor, *Bulletin No. 95* (Washington: GPO, July 1911), 191.

11. Alice Hamilton to Mr. Verrill (February 12, 1913), Alice Hamilton Papers, A-22, no. 29, Schlesinger Library, Radcliffe College.

12. Alice Hamilton, "Recent Changes in the Painters Trade," in U.S. Department of Labor, Division of Labor Standards, *Bulletin No. 7* (Washington: GPO, 1936), 27.

13. Alice Hamilton, "Hygiene of the Painters' Trade," in U.S. Bureau of Labor Statistics, *Bulletin No. 120,* Industrial Accidents and Hygiene Series No. 2 (Washington: GPO, May 13, 1913), 65.

14. Ibid., 66.

15. U.S. Congress, House, Interstate and Foreign Commerce Committee, *Hearings on H.R. 21901,* 61 Cong., 2 sess. (May 31, 1910), 20.

16. See, for example, Alice Hamilton, "Leadless Glaze: What It Means to Pottery and Tile Workers," *The Survey* 31 (October 4, 1913), 22–26; Alice Hamilton, "Lead Poisoning in the Smelting and Refining of Lead," U.S. Department of Labor, Bureau of Labor Statistics, *Bulletin No. 141,* Industrial Accidents and Hygiene Series No. 4, February 17, 1914 (Washington: GPO, 1914); Alice Hamilton, "Lead Poisoning in the Manufacture of Storage Batteries," U.S. Department of Labor, Bureau of Labor Statistics, *Bulletin No. 165* (Washington: GPO, December 15, 1914); "Precautions Necessary to Safeguard the Health of Printers," *Monthly Labor Review* 1 (December 1915), 22: "Do not eat food.... While at work unless your hands are first carefully washed, because of the danger of getting lead into the mouth"; "Industrial Diseases in New Jersey," *Monthly Labor Review* 3 (November 1916), 643–44; "Prevention of Lead Poisoning in the Manufacture of Storage Batteries," *American Journal*

of Public Health 9 (November 1919), 905; Alice Hamilton, "Women in the Lead Industries," U.S. Department of Labor, Bureau of Labor Statistics, *Bulletin No. 253* (Washington: GPO, February 1919); Alice Hamilton, "Lead Poisoning in the United States," *American Journal of Public Health* 4 (June 1914), 477–80; Alice Hamilton, "Industrial Lead-Poisoning in the Light of Recent Studies," *JAMA* 59 (September 7, 1912), 777–82.

17. Gordon Thayer, "The Lead Menace," *Everybody's* 28 (March 1913), 325.

18. [Summary on Factory Commission Report], *The Survey* 29 (November 23, 1912), 229.

19. Alice Hamilton, "Lead Poisoning in American Industry," *Journal of Industrial Hygiene* 1 (May 1919), 12–13.

20. National Lead Company, Annual Report (December 31, 1912), 7, Lead Industries Association, hereafter LIA Papers.

21. Ibid., 9.

22. Mr. F. V. Hammar, President of Hammar Brothers White-Lead Company, East St. Louis, Illinois, "Discussion of Edward Ewing Pratt, Lead Poisoning in New York City," *American Labor Legislation Review* 2 (June 1912), 282.

23. Henry A. Gardner, "The Toxic and Antiseptic Properties of Paints," Bulletin No. 41 of the Educational Bureau of the Paint Manufacturers' Association, 1914, p. 12 reprinted in *Paint Researches and Their Practical Application* (Washington: Judd and Detweiler, 1917).

24. George B. Heckel, *The Paint Industry: Reminiscences and Comments* (St. Louis: American Paint Journal Company, 1928), 6–7. He argues elsewhere, "The history of zinc oxide as a pigment is unique. Its substitution as a non-poisonous pigment for white lead, was proposed in France and other European countries, during the last half of the eighteenth century." It was first produced by the New Jersey Zinc Company in the 1850s. See G. B. Heckel, "Zinc Oxide in the Paint Industry," *Drugs, Oils and Paints* 35 (November 1919), 212.

25. R. M. Hutton, *Lead Poisoning: A Compilation of Present Knowledge* (Toronto: Provincial Board of Health of Ontario, 1923), 59.

26. Edward Ewing Pratt, "Occupational Diseases, a Preliminary Report on Lead Poisoning in the City of New York" in New York [State], Factory Investigating Commission, *Preliminary Report of the Factory Investigating Commission* (Albany: Argus Co., 1912), 375.

27. Ibid. See also Thomas Oliver, *Lead Poisoning: From the Industrial, Medical, and Social Points of View* (New York: Paul B. Hoeber, 1914); F. L. Hoffman, *Lead-Poisoning Legislation and Statistics* (Newark: Prudential Insurance of America, 1933); International Labour Office, *White Lead: Data Collected by the International Labour Office in Regard to the Use of White Lead in the Painting Industry*, Studies and Reports, Series F, Industrial Hygiene, No. 11 (Geneva, 1927); ILO, Legislative Series, 1922, 1926, 1927, 1931, 1934.

28. "Prohibition of White Lead in Belgium," *American Journal of Public Health* 13 (April 1923), 337: The pigment and paint manufacturers watched

these events with concern, noting that it was not just the Europeans who were acting but Argentina and Chile as well. "The present tendency is towards the internationalization of the white lead question, in that it is proposed absolutely to prohibit the use of white lead for painting in all countries; such interdiction to be affected by international convention after the manner of that of January 26, 1906, prohibiting the use of white (yellow) phosphorous in the match industry."

29. "White Lead in Outside Paints Limited to 2%," *Drugs, Oils and Paints* 37 (December 1921), 249.

30. "Health Conditions in the Painting Industry," *American Journal of Public Health* 14 (September 1924), 804. See also W. H. Rand, "Occupational Lead Poisoning," *Monthly Labor Review* 12 (February 1921), 135–47.

31. International Labour Office, *White Lead* (Geneva, 1927), 30.

32. Workers Health Bureau, *Dangerous Work Materials Cause Occupational Diseases* (pamphlet) (1924). See David Rosner and Gerald Markowitz, "Safety and Health as a Class Issue: The Workers' Health Bureau of America During the 1920s," in David Rosner and Gerald Markowitz, eds., *Dying for Work: Workers' Safety and Health in Twentieth Century America* (Bloomington: Indiana University Press, 1987), 53–64.

33. *Drugs, Oils and Paints* 39 (February 1924), 334.

34. "Health Safeguards for Painter," *Drugs, Oils and Paints* 39 (April 1924), 399–400.

35. C. O. Sappington, "The Prevalence of Lead Poisoning," *National Safety News* 20 (September 1929), 70.

36. Benjamin Joachim, *Lithopone in Paint Formulation* (pamphlet) (1931), 3.

37. William Kovarik, "Henry Ford, Charles Kettering and the 'Fuel of the Future,'" *Automotive History Review* (Spring 1998); Hal Bernston, William Kovarik, and Scott Scklar, *The Forbidden Fuel: Power Alcohol in the Twentieth Century* (New York: Boyd Griffin, 1982); and Kovarik's Web site: <http://www.radford.edu/~wkovarik/lead>.

38. Kovarik, "Henry Ford, Charles Kettering and the 'Fuel of the Future'; Alan P. Loeb, "Birth of the Kettering Doctrine: Fordism, Sloanism and the Discovery of Tetraethyl Lead," *Business and Economic History* 24 (Fall 1995), 72–87. Much of this argument first appeared in David Rosner and Gerald Markowitz, "'Gift of God'? The Public Health Controversy over Leaded Gasoline during the 1920s," *American Journal of Public Health* 75 (April 1985), 344–52. Others have built on this work. See Jamie Kitman, "The Secret History of Lead," *Nation* (March 20, 2000).

39. Joseph C. Robert, *Ethyl: A History of the Corporation and the People Who Made It* (Charlottesville, VA: University of Virginia Press, 1983).

40. William Mansfield Clark to Assistant Surgeon General A. M. Stimson (through Acting Director, Hygienic Laboratory), memorandum (October 11, 1922), National Archives, Record Group 90 (hereafter referred to as NARG 90), U.S. Public Health Service (hereafter USPHS); N. Roberts to Surgeon

General (November 13, 1922), National Archives, Record Group 443 (hereafter NARG 443), National Institutes of Health, General Records, 0425T Box 23 for further statements on the fears of tetraethyl lead contamination.

41. A. M. Stimson to R. N. Dyer (October 13, 1922), NARG 90; Dyer to Surgeon General (October 18, 1922), NARG 90.

42. G. W. McCoy to Surgeon General, memorandum (November 23, 1922), NARG 90.

43. H. S. Cumming to P. S. DuPont (December 20, 1922), NARG 90; Thomas Midgley Jr. to Cumming (December 30, 1922), NARG 90.

44. A. C. Fieldner to Dr. H. Foster Bain (September 24, 1923), National Archives, Record Group 70 (hereafter NARG 70), 101869, File 725.

45. S. C. Lind, Chief Chemist, to Superintendent Fieldner, Pittsburgh (November 3, 1923), NARG 70, 101869, File 725; Reply, A. C. Fieldner to Lind (November 5, 1923), NARG 70, 101869, File 725.

46. A. C. Fieldner to Dr. H. Foster Bain (September 24, 1923), NARG 70, Bureau of Mines, 101869, File 725.

47. Agreement between the Department of Interior and General Motors Chemical Company, Dayton, Ohio, NARG 70, 101869, File 725.

48. C. A. Straw to R. R. Sayers (August 22, 1924), NARG 70, 101869, File 725.

49. Graham Edgar to Dr. Paul Nicholas Leech (July 18, 1924), NARG 70, 101869, File 725.

50. Yandell Henderson to R. R. Sayers (September 27, 1924), NARG 70, 101869, File 725. He continued that he felt "very strongly that there is the most urgent need for an absolutely unbiased investigation."

51. C. W. Deppe to Hubert Work (October 31, 1924), NARG 70, 101869, File 775.

52. "Odd Gas Kills One, Makes Four Insane," *New York Times* (October 27, 1924), 1; "Gas Madness Stalks Plant," *New York World* (October 27, 1924), 1, 6: "When M. D. Mann, head of the research department . . . was asked . . . he denied the men had been affected by the gas."

53. Ibid. New York State Department of Health, "Health News" (February 2, 1925), NARG 90, General Files, 1924–1935, 1340–216, Tetraethyl Lead; *New York Times* (October 31, 1924), 1; *New York World* (October 31, 1924), 1; "No Peril to Public Seen in Ethyl Gas," *New York Times* (November 1, 1924), 1.

54. Roland Marchand, *Creating the Corporate Soul: The Rise of Public Relations in Corporate Imagery in American Big Business* (Berkeley and Los Angeles: University of California Press, 1998), 7–8.

55. *New York Times* (October 28, 1924), 1.

56. *New York Times* (October 31, 1924), 15.

57. *New York World* (October 29, 1924), 1.

58. *New York Times* (October 30, 1924), 1.

59. *New York Times* (October 31, 1924), 1.

60. *New York Times* (November 1, 1924), 1.

61. E. E. Free to R. R. Sayers (October 21, 1924), NARG 70, 5445, File 437; R. R. Sayers et al., "Exhaust Gases from Engines Using Ethyl Gasoline," NARG 443, General Records, 0425T.

62. C. K. Drinker to R. R. Sayers (January 12, 1925), NARG 70, 101869, File 725; Sayers to Drinker (January 15, 1925), NARG 70, 101869, File 725; Drinker to Sayers (January 19, 1925), NARG 70, 101869, File 725.

63. A. Hamilton to Surgeon General Cumming (February 12, 1925), NARG 90, General Files, 1924–1935, 1340–216, Tetraethyl Lead.

64. E. Hayhurst to Sayers (September 29, 1924), NARG 70, 101869, File 725, in which he identifies himself as "Consultant to Ethyl Gasoline Corporation."

65. Hayhurst to William P. Yant, Bureau of Mines (October 4, 1924), NARG 70, 101869, File 725.

66. Hayhurst to Sayers (February 7, 1925), NARG 70, 101869, File 725; Sayers to Hayhurst (February 13, 1925), NARG 70, 101869, File 725; Hayhurst to Sayers (February 13, 1925), NARG 70, 101869, File 725; C.-E. A. Winslow, "The Workers' Health Bureau Report on the Hazards Involved in the Manufacture, Distribution and Sale of Tetra-Ethyl Lead" (April 1925), Winslow manuscripts, Yale University, Box 102, Folder 1838.

67. "Ethyl Gasoline" (editorial), *American Journal of Public Health* 15 (1925), 239–40.

68. *New York Times* (October 30, 1924), 1; C.-E. A. Winslow "The Workers' Health Bureau Report on the Hazards Involved in the Manufacture, Distribution and Sale of Tetra-Ethyl Lead" (April 1925), manuscript, Winslow mss., Box 102, Folder 1838.

69. *New York Times* (June 22, 1925), 3. The *Times* reported that eight workers had died in the Deepwater plant.

70. Haven Emerson to Cumming (February 9, 1925), NARG 90, General Files, 1924–1935, 1340–216, Tetraethyl Lead.

71. *New York World* (May 1, 1925), 1.

72. Ibid.

73. U.S. Public Health Service, "Proceedings of a Conference to Determine Whether or Not There Is a Public Health Question in the Manufacture, Distribution or Use of Tetraethyl Lead Gasoline," in *Public Health Bulletin No. 158* (Washington: GPO, 1925), 62.

74. Ibid., 4, 69, 105–07.

75. *New York Times* (May 7, 1925); *New York Times* (October 28, 1924); "Sober Facts about Tetra-ethyl Lead," *Literary Digest* 83 (1924), 25–26.

76. *New York Times* (October 28, 1924); USPHS, *Bulletin No. 158* (Washington: GPO), 12; *New York World* (May 9, 1925); see also *New York Times* (November 27, 1924), 14, for this statement by the American Chemical Society: "Perhaps the greatest hazard is the indifference which not only workmen but even chemists come to have for dangerous work with which they are familiar."

77. USPHS, *Bulletin No. 158*, 62; *New York Times* (April 22, 1925); Henderson to Sayers (January 20, 1925), NARG 70, 101869, File 725.

78. USPHS, *Bulletin No. 158*, 60, 109; "American Federation of Labor's Concern," *American Federationist* 30 (August 1923), 632–33.

79. USPHS, *Bulletin No. 158*, 108, 96.

80. Ibid., 98.

81. Alice Hamilton, "What Price Safety, Tetraethyl Lead Reveals a Flaw in Our Defenses," *The Survey Mid-Monthly* 54 (June 15, 1925), 333–34.

82. USPHS, *Bulletin No. 158*, 86–87, 91; "Perils and Benefits of Ethyl Gas," *Literary Digest* 85 (1925), 17; J. H. Shrader, "Tetra-ethyl Lead and the Public Health," *American Journal of Public Health* 15 (1925), 213–14.

83. Flinn to Sayers (May 11, 1925), NARG 70, 101869, File 725.

84. Hayhurst to Sayers (May 14, 1925), NARG 70, 101869, File 725.

85. Alice Hamilton, "What Price Safety, Tetraethyl Lead Reveals a Flaw in Our Defenses," *The Survey Mid-Monthly* 54 (June 15, 1925), 333.

86. For further elaboration of the committee members' positions, see "Conference of Tetraethyl Lead," *Automotive Industries* 52 (May 7, 1925), 835; "Tetraethyl Lead Sales Are Suspended," *National Petroleum News* (May 27, 1925); 17–37; "Ethyl Gasoline Given Clean Bill Thus Far" (editorial), *American Journal of Public Health* 16 (1926), 295–96.

87. *New York Times* (January 20, 1926), 13. For a copy of this report, see Treasury Department, USPHS, "The Use of Tetraethyl Lead Gasoline in Its Relation to Public Health" in *Public Health Bulletin No. 163* (Washington: GPO, 1926); Winslow's handwritten comments on the draft of the committee's report: He wanted a specific statement that "a more extensive study was not possible in view of the limited time allowed to the committee." Winslow MSS, Box 101, Folder 1805, Yale University. See also other committee members' responses on the draft. Winslow MSS, Box 101, Folder 1805, Yale University, Folders 1800 and 1801.

88. Kehoe et al., *A Study of the Health Hazards Associated with the Distribution and Use of Ethyl Gasoline* (April 1928), from the Eichberg Laboratory of Physiology, University of Cincinnati, Cincinnati, OH, NARG 70, 101869, File 725.

CHAPTER 2: A CHILD LIVES IN A LEAD WORLD

1. The early trade journal aimed at the nascent paint industry was founded in the 1880s and was called *Drugs, Oils and Paints*.

2. Quoted in Teresa Osterman Green, "The Birth of the American Paint Industry" (master's thesis, University of Delaware, 1965), 71.

3. Oliver Zunz, *The Changing Face of Inequality: Urbanization, Industrial Development, and Immigrants in Detroit, 1880–1920* (Chicago: University of Chicago Press, 1982), 161, quoted in Margaret Garb, "Building the American Dream: A History of Home Ownership and Housing Reform, Chicago, 1871–1919" (Ph.D. diss., Columbia University, 2000), 4.

4. Margaret Garb, "Building the American Dream."

5. Kenneth T. Jackson, *Crabgrass Frontier: The Suburbanization of the United States* (New York: Oxford University Press, 1985), 175.

6. Margaret Garb, "Building the American Dream," 8.

7. Because relatively little lead leached from lead pipes or lead solder into the water supply, lead pigments emerged as the primary source of childhood lead poisoning.

8. Garb, "Building the American Dream," 177.

9. Ruth Schwartz Cowan, *More Work for Mother: The Ironies of Household Technology from the Open Hearth to the Microwave* (New York: Basic Books, 1983), 69–101.

10. "A Living Room Decorated in Lead and Oil," *Dutch Boy Painter* 3 (1910), 27.

11. Douglas Knerr, *Eagle-Picher Industries: Strategies for Survival in the Industrial Marketplace, 1840–1980* (Columbus: Ohio State University Press, 1992), 18–19.

12. Ibid.

13. Christian Warren, *Brush with Death: A Social History of Lead Poisoning* (Baltimore: The Johns Hopkins University Press, 2000), 46. Douglas Knerr, *Eagle-Picher Industries*.

14. Hans Thorelli, *The Federal Anti-Trust Policy: Organization of an American Tradition* (Stockholm, 1954), 79, quoted in Douglas Knerr, *Eagle-Picher Industries*, 33.

15. Douglas Knerr, *Eagle-Picher Industries*, 33.

16. Warren, *Brush with Death*, 46.

17. Knerr, *Eagle-Picher*, 36.

18. Ibid., 2.

19. Charles R. King, *Children's Health in America: A History* (New York: Twayne Publishers, 1993), 127, 97.

20. David Rosner, "Hives of Sickness and Vice," in David Rosner, ed., *Hives of Sickness: Epidemics and Public Health in New York* (New Brunswick: Rutgers University Press, 1985).

21. Julie Miller, "To Stop the Slaughter of the Babies: Nathan Straus and the Drive for Pasteurized Milk, 1893–1920," *New York History* 74 (April 1993), 158–84.

22. David Rosner, *A Once Charitable Enterprise: Hospitals and Health Care in Brooklyn and New York, 1895–1915* (Cambridge: Cambridge University Press, 1982).

23. Warren, *Brush with Death*, 39, suggests that as many as three hundred children a year had been killed by being lead poisoned in the early decades of the twentieth century.

24. See Samuel L. Dana, trans. *Lead Diseases: A Treatise from the French of L. Tanqueral des Planches* (Lowell: Daniel Bixby & Company, 1848). For a review of the 19th and 20th century medical literature, see Peter Reich, "The Teacup and the Sponge: Lead Paint Poisoning of Children, 1900–1971," mimeo (September 1988), and Richard Rabin, "Warnings Unheeded: A History of

Child Lead Poisoning," *American Journal of Public Health* 79 (December 1989).

25. David Dennison Stewart, M.D., "Notes on Some Obscure Cases of Poisoning by Lead Chromate Manifested Chiefly by Encephalopathy," *Medical News* 45 (June 18, 1887), 676–81.

26. William Glenn, "Chrome Yellow Considered as a Poison," *Science* 13 (January 1, 1889), 347–49.

27. Lockhart Gibson, Wilton Love, David Hardie, Peter Bancroft, and A. Jefferis Turner, "Notes on Lead-Poisoning as Observed among Children in Brisbane," *Intercolonial Medical Congress of Australia* (1892), 76–83.

28. R. Abrahams, "Acute Lead Poisoning in an Infant with Report of Two Other Interesting Cases," *American Medico-Surgical Bulletin* 10 (November 7, 1896), 531–32.

29. Ibid.

30. A. Jefferis Turner, "Lead Poisoning among Queensland Children," *Australasian Medical Gazette* (1897), 475–79.

31. J. Lockhart Gibson, "A Plea for Painted Railings and Painted Walls of Rooms as the Source of Lead Poisoning amongst Queensland Children," *Australasian Medical Gazette* 23 (April 20, 1904), 149–53.

32. J. Lockhart Gibson, "The Importance of Lumbar Puncture in the Plumbic Ocular Neuritis of Children," *Australasian Medical Congress Transactions* 2 (1911), 750–54.

33. David L. Edsall, "Chronic Lead Poisoning" in William Osler, ed., *Modern Medicine*, vol. 1 (1907), 87, 92, 108. Edsall noted the "wholesale poisoning in the Queensland children" by "ingestion of lead from painted wood work of houses."

34. A. Jefferis Turner, "Lead Poisoning in Childhood," *Australasian Medical Congress* (1908), 2–9; J. Lockhart Gibson, "Plumbic Ocular Neuritis in Queensland Children," *British Medical Journal* 2 (November 14, 1908), 1488–90. Even before the first cases of lead poisoning documented among children in America, Henry Gardner, who headed the educational bureau of the Paint Manufacturers Association, a trade group of manufacturers of both leaded and nonleaded paint, suggested that the lead paint being placed on interior surfaces represented a hazard. "Should we not exercise similar care in guarding against lead dust in our public buildings? The many tons of corroded white lead flatted with turpentine once applied to the walls and ceilings of school rooms and hospitals would gradually disintegrate and cause the formation of dried particles of white lead dust very dangerous to those who breathed it. Fortunately," he erroneously asserted, "the use of flatted white lead has been largely abandoned for wall and ceiling decoration, and its place has been taken by the more sanitary leadless Flat Wall Paints." He predicted that "with the adoption of preventive measures...lead poisoning will be done away with almost entirely." Henry A. Gardner, *The Toxic and Antiseptic Properties of Paints* (Philadelphia: Educational Bureau, Paint Manufacturers' Association of the U.S., February 12, 1914), 11–12.

35. Henry Thomas and Kenneth Blackfan, "Recurrent Meningitis, Due to Lead, in a Child of Five Years," *American Journal of Diseases of Children* 8 (November 1, 1914), 377; A. Brent and W. J. Young, "The Occurrence of Lead Poisoning amongst North Queensland Children," *Annals of Tropical Medicine and Parasitology* 8 (January 1914), 575–90.

36. Kenneth D. Blackfan, "Lead Poisoning in Children with Especial Reference to Lead as a Cause of Convulsions," *American Journal of the Medical Sciences* 153 (June 1917), 877–87.

37. See, for example, Robert Strong, "Meningitis Caused by Lead Poisoning in a Child of Nineteen Months," *Archives of Pediatrics* 37 (January 1920), 532–37; L. Emmett Holt, "General Function and Nervous Diseases" in *The Diseases of Infancy and Childhood for the Case of Students and Practitioners of Medicine*, chapter 11, 8th ed. (New York: D. Appleton, 1923), 645–94; L. Emmett Holt, "Lead Poisoning in Infancy," *American Journal of Diseases of Children* 25 (March 1923), 229–33; Council of Queensland Branch of the British Medical Association, "An Historical Account of the Occurrence and Causation of Lead Poisoning among Queensland Children," *Medical Journal of Australia* 1 (February 11, 1922), 148–52; Stafford McLean and Ruston McIntosh, "Studies of the Cerebral Spinal Fluid in Infants and Young Children" in *The Human Cerebrospinal Fluid* (New York: P. B. Hoeber, 1926), 299–300; Carl Vernon Weller, "Some Clinical Aspects of Lead Meningo-Encephalopathy," *Annals of Clinical Medicine* 3 (1925), 604–13; Joseph Aub, Lawrence Fairhall, A.S. Minot, Paul Reznikoff, and Alice Hamilton, *Lead Poisoning* (Baltimore: Williams and Wilkins, 1926), 70 and preface; L. Emmett Holt and John Howland, *The Diseases of Infancy and Childhood*, 9th ed. (New York: D. Appleton, 1926), 542; Frederick L. Hoffman, *Deaths from Lead Poisoning*, U.S. Department of Labor, Bureau of Labor Statistics, *Bulletin No. 426* (Washington: GPO, February 1927), 33–34; Boston, Health Department, "Lead Poisoning in Early Childhood," *Monthly Bulletin* 16 (November 1927), 266.

38. Issac Abt, ed., *Pediatrics*, vol. VII (Philadelphia, 1925), 246.

39. John Ruddock, "Lead Poisoning in Children with Special Reference to Pica," *Journal of the American Medical Association* (hereafter *JAMA*) 82 (May 24, 1924), 1684. In 1926 another American researcher, in an article titled, "Lead Poisoning in Children," noted that lead paint was dangerous to children and that "many cases of lead poisoning are overlooked" by physicians and parents. He suggested that the first thing to do was to make parents aware "of the hazards of painted articles to little children." See L. W. Holloway, "Lead Poisoning in Children," *Journal of the Florida Medical Association* 13 (1926), 94–100; Frederick Hoffman, *Deaths from Lead Poisoning*, U.S. Bureau of Labor Statistics, *Bulletin No. 426*, in which he lists eleven boys and eight girls under the age of eighteen who died from lead poisoning, a number of whom were poisoned from eating the paint from windows, walls, toys, and cribs.

40. Charles F. McKhann, "Lead Poisoning in Children," *American Journal of Diseases of Children* 32 (1926), 386–92.

41. See, "Affidavit of Peter C. English," City of New York et al. against Lead Industries Association, Inc., et al. Index Number 14365/89, 1999.

42. L. Emmett Holt and Rustin McIntosh, "Lead Poisoning," *Holt's Diseases of Infancy and Childhood,* 10th ed. (New York: D. Appleton, 1933), 1188; 11th edition, 1940, 1368.

43. Charles McKhann and Edward Vogt, "Lead Poisoning in Children," *JAMA* 101 (October 7, 1933), 1131. See also Charles F. McKhann, "Lead Poisoning in Children," *The Archives of Neurology and Psychiatry* 27 (February 1932), 294–95. McKhann acknowledged that some children chewed paint because they were anemic, had "certain intestinal parasites," or were prone to pica as a result of mental defects, but that most "do not fit into any of these groups, but appear normal children who have merely a pernicious habit."

44. Charles McKhann and Edward Vogt, "Lead Poisoning in Children," *JAMA* 101 (October 7, 1933), 1131.

45. John Ruddock, "Lead Poisoning in Children with Special Reference to Pica," *JAMA* 82 (May 24, 1924), 1682; Carl Vernon Weller, "Some Clinical Aspects of Lead Meningo-Encephalopathy, *Annals of Clinical Medicine* 3 (1925), 604–13. See also Stafford McLean and Rustin McIntosh, "Studies of the Cerebrospinal Fluids in Infants and Young Children," in *The Human Cerebrospinal Fluid* (New York: Paul Hoeber, 1924), 299–300; T. Suzuki and J. Kaneko, "Serious Meningitis in Infants Caused by Lead Poisoning from White Powders," *Journal of Oriental Medicine* (January 1924).

46. See Roland Marchand, *Creating the Corporate Soul: The Rise of Public Relations and Corporate Imagery in American Big Business* (Berkeley and Los Angeles: University of California Press, 1998).

47. [Wormser?] to William J. Donovan (September 21, 1928), National Archives, Federal Trade Commission Documents, in Papers of the Lead Industries Association and Associated Companies, New York City Law Department, Affirmative Litigation Division, New York (hereafter LIA Papers). See also "Constitution of the Lead Industries Association" for Article II, "Objects" of the LIA. While the "welfare of those engaged in the lead industries" is one objective, there is no specific mention of industrial disease or the need to "combat the substitution of other metals." See also "First and Organization Meeting of the Members of the Lead Industries Association" (November 14, 1928), FTC Records, LIA Papers.

48. Wormser to Edward McCready, Esq., Grand Rapids Store Equipment Corporation (July 7, 1930), LIA Papers.

49. See John C. Burnham, John E. Sauer, and Ronald Gibbs, "Peer-Reviewed Grants in U.S. Trade Association Research," *Science, Technology, & Human Values* 12 (Spring 1987), 42–51, in which they point out "much of the trade association research was defensive, designed to protect existing markets by attempting to counter bad publicity or changed conditions that could lessen the demand for the product." Most of that research was not health related, although they do cite the Meat Institute and the National Dairy Council as having "spent large

sums attempting to counter the effects of new health beliefs that caused many consumers to look unfavorably upon fats of various kinds."

50. [Wormser?] to William J. Donovan (September 21, 1928), National Archives, Federal Trade Commission Documents, LIA Papers. See also "Constitution of the Lead Industries Association" for Article II, "Objects" of the LIA. Sherwin-Williams, Glidden, and Eagle-Picher were among the first companies to join, also in 1928. The International Smelting and Refining Company joined in 1929.

51. *Drugs, Oils and Paints* 48 (April 1933), 140.

52. Report of the President, LIA, Annual Meeting of the Members of the Lead Industries Association (April 12, 1933), LIA Papers.

53. Felix Edgar Wormser, curriculum vitae, Wormser MSS, American Heritage Center, University of Wyoming, Cheyenne.

54. LIA, Directors Meeting (May 29, 1929), LIA Papers.

55. LIA, Directors Meeting (September 11, 1929), LIA Papers. Before the LIA was formed, Alice Hamilton had initiated Harvard's relationship with the lead industry.

56. Edward J. Cornish to David Edsall (May 12, 1921), courtesy of Christopher Sellers.

57. Edward J. Cornish to David Edsall (March 29, 1923), courtesy of Christopher Sellers. The Eagle-Picher Lead Company contributed $3,141 to Harvard's lead studies in 1921. Thomas S. Brown to David Edsall (November 12, 1921), courtesy of Christopher Sellers.

58. "In 1925 Dr. Aub and his associates at the Massachusetts General Hospital, who had been investigating lead poisoning with the support of lead mining, smelting, and fabricating companies, published the results of the early part of their medical research, in a volume entitled 'Lead Poisoning.'" See LIA, "Lead Poisoning Research by Drs. Aub and Others" (November 1, 1929), LIA Papers.

59. LIA, Directors Meeting (May 28, 1930), LIA Papers. See also Wormser to Edward McCready (July 7, 1930), LIA Papers. The LIA also disbursed $5,000 for medical research. "Last Spring I [Wormser] visited Boston for the purpose of discussing the subject of lead poisoning in infants with some of the medical profession there who have caused us to receive some unfavorable publicity about lead and I believe the visit was worthwhile." LIA, Directors Meeting (September 30, 1931), LIA Papers.

60. Joseph Aub, "The Biochemical Behavior of Lead in the Body," *JAMA* 104 (January 12, 1935), 87. See also Christopher Sellers, *Hazards of the Job: From Industrial Disease to Environmental Health* (Chapel Hill: University of North Carolina Press, 1997), 197. LIA, Directors Meeting (September 30, 1931), LIA Papers. In 1929, the LIA gave Aub and the Harvard School of Public Health $10,000 for research into the physiological effects of lead; at the next year's meeting the LIA earmarked another $2,000 for "Medical Research" at Harvard. In 1931, another $5,000 was given to "Harvard College." When Felix Wormser learned that Aub "was planning to write an article on the treatment

of lead poisoning for the *Journal of Industrial Hygiene*, he urged members to develop a plan for the distribution and use of its results "at the time Dr. Aub's results become public." See LIA, Directors Meeting (May 28, 1930), LIA Papers.

61. LIA, Directors Meeting (June 15, 1933), LIA Papers.

62. LIA, Executive Committee Minutes (January 15, 1943), LIA Papers.

63. LIA, Minutes (May 11, 1942), LIA Papers.

64. "Lead-free Paint on Furniture and Toys to Protect Children," *United States Daily* (November 20, 1930), 1.

65. LIA, Directors Meeting (December 12, 1930), LIA Papers.

66. "Chronic Lead Poisoning in Infancy and Early Childhood," [mimeo] Metropolitan Life Insurance Company, *Statistical Bulletin* (October 1930), LIA Papers; quoted in "Chronic Lead Poisoning in Infancy and Early Childhood," *American Journal of Public Health* 21 (January 1931), 18.

67. "Chronic Lead Poisoning in Infancy and Early Childhood," [mimeo] Metropolitan Life Insurance Company, *Statistical Bulletin* (October 1930), LIA Papers.

68. Louis Dublin to Ella Oppenheimer (September 14, 1933), courtesy of Christian Warren.

69. Frederick L. Hoffman, *Lead Poisoning Legislation and Statistics* (Newark: Prudential Insurance Company of America, 1933), 19.

70. Ibid.

71. Charles McKhann and E. C. Vogt, "Lead Poisoning in Children," *JAMA* 149 (1933), 1131. McKhann and Vogt had depended upon a "personal communication to the authors of a survey of crib and toy manufacturers made by the Lead Industries Association, Secretary, F. E. Wormser."

72. A. Schoenhut Company to Ella Oppenheimer (April 17, 1935), LIA Papers.

73. Newark Varnish Works to Ella Oppenheimer (April 25, 1935), LIA Papers. See also Robert Kehoe to A. J. Lanza (March 18, 1938), LIA Papers: "In the course of the past several years I have seen several fatal cases of lead poisoning in children as the result of ingesting lead from toys, play pens, and in one instance contaminated food."

74. "Lead Hazard in Toys," *Consumers Union Report* (May 1936), 11.

75. George Rice, "Painting and Gilding Wooden Toys," *Painter and Decorator* 47 (July 1933), 12–14.

76. Charles F. McKhann, "Lead Poisoning in Children," *The Archives of Neurology and Psychiatry* 27 (February 1932), 294–95; Norman Porritt, "Cumulative Effects of Infinitesimal Doses of Lead," *British Medical Journal* (July 18, 1931), 92–94. An article by a British physician documented lead poisoning from "the slow, subtle, insidious saturation of the system by infinitesimal doses of lead extending over a long period of time."

77. Edward Vogt, "Roentgenologic Diagnosis of Lead Poisoning in Infants and Children," *JAMA* 98 (January 9, 1932), 125.

78. LIA Directors Meeting (September 30, 1931), LIA Papers.

79. Louis Dublin to Ella Oppenheimer (September 14, 1933), courtesy of Christian Warren.

80. Transcript of Norton's confirmation hearing before the Senate Energy and Natural Resources Committee: <http://web.lexis-nexis.com/congcomp /docume...SIAA&_md5=41383eb56ed09fcfa2c2e9cf9248d2e2>

81. "Of late the lead industries have been receiving much undesirable publicity regarding lead poisoning," Wormser told his board of directors. LIA, Annual Meeting of the Members of the Lead Industries Association (April 12, 1933), LIA Papers. In November 1933 the Massachusetts Department of Labor and Industries picked up on the issue, noting in a bulletin focused on occupational hazards that "many serious and even fatal cases of lead poisoning among infants have been traced to the sucking or chewing of lead-painted surfaces. Toys, cribs, furniture and other objects with which infants may come in contact should not be painted with lead colors." Massachusetts, Department of Labor and Industries, Division of Industrial Safety, "Revised Rules, Regulations, and Recommendations Pertaining to Structural Painting," *Industrial Bulletin No. 13* (November 1, 1933), 8, LIA Papers. Manfred Bowditch was the occupational hygienist in the Division of Industrial Safety and in the 1950s became the LIA's health and safety director. Also in 1933 a paper delivered at the American Congress of Radiology by E. C. Vogt and Charles F. McKhann was abstracted in *Scientific American* under the title "If Your Children Chew Paint." It reported, "Unfortunately, infants and children very often eat or swallow enough lead to be poisoned by it and in a large percentage of cases they die. Ninety-five cases of lead poisoning have been observed at the Infants' and Children's Hospital, Boston, during the past nine years." The article continued by noting that "most children suffering from lead poisoning seem to have ingested the lead by chewing the paint from woodwork, furniture, or toys." "If Your Children Chew Paint," *Scientific American* 149 (December 1933), 291.

82. LIA, Annual Meeting (June 13, 1935), LIA Papers. Meanwhile, the information from physicians documenting lead poisoning in children pointed increasingly to lead as an even more dangerous substance than previously understood. The John Hopkins *Hospital Bulletin* reported on lead poisoning in Baltimore, including one child who "ate flakes of dry paint from the walls." S. S. Blackman Jr., "Intranuclear Inclusion Bodies in the Kidney and Liver Caused by Lead Poisoning," *Bulletin of the Johns Hopkins Hospital* 58 (1936), 384–97. See also, S. S. Blackman Jr., "The Lesions of Lead Encephalitis in Children," *Bulletin of the Johns Hopkins Hospital* 61 (1937), 40.

83. Robert Kehoe, abstract of discussion in Charles F. McKhann and E. C. Vogt, "Lead Poisoning in Children," *JAMA* 101 (October 7, 1933), 1135. Elsewhere, Kehoe wrote, "There is every reason for suspecting the existence of significant and dangerous lead exposure in the case of children with a history of pica. The occurrence of lead-containing commodities and the use of lead paints on furniture, toys, and other objects within the reach of small children is much

too common to ignore. The existence of symptoms even slightly suggestive of plumbism should result in prompt investigation of the child and his surroundings." See Kehoe, "The Diagnosis of Lead Poisoning in the Light of Recent Information," reprint from *Journal of Medicine* (December 1935), 3–8. See also Kehoe, "My experience, and that of my colleagues at Harvard, leads me to believe that most cases of lead poisoning in infants and children come from chewing objects coated with metallic lead and lead pigment. I am not quite sure, but I believe that every case, except one, in our list of children has had such a causative factor." In Kehoe to Hoffman (June 26, 1937), LIA Papers.

84. John R. Ross and Alan Brown, "Symposium on Common Poisonings: III. Poisonings Common in Children," *Canadian Public Health Journal* 26 (1935), 237–43. See A. S. Minot, "The Physiological Effects of Small Amounts of Lead: An Evaluation of the Lead Hazard of the Average Individual," *Physiological Review* 18 (1938), 554–57.

85. "Chronic Lead Poisoning in Infancy and Early Childhood," *American Journal of Public Health* (January 1931), 18

86. Williams Haynes, *American Chemical Industry*, vol. 4, (New York: Van Nostrand, 1954), 367.

87. National Safety Council, *Proposed Revision LEAD Health Practices Pamphlet No. 3* (Final Draft) (1942), LIA Papers.

88. LIA, Annual Meeting of the Members of the Lead Industries Association (April 12, 1933), LIA Papers.

89. LIA, Annual Meeting, Minutes (June 4, 1943), LIA Papers.

90. LIA, Annual Meeting of the Members of the Lead Industries Association, Report of Secretary (June 5, 1934), LIA Papers.

91. LIA, Board of Directors Meeting, "Report Summarizing the Activities of the Lead Industries Association and Furnishing Data to Draft the Budget for 1937" (December 23, 1936), LIA Papers.

92. Haynes, *American Chemical Industry*, 367–69.

93. Elizabeth Fee, "Public Health in Practice: An Early Confrontation with the 'Silent Epidemic' of Childhood Lead Paint Poisoning," *Journal of the History of Medicine and Allied Sciences* 45 (October 1990), 570. This section on the Baltimore experience is drawn largely from Fee's pioneering work.

94. LIA Directors Meeting (September 28, 1932), LIA Papers.

95. "Paint Eating Children," *Baltimore Health News* (1932), 83.

96. Fee, "Public Health in Practice," 581.

97. Baltimore Health Department, radio broadcast (October 15, 1935), LIA Papers.

98. Randolph K. Byers, "Introduction," in Herbert L. Needleman, ed., *Low Level Lead Exposure: The Clinical Implications of Current Research* (New York: Raven Press, 1980), 1.

99. Ibid.

100. Ibid.

101. Jane S. Lin-Fu, "Lead Poisoning and Undue Lead Exposure in Children: History and Current Status," in Herbert L. Needleman, ed., *Low Level*

Lead Exposure: The Clinical Implications of Current Research (New York: Raven Press, 1980), 9; Jane S. Lin-Fu, "Modern History of Lead Poisoning: A Century of Discovery and Re-Discovery," in Herbert L. Needleman, *Human Lead Exposure* (Boca Raton, FL: CRC Press, 1992), 35.

102. Fee, "Public Health in Practice," 584.

103. Ibid., 585.

104. J. M. McDonald and E. Kaplan, "Incidence of Lead Poisoning in the City of Baltimore," *JAMA* 119 (July 11, 1942), 871.

105. Edward A. Park to Marian M. Crane (May 14, 1947), National Archives Record Group 102, Records of the Children's Bureau, Central Files, 1945–48, Box 104, Folder: 4-5-17.

106. LIA, Board of Directors Meeting (June 6, 1940), LIA Papers. Wormser told the directors that "the lead industry received two blasts in the press recently" and that "as usual the Association investigated these attacks." See LIA, Board of Directors Meeting (May 16, 1939), LIA Papers. In January 1940 the directors were informed that "attacks against the use of lead on the ground of lead poisoning continued to be made." See LIA, Board of Directors Meeting (January 17, 1940), LIA Papers.

107. LIA, Board of Directors Meeting (January 7, 1941), LIA Papers. By 1936, some outside the professions were noting the dangers of lead. In May 1936, *Consumers Union* told its readers that "lead paint used on floors, porches, cribs, and other furniture sometimes causes acute lead poisoning of children." See "Lead Hazard in Toys," *Consumers Union* (May 1936), 11.

108. LIA, Board of Directors Meeting (June 4, 1943), LIA Papers.

109. L. Emmett Holt and Rustin McIntosh, *Holt's Diseases of Infancy and Childhood* (New York: Appleton-Century-Crofts, 1940), 1368–72.

110. "Paint Eaters," *Time* (December 20, 1943), 49.

111. LIA, "Preliminary Report of Investigation of 'Time' Article 'Paint Eaters,'" in Lead Hygiene and Safety Bulletin No. 40 (January 1945), LIA Papers.

112. Wormser to Members of the Lead Industries Association (December 8, 1944), "Exhibit A to LIA Executive Committee Minutes," January 13, 1945; LIA Papers; "Preliminary Report...," Lead Hygiene and Safety Bulletin, No. 40 (January 1945), LIA Papers.

113. Ibid.

114. "Preliminary Report..." Lead Hygiene and Safety Bulletin, No. 40, LIA Papers. Note that Wormser also visits a Dr. Mayer, questioning his findings of lead as a factor in the death of a child in Philadelphia. He reports that the LIA's executive committee is providing a grant to Dr. Byers. Wormser to Aub (January 4, 1945), LIA Papers.

115. Randolph K. Byers, "Introduction," in Herbert L. Needleman, ed., *Low Level Lead Exposure: The Clinical Implications of Current Research* (New York: Raven Press, 1980), 2.

116. Warren, 149–50.

117. Kim N. Dietrich, "Environmental Neurotoxicants and Psychological Development," in G. Taylor, K. O. Yeats, M. D. Ris, eds., *Pediatric Neuropsychology: Research, Theory and Practice* (New York: Guilford Press, 1999), 222.

118. Warren, 150.

119. J. H. Schaefer to Wormser (June 27, 1944), LIA Papers.

120. Wormser to Kehoe (January 19, 1944), LIA Papers.

121. Kehoe to Wormser (February 7, 1944), LIA Papers.

122. Kehoe to R. L. Gorrell (September 5, 1945), LIA Papers. Kehoe's position on the danger of paint to children was consistent with statements he had made before and after this communication with the LIA. As early as 1930 Kehoe had noted lead poisoning among children who "sucked the paint from toys and beds from inside the house." He also cited the danger of "leaded" dust on windowsills from crumbling paint. See Kehoe to Worth (September 25, 1930), LIA Papers. In 1938 Kehoe wrote to Metropolitan Life's Anthony Lanza that he had "seen several fatal cases of lead poisoning in children as the result of ingesting lead from toys [and] playpens." See Kehoe to Lanza (March 18, 1938), LIA Papers. About this time Kehoe noted, "There is every reason for suspecting the existence of significant and dangerous lead exposure in the case of children with a history of pica. The occurrence of lead-containing commodities and the use of lead paints on furniture, toys, and other objects, within the reach of small children is much too common to ignore." Kehoe, *The Diagnosis of Lead Poisoning in the Light of Recent Information* (n.d.), LIA Papers.

123. LIA Executive Committee Meeting, Exhibit D, "A Safety and Hygiene Program for the Lead Industries Association, "December 28, 1945, LIA Papers, and LIA, Annual Meeting, Minutes (May 15, 1944), LIA Papers. Felix Wormser argued, "Our industry continues to be plagued unfairly by attacks made upon lead products because of their toxicity. It seems to me that we must be losing a vast amount of business each year because of the fact that lead has such unpleasant connections in the minds of so many Americans." See also Roland Marchand, *Creating the Corporate Soul: The Rise of Public Relations and Corporate Imagery in American Big Business* (Berkeley and Los Angeles: University of California Press, 1998), for a detailed analysis of the broader public relations campaigns by corporations.

124. LIA, Executive Committee, Minutes (January 12, 1945), LIA Papers. Wormser, arguing in early 1945 that "grave doubt existed as to [lead poisoning's] prevalence," suggested that "the Association contemplated an investigation of statistics of death from lead poisoning which, from a preliminary examination, were believed to be seriously faulty." He suggested to the directors that the organization take "a more aggressive attitude in meeting the attacks frequently made on the lead industry."

125. LIA, Executive Committee Meeting, Exhibit D (December 28, 1945), LIA Papers.

126. Wormser, "Facts and Fallacies of Lead Exposure," Kehoe Manuscripts, Box 90; See also, Philip Drinker, "Public Exposure to Lead" in *Occupational*

Medicine 3 (1947), 146, in which Drinker says: "In the United States [lead poisoning of children] is becoming rare because lead-painted toys and furniture are rare—toy manufacturers are advised not to use lead paint for these purposes, and compliance with this advice is good. Certainly, such poisoning today is not common."

127. Kehoe to J. H. Schaefer (January 29, 1945), Kehoe Manuscripts, Box 90.

128. Wormser, "Facts and Fallacies of Lead Exposure," 12.

129. Kehoe to J. H. Schaefer (January 29, 1945), Kehoe Papers, Box 90.

130. Wormser, "Facts and Fallacies Concerning Exposure to Lead," and Discussion, in "Symposium on Lead Poisoning," at Seventh Annual Congress on Industrial Health, Boston, September 30, 1946, 51, also published in *Occupational Medicine* 3 (January 1947), 13–19.

131. F. J. Schlink to LIA (June 28, 1948), LIA Papers.

132. National Lead, "Versatile" (ad), in *American Painter and Decorator* (June 1949) and in *National Painters Magazine* (October 1949).

133. Robert Kehoe, Discussion in Conference on Lead Poisoning, at the Seventh Annual Congress on Industrial Health, American Medical Association (September 30–October 2, 1946), 52.

134. Robert L. Zeigfield, Secretary, to Members of LIA (January 15, 1948), LIA Papers.

135. "Alumni Trustee Chosen by Columbia University," *New York Times* (October 6, 1953), 31; "Wormser Resumes Old Post," *New York Times* (June 18, 1957), 48.

136. Kehoe to Manfred Bowditch (February 11, 1948), courtesy of Warren.

137. See Marchand, *Creating the Corporate Soul.*

138. LIA, Annual Meeting, Report of the Secretary (April 13–14, 1950), LIA Papers.

139. Robert L. Ziegfeld to E. V. Gent (April 9, 1948), LIA Papers; LIA, Executive Committee Minutes (April 2, 1948), and attachment, "Abstract" from minutes of meeting of the Industry Development Committee of the American Zinc Institute (December 18, 1947), LIA Papers.

140. See Christian Warren, "The Silenced Epidemic: A Social History of Lead Poisoning in the United States since 1900," (Ph.D. diss., Brandeis University, 1997).

CHAPTER 3: CATER TO THE CHILDREN

1. "Cater to the Children" (ad), *Dutch Boy Painter* (January/February 1918), advertising section.

2. "How Lead Keeps the Wolf from Your Door" (ad), *National Geographic* (ca. 1923), LIA Papers.

3. "What Lead Does in a Motor Car" (ad), *National Geographic* (ca. 1923), LIA Papers.

4. "How Lead Helps You See" (ad), *National Geographic* (ca. 1923), LIA Papers.

5. "For Bull's-Eyes—Lead!" (ad), *National Geographic* (ca. 1923), LIA Papers.

6. Ruth Schwartz Cowan, *More Work for Mother: The Ironies of Household Technology from the Open Hearth to the Microwave* (New York: Basic Books, 1983).

7. [National Lead Company], *Decorating the Home: Illustrating Up-to-the-Minute Effects Obtainable with White Lead Paint* (1926).

8. Ibid., 4–5.

9. Ibid., 11, 13.

10. "Interior Finishes Once Found Only in the Houses of the Rich" (ad), *Saturday Evening Post* (April 25, 1925).

11. "Interior of Rare Beauty Now Within the Means of All" (ad), *National Geographic* 47 (May 1925). See also "Four Walls—a Roof—and LEAD" (ad), *National Geographic* 48 (November 1925) and *Drugs, Oils and Paints* 41 (November 1925), 189.

12. "If You Could Turn This Room Inside-Out," National Lead, Advertising Copy, LIA Papers.

13. Susan Strasser, *Satisfaction Guaranteed: The Making of American Mass Marketing* (Washington, DC: Smithsonian Institution Press, 1989), 189.

14. [National Lead Company], *The House We Live In: Its Decoration, Its Protection*, 5th ed. (1936).

15. [National Lead Company], *So You're Going to Paint!* (1938).

16. "Something Worth Thinking About" (ad), *Hardware Retailer* 59 (November 1940), 7. Other ads sought to convince consumers that the use of lead-based color paints conformed to the latest ideas about modern style. "Leading architects recommend white lead paint for modern interior paint styling because of the rich colors and beautiful finish it offers . . . easily and safely cleaned by washing." See also "White Lead Paint Economical for Interiors" (ad), *Lead* 8 (January 1938), 7: Lead paint was touted as the most "versatile, decorative medium" because of its unlimited "number of shades and tints that you can secure" and the "wide choice of wall effects or finishes." The LIA's *Lead* magazine asserted that "pure white lead paints gain the continued good will of apartment owners. Their long life eliminates frequent repainting which is so annoying and bothersome to tenants. Walls and ceilings painted with white lead may be washed often, removing dust and dirt with no other effect other than regaining the original luster and beauty of these surfaces."

17. Nancy Tomes, *The Gospel of Germs: Men, Women, and the Microbe in American Life* (Cambridge: Harvard University Press, 1998), 168.

18. Ibid, 192.

19. "The White Plumber," *The Carter Times* (August 1913), 10, Warshaw Collection, Smithsonian Institution, Washington, Paint, file #60, Box 2, Folder: Carter.

20. "This Colorful Language of Ours," General Printing Ink Corporation, National Archives, Record Group 102 (Children's Bureau), Central Files, 1941–44, File 4-5-17, Box 103.

21. *Handy Book on Painting* (Pittsburgh, PA: National Lead and Oil Co. of Penna., 1924), 23–37; and "Lead Paint, the Fire Extinguisher" (ad), *National Geographic* 47 (April 1925). See also, for example, ad, *Hospital Progress* (July 1931), n.p.

22. Ad, *Drugs, Oils and Paints* 51 (December 1936), 497. See also *Drugs, Oils and Paints* 52 (June 1937), 229; and ad, *Drugs, Oils and Paints* 53 (April 1938), 125.

23. Ad, *Drugs, Oils and Paints* 54 (January 1939), 5.

24. Harvey W. Wiley, "Paints vs. Wall-Papers," *Good Housekeeping* (August 1915), 222–23.

25. See, for example, "Advertising to Children to Increase Wall Paint Sales," *Printers' Ink Monthly* (June 1929), 81.

26. "Lead Takes Part in Many Games" (ad), *National Geographic* (ca. 1923), LIA Papers. National Lead was proud that "toy makers use lead extensively because it can be easily shaped and moulded [*sic*] into many forms."

27. "For Bull's-Eyes—Lead!" (ad), *National Geographic* (ca. 1923), LIA Papers.

28. "Painting the House that Jack Built; Do Not Forget the Children—Some Day They May Be Customers" (ad), *Dutch Boy Painter* (1920), 126.

29. Ibid., 126–27.

30. *Dutch Boy's Jingle Paint Book* (1922).

31. [National Lead Company], *The Dutch Boy's Lead Party* (ca. 1923).

32. "Insuring Business for the Years Ahead," *Dutch Boy Painter* (July 1924), 139.

33. [National Lead Company], *Dutch Boy in Story Land* (1925).

34. [National Lead Company], *The Dutch Boy's Hobby, a Paint Book for Girls and Boys* (1928).

35. [National Lead Company], *The Dutch Boy Conquers Old Man Gloom* (1929).

36. Ibid. See also *Dutch Boy Painter* (July–August 1930), 114.

37. "Reaching Out for Business," *Dutch Boy Painter* (1927), 117.

38. "Takes a Scrubbing with a Smile," *The Modern Hospital* (April 1937).

39. "Smashing 4-Color Advertising Campaign." *Dutch Boy Painter—Carter Times* (January–February 1930), 199.

40. "Stencils—How to Use Them . . . ," *Dutch Boy Painter* (1933), 77.

41. "A Unique Travelling Lumber and Paint Display," *Lead* 7 (July 1937), 7.

42. "When the School Room is Empty," *Dutch Boy Painter* (July 1924), back cover.

43. [National Lead Company], "Our Company . . . Its Past, Present and Future," *Dutch Boy Paint Salesmen's Manual* (n.d.) [post-World War II], 8–9.

44. "Dutch Boy Nominated for Packaging's Hall of Fame Because:" *Modern Packaging* (April 1949), 126–30, 266, 268.

45. National Lead Company, "Important" (1949), LIA Papers.

46. "How Paint Promotes Public Health," *Dutch Boy Painter* (ca. 1918), LIA Papers.

47. "Dutch Boy White Lead + Dutch Boy Flatting Oil = " (ad), *Drugs, Oils and Paints* (May 1919), 439.

48. "Lead Helps to Guard Your Health" (ad), *National Geographic* 44 (November 1923).

49. "Clean and Bright Hospital Walls" (ad), *The Modern Hospital* (July 1921); also see, for example, "Color—the Doctor's Assistant" (ad), *The Modern Hospital* (July 1922).

50. "Color—Yes . . . for Every Part of the Hospital" (ad), *The Modern Hospital* 30 (June 1928). See also "Quieting Color Can Be Peaceful as a Hillside at Dawn" (ad), *The Modern Hospital* (July 1930).

51. "Color—the Doctor's Assistant" (ad), *The Modern Hospital* (July 1922).

52. Ibid.

53. "Color—Yes . . . for Every Part of the Hospital" (ad), *The Modern Hospital* 30 (June 1928). See also "Quieting Color Can Be Peaceful as a Hillside at Dawn" (ad), *The Modern Hospital* (July 1930).

54. Christian Warren, *Brush with Death: A Social History of Lead Poisoning* (Baltimore: Johns Hopkins University Press, 2000), 48. Heckel was also an official of the National Paint, Oil and Varnish Association.

55. George B. Heckel, "Painting the Hospital, II. The Inside of the Cup," *Drugs, Oils and Paints* 37 (September 1921), 126–27.

56. "Why Paint Saves Lives," *Dutch Boy Painter* (May 1923), 54–55. See also "Every Room in a Modern Hospital Deserves a Dutch Boy Quality Painting Job," *The Modern Hospital* (July 1930); and National Lead Company, *The Handbook on Painting* (1930).

57. "How Paint Promotes Public Health," *Dutch Boy Painter* (ca. 1918), LIA Papers.

58. [Eagle-Picher], "These 4 Points Will Help You Sell Paint Jobs Today," *National Painters Magazine* (1943), LIA Papers.

59. LIA, Board of Directors Meeting, *Report Summarizing the Activities of the Lead Industries Association and Furnishing Data to Draft the Budget for 1937* (December 23, 1936), LIA Papers.

60. *Drugs, Oils and Paints* 44 (August 1928), 94.

61. LIA, Advisory Committee of White Lead Promotion, "White Lead Promotion Program," Minutes of 10th Meeting (October 20, 1941), slide presentation, LIA Papers.

62. Ibid. The market for white lead in 1939 was "about half as big (100,000 tons) as it had [been] in 1922 (195,000 tons)." LIA, "Bulletin No. 1, Reasons for the White-Lead Promotion Program" (February 20, 1939), LIA Papers.

63. LIA, "Bulletin No. 1, Reasons for the White Lead Promotion Program" (February 20, 1939), LIA Papers.

64. Roland Marchand, *Creating the Corporate Soul: The Rise of Public Relations and Corporate Imagery in American Big Business* (Berkeley and Los Angeles: University of California Press, 1998).

65. LIA, Advisory Committee of White Lead Promotion, "White Lead Promotion Program," Minutes of 10th Meeting (October 20, 1941), Exhibit C, LIA Papers.

66. LIA, "Bulletin No. 1, Reasons for the White-Lead Promotion Program" (February 20, 1939), Exhibit C, LIA Papers.

67. LIA, Board of Directors Meeting, Minutes (January 17, 1940), LIA Papers.

68. LIA, Advisory Committee of White Lead Promotion, "White Lead Promotion Program," Minutes of 10th Meeting (October 20, 1941), Exhibit C, LIA Papers.

69. Members included National Lead, Sherwin-Williams, and Glidden.

70. NPVLA, Executive Committee, Minutes (July 11, 1939), LIA Papers.

71. Ibid. NPVLA, Letter "To Class 'A' Members" (July 18, 1939), LIA Papers.

72. NPVLA, Letter "To Class 'A' Members" (July 18, 1939), LIA Papers.

73. "Safety and Health Hazards," *Paint Industry Magazine* 55 (December 1940), 18–20.

74. LIA, Advisory Committee of White Lead Promotion, Minutes of 2nd Meeting (April 12, 1939), LIA Papers.

75. LIA, Advisory Committee of White Lead Promotion, Minutes of 4th Meeting (September 27, 1939), LIA Papers. See also Minutes of 6th Meeting (December 14, 1939), in which members found that their efforts had generated so much interest that "steps had been taken to expand the project in Iowa as quickly as possible."

76. LIA, Advisory Committee of White Lead Promotion, Minutes of 8th Meeting (October 18, 1940), LIA Papers.

77. LIA, White Lead Promotion Campaign, Bulletin 37 (May 23, 1941), LIA Papers.

78. LIA, White Lead Promotion Campaign, "Review of Painting Practices of Municipalities, Counties and States" (October 11, 1939?), LIA Papers.

79. LIA, White Lead Promotion Campaign, Bulletin 47 (May 20, 1942), LIA Papers.

80. Ibid.

81. LIA, White Lead Promotion Campaign, Bulletin 40 (October 2, 1941), LIA Papers.

82. Ibid.

83. LIA, White Lead Promotion Campaign, Bulletin 32 (January 15, 1941), LIA Papers; LIA, Advisory Committee of White Lead Promotion, Minutes of 8th Meeting (October 18, 1940), LIA Papers. See also "Schenectady Schools Modernize with Paint," which shows an illustration of interiors of a school painted with white lead. It describes the use of Dutch Boy "white lead and lead mixing oil" at the Howe School. "Perhaps this Schenectady modernization project

may put a bee in the bonnets of those of our painter friends who are acquainted with or have access to members of their local school boards." *Dutch Boy Painter* 38 (1945).

84. LIA, White Lead Promotion Campaign, Bulletin 25 (Poplar Bluff, Mo.) (October 11, 1940), LIA Papers.

85. LIA, White Lead Promotion Campaign, Bulletin 32 (January 15, 1941), LIA Papers.

86. LIA, White Lead Promotion Campaign, "Review of Painting Practices of Municipalities, Counties and States" (October 11, 1939?), LIA Papers.

87. "Lead Industry Begins Campaign to Advertise White-Lead Campaign," *Dutch Boy Painter* 32 (1939), 27.

88. Advertising appeared in the following general readership magazines: *Saturday Evening Post* (from spring 1939 to October 1941—nineteen full-page and six half-page ads); *Colliers* (fifteen full and seven half); *Better Homes and Gardens* (twenty half); *American Home* (twenty half); *Country Gentleman* (twelve full, six half); and *Successful Farming* (three half, all in 1941). Total circulation of these magazines was put at 13,881,000. The LIA also advertised in trade journals and farm and agricultural magazines.

The LIA also placed at least seventy-five articles about white lead in the first two years in *Painter and Decorator*, the official publication of the Brotherhood of Painters, Decorators and Paperhangers of America, and other trade publications. In the first two years, they released ninety-one columns of "Home Owner's Forum" to eight hundred newspapers and eleven "House of the Month" features to five hundred newspapers. They also helped write the Iowa State College circular "Selecting and Applying Paints," with 110,000 copies distributed in the first two years. The LIA also worked with a variety of other associations to produce small publications that extolled the value of white lead. At the Golden Gate International Exposition in 1939 the LIA painted a home with white lead inside and out for the Western Pine Association Model Home.

The White Lead Promotion Campaign was initially intended as a three-year effort. But it was extended at the end of the third year for a fourth (into 1942). At the eleventh meeting of the advisory board, held November 10, 1942, members voted to extend the campaign yet another year. Activity in the later war years and postwar period was minimal (in part due to wartime material shortages of lead and other essential paint components). However, there is no evidence that the campaign was ever formally abandoned. It was officially revived in 1950 and then discontinued at the end of 1952. At least through 1942, the campaign was run by an advisory committee, which met with varying frequency: at least five times in 1939, three times in 1940, once in 1941, and at least once in 1942. Companies that sent representatives to the meetings were Eagle-Picher, National Lead, St. Joseph Lead, International Smelting and Refining, United States Smelting, Refining and Mining. Committee members included E. V. Peters, chairman (St. Joseph Lead); F. F. Wormser, secretary; F. L. Ziegfield, assistant secretary; and J. L. Cobbs, of the advertising agency Arthur

Kudner. See various White Lead Promotion Campaign minutes and LIA Annual Meeting minutes, 1932–1952, LIA Papers.

89. *Report of the Secretary,* Annual Meeting (June 6, 1940), LIA Papers.

90. LIA, Advisory Committee of White Lead Promotion, Minutes of 8th Meeting (October 18, 1940), LIA Papers.

91. LIA, Advisory Committee of White Lead Promotion, Minutes of 10th Meeting (Slide Presentation) (October 20, 1941), LIA Papers.

92. LIA, Annual Meeting (September 22, 1941), LIA Papers.

93. A war production order, M-384, restricted the nonmilitary uses of lead, including the amount of white lead that the paint manufacturers could use in paint. See "White Lead Is Back from the War," *Paint, Oil, and Chemical Review* (October 4, 1945); and Wormser to Members Manufacturing White Lead, "Subject: Modification of White Lead Restrictions" (August 30, 1945), LIA Papers. In 1942, in the midst of the Second World War, the LIA decided to concentrate on influencing 4-H Club members, primarily children and young adults in Iowa, Wisconsin, Kansas, Oklahoma, and Georgia. In 1942 the LIA published a booklet, "What to Expect from White Lead Paint," which suggested that white lead paint "has many of the same advantages for painting interiors that it has for exteriors. Of course, interior paint is not subjected to weathering and hard wear to the same extent that exterior paint is. But the ability to stand wear *is* important."

94. LIA, *Lead in Modern Industry* (1952), 153–54.

95. Ibid., 174. See also National Lead Company, "How to Paint Right: The Inside about Painting Inside and Outside" (1951), 45.

96. Bowditch to Kehoe (August 13, 1952), LIA Papers.

97. Secretary, LIA, to Members of the White Lead Divisions, "Subject: Discontinuance of White Lead Program" (January 8, 1953), LIA Papers.

98. M. Q. McDonald, "Maryland—Toxic Finishes" (July 14, 1949), LIA Papers. McDonald was on the staff of the National Paint, Varnish and Lacquer Association.

99. LIA, "Lead Hygiene and Safety Bulletin #79" (December 1, 1950), LIA Papers.

100. LIA, Annual Meeting, *Report of the Secretary* (April 13–14, 1950), LIA Papers.

101. LIA, "Lead Hygiene and Safety Bulletin #79" (December 1, 1950), LIA Papers.

102. Elizabeth Fee, "Public Health in Practice: An Early Confrontation with the 'Silent Epidemic' of Childhood Lead Paint Poisoning," *Journal of the History of Medicine and Allied Sciences* 45 (October 1990), 588.

103. LIA, "State and Territorial Warning Labeling Laws" (June 1952), LIA Papers.

104. LIA, Annual Meeting, *Report of the Secretary* (April 13–14, 1950), LIA Papers.

105. J. Julian Chisolm Jr. and Harold Harrison, "The Exposure of Children to Lead," *Pediatrics* 18 (1956), 943–57.

106. Huntington Williams, Emanuel Kaplan, Charles Couchman, and R. R. Sayers, *Public Health Reports* 67 (March 1952), 230–36.

107. LIA, Annual Meeting, *Report of the Secretary* (April 13–14, 1950), LIA Papers.

108. LIA, Annual Meeting, "Lead Hygiene" (April 9–10, 1953), LIA Papers.

109. Bowditch to Joseph Aub (December 21, 1949), LIA Papers.

110. LIA, Board of Directors Meeting, Minutes (December 16, 1952), LIA Papers; LIA, Annual Meeting, "Lead Hygiene" (April 9–10, 1953), LIA Papers.

111. Bowditch to Ziegfield (December 16, 1952), LIA Papers.

112. *New York Times* (November 9, 1954), 26.

113. Bowditch to Ziegfield (December 16, 1952), LIA Papers.

114. Ibid.

115. Kehoe to Herbert Hillman (September 4, 1953), LIA Papers.

116. Articles in the popular and professional press continued to document new sources of lead in the environment and the dangers it posed to children and the broader population. Nevertheless, the LIA continued to minimize the dangers of lead to children. As late as 1955, the LIA was still referring to this problem as a "headache" for the industry, claiming that many other common substances were "responsible for many more child poisoning than lead." LIA, Annual Meeting (April 27–28, 1955), LIA Papers. Again, in 1956, childhood lead poisonings continued to be seen as a "major problem and source of adverse publicity." The LIA noted a headline from the New York *Daily News,* "Lead Poisoning Killed 10 Kids in Brooklyn in '55, Highest Toll in the City," that was "based largely on data from the Health Department." LIA, *Quarterly Report of the Secretary* (April 2, 1956), LIA Papers. In addition to "the common run of newspaper studies on childhood and other types of plumbism," the LIA noted two "items of adverse publicity transcending [them] in importance: In July 1956 *Parade* magazine, which reached over seven million readers in fifty newspapers across the country, ran an article titled "Don't Let YOUR Child Get Lead Poisoning," and the CBS television network also carried a broadcast on childhood lead poisoning. LIA, *Quarterly Report of the Secretary* (October 1, 1956), LIA Papers. In response to all of this information, the LIA "virtually prepared a talk on lead poisoning that a New York doctor delivered before a group of pediatricians in that city." LIA, *Quarterly Report of the Secretary* (April 2, 1956), LIA Papers.

117. National Lead Company, "Important" [sales manual] (ca. 1949), LIA Papers.

118. Felix Wormser, "Discussion in Conference on Lead Poisoning," Seventh Annual Conference on Industrial Health, American Medical Association (September 30–October 2, 1946), 51.

119. Sherwin-Williams, file: "High Standard House Paints," "Super One Coat House Paint," sold under the Lowe Brothers label, an affiliate of S-W, February 12, 1954, "Lowe Brothers High Standard House Paint" label, Basic Carbonate White Lead, Primer white 260: 62% pigment, 23% lead "for Exterior

or Interior Use"; "Lowe Brothers High Standard House Paint" label, Basic Carbonate White Lead, Colony Yellow 317: 65% pigment, 14% lead "for Exterior or Interior Use," LIA Papers.

120. LIA, Annual Meeting, *Report of the Secretary* (April 13–14, 1950), LIA Papers.

121. American Standards Association, "American Standards Specifications to Minimize Hazards to Children from Residual Surface Coating Materials," (Z66.1-1955) ASA, approved February 16, 1955, LIA papers; NPVLA, "Subcommittee on Model Labeling, "Minutes of Meeting," August 12, 1954.

122. Ibid.

123. NPVLA, Subcommittee on Model Labeling, "Minutes of Meeting" (August 12, 1954), LIA Papers. He noted that "considerable change from the original proposal had resulted."

124. "New Label to Warn of Paint Poison Risk," *New York Times* (September 9, 1954), 45.

125. Jerome Trichter to C. W. Slocum (August 24, 1954), LIA Papers.

126. LIA, "Report of the Secretary Summarizing the Activities of the Lead Industries Association for the Year 1953," Annual Meeting (April 22–23, 1954), in Robert Zeigler to Members of the LIA (April 12, 1954), 5, LIA Papers.

127. Paul Whitford to John C. Moore (September 2, 1954), LIA Papers.

128. Paul Whitford to Joseph F. Battley (May 27, 1958), LIA Papers.

129. "Precautionary Labels Recommended by the National Paint, Varnish and Lacquer Association" in Battley, President, NPVLA, to Members of the Executive Committee (October 6, 1954), LIA Papers.

130. Bernard E. Conley to Jerome Trichter (September 9, 1954), LIA Papers.

131. "Paint Edict Here to Cut Lead Peril," *New York Times* (October 30, 1954), 19; NPVLA, Toxic Materials Committee Meeting, Minutes (October 27, 1954), "Confidential"; New York City Department of Health, Press Release, (November 10, 1954), LIA Papers.

132. LIA, *Annual Report for the Year 1955* (1955), 6, LIA Papers.

133. LIA, *Report of Health and Safety Division*, 28th Annual Meeting (April 24-25, 1956), LIA Papers. See also LIA, *Annual Report for the Year 1956* (1956), LIA Papers: "Publications relative to lead hazards have been watched and, where warranted, the attention of authors has been called to unduly adverse statements."

134. NPVLA, Subcommittee on Model Labeling, Minutes (June 15, 1954), LIA Papers.

135. T. J. McDowell, "Suggested Course of Action for NPVL Association Re: Labeling Laws" (ca. July 1954) in NPVLA, Subcommittee on Model Labeling, Minutes (July 15, 1954), LIA Papers.

136. Bowditch to Wormser (July 11, 1956), LIA Papers. Supported by officials such as Gale Norton, the secretary of the interior in the George W. Bush administration, the lead interests have been well represented in government

and in those agencies that regulate it. In 1947 Wormser had assumed the role of president of the LIA, but he had also assumed the more remunerative role of vice president of the St. Joseph Lead Company, engaging in public relations and "Washington legislative matters," that is, lobbying. In 1953 he resigned from St. Joseph Lead to join the Eisenhower administration where he supervised the Bureau of Mines, the Defense Minerals Exploration Administration, and the Office of Oil and Gas. Douglas McKay, "Memorandum to the President" (March 17, 1953), Dwight D. Eisenhower: Records as President (White House Central Files), Official File, Box 115, 4 April 1953, Dwight D. Eisenhower Library Abilene, Kansas.

137. Wormser to Clinton H. Crane, Chair of the Board, St. Joseph Lead Company (March 18, 1953), Wormser MSS, American Heritage Center, University of Wyoming, Cheyenne.

138. Felix Edgar Wormser, curriculum vitae (ca. 1961), Wormser MSS; Marquis W. Childs, "Senators Continuing Inquiry into Grants to Missouri Firm, Committee Still Exploring Possible Conflict of Interest in $345,185 in Advances to St. Joseph Lead Company," *St. Louis Post-Dispatch* (August 28, 1957), Wormser MSS; George Clifford, "Company Ties to U.S. Buying of Lead Bared," *Washington Daily News* (June 15, 1962), 5, Wormser MSS.

139. E. P. Hubschmitt, "A Review of the Second Draft Copy of Title IV: Dealing with the Sanitary Code, New York City," in Hubschmitt to members of the Subcommittee on Uniform Labeling, Subject: Ref. File Misc. #44E-Uniform Paint Labeling Law (September 15, 1958), LIA Papers. By 1960 even consultants for the NPVLA acknowledged that "the dried film of paint may present a hazard during removal by sanding or burning, if chewed by children, or if the loose paint is eaten by children." This conclusion was circulated by the NPVLA to the members of the Subcommittee on Toxicology and Labeling and was approved by them for circulation to the Scientific Committee. This was done because it "summarize[d] the present state of knowledge as to the toxicity of our industry's products." A. E. Van Wirt, "Suggestions on Toxicological Study" (June 14, 1960), LIA Papers; and Francis Scofield to Members of the Scientific Committee: Toxicological Study (June 14, 1960), LIA Papers.

140. LIA, *Quarterly Report of the Secretary, January 1 to March 31, 1956* (April 2, 1956), LIA Papers: "A protest was filed with the proper legislative committee in New York State against a bill dealing with paint that would be unnecessarily harmful to both the paint and lead industries." The association proudly informed its members that "the bill did not come out of committee."

141. LIA, *Quarterly Report of the Secretary, October 1 to December 31, 1957* (January 10, 1958), LIA Papers.

142. LIA, *Report of Health and Safety Division*, 30th Annual Meeting (April 15–16, 1958), LIA Papers.

143. Bowditch to Wormser (July 11, 1956), LIA Papers.

144. LIA, *Report of Health and Safety Division*, Manfred Bowditch, Director, 29th Annual Meeting (April 24–25, 1957), LIA Papers.

145. LIA, *Report of Health and Safety Division*, 29th Annual Meeting (April 24–25, 1957), LIA Papers.

146. Bowditch to Kehoe (December 26, 1957), LIA Papers.

147. Vincent F. Guinee, M.D. [New York City Department of Health], to Naomi Feigelson (January 5, 1973), "Subject: News Release—Illegal Paint," LIA Papers.

148. Folder: "Lead in Paint on Children's Toys" (1957), Kehoe Papers, Box 39.

149. LIA, *Quarterly Report of the Secretary, July 1 to September 30, 1959* (October 8, 1959). LIA, *Annual Report for 1959* (1959), LIA Papers.

150. Ibid.

151. Ibid.

152. LIA, *Quarterly Report of the Secretary, April 1 to June 30, 1960* (July 1, 1960), LIA Papers.

153. Christian Warren, *Brush with Death: A Social History of Lead Poisoning* (Baltimore: Johns Hopkins University Press, 2000), 186–87.

154. We are indebted to Christian Warren's book, *Brush with Death*, for his excellent discussion of this period.

155. Noted in Warren, *Brush with Death*, 191–97.

156. Don G. Fowler to All Members of the Lead Health and Safety Committee, "Table 6 Number of Deaths Due to Accidental Poisoning by Type of Solid and Liquid Substances for Children under 5 Years of Age, United States 1960–1964" (June 28, 1966), LIA Papers.

157. Warren, *Brush with Death*, 199–200.

158. Ibid., 200.

159. Ibid., 198.

160. National Academy of Sciences, "Report of the Ad-Hoc Committee to Evaluate the Hazard of Lead in Paint," prepared for the Consumer Product Safety Commission (November 1973), 17, 11, in Jerome F. Smith to Official Members of the Lead Industries Association, Inc. (March 5, 1974).

161. LIA, Environmental Health Committee, "Minutes of the 1972 Autumn Meeting," in J. F. Cole to Members of the Lead Environmental Health Committee, (November 19, 1971), LIA Papers.

162. Warren, *Brush with Death*, 201.

163. Ibid., 202.

164. Ibid.

165. Ibid.

166. Carmel McCoubrey, "J. J. Chisolm, 79, Dies: Lead Poison Crusader," *New York Times* (June 26, 2001), C15. See also J. Julian Chisolm Jr. and David M. O'Hara, *Lead Absorption in Children: Management, Clinical, and Environmental Aspects* (Baltimore: Urban and Schwarzenberg, 1982).

167. Warren, *Brush with Death*, 229. Chisolm had begun to receive funds from the LIA following the first of his publications on lead poisoning and children. This was in the mid-1950s when the industry had virtually given up on large amounts of lead pigments in interior paints.

168. Ibid., 227.

169. J. S. Lin-Fu, "Modern History of Lead Poisoning: A Century of Discovery and Rediscovery," in H. L. Needleman, ed., *Human Lead Exposure* (Boca Raton, FL: CRC Press, 1992), 23–43. In 1982 *Science News* reported that over 12 percent of African American children six months to five years old and 2 percent of all white children had blood-lead levels of 30 micrograms per deciliter. In families with incomes below $6,000, 18.5 percent of black children and 5.9 percent of white children had these levels. In urban centers of 1,000,000 or more, 18.6 percent of black children and 4.5 percent of white children had such levels. "The biggest problem is still leaded paint and soil or dust saturated with lead deposited by auto exhaust and industrial emissions." J. Raloff, "Childhood Lead: Worrisome National Levels," *Science News* 121 (February 1982), 88.

CHAPTER 4. OLD POISONS, NEW PROBLEMS

1. LIA, *Report of Health and Safety Division*, Manfred Bowditch, Director (April 24–25, 1956), LIA Papers.

2. LIA, *Quarterly Report of the Secretary* (October 1, 1956), LIA Papers.

3. Quoted in Christian Warren, *Brush with Death: A Social History of Lead Poisoning* (Baltimore: Johns Hopkins University Press, 2000), 205. This section is based upon the research and insights of Warren, especially on pp. 203–23.

4. Kehoe to R. E. Eckardt, Esso (March 10, 1955), Kehoe Manuscripts, Box 99.

5. Warren, 208.

6. U.S. Public Health Service, *Symposium on Environmental Lead Contamination* (Washington: GPO, March 1966), Table 1, 32.

7. Quoted in Warren, 209.

8. Robert A. Kehoe, "The Fate of Inhaled Particulate Lead Compounds," Grant Application to the U.S. Public Health Service (May 29, 1964), Kehoe Manuscripts, University of Cincinnati, Box 34, Folder: "Experimental Subjects—Inhalation of Lead."

9. Robert A. Kehoe, "The Administration and Elimination of Lead from Adult Human Subjects under Natural and Experimentally Induced Conditions over Extended Periods of Time," Kehoe Manuscripts, Box 83, Folder: Dr. Kehoe's Manuscript (August 2, 1983), 11.

10. See David Rothman, *Strangers at the Bedside: A History of How Law and Bioethics Transformed Medical Decision Making* (New York: Basic Books, 1991), for a history of human experimentation during this period.

11. LIA, *Quarterly Report of the Secretary, October 1 to December 31, 1961* (January 3, 1962), LIA Papers.

12. LIA, *Members Quarterly Report, January 1 to March 31, 1962* (April 30, 1962), LIA Papers; LIA, *Report of Association Activities—1962* (April 8, 1963), LIA Papers.

13. Warren, *Brush with Death*, 207–10.

14. Clair C. Patterson, "Contaminated and Natural Lead Environments of Man," *Archives of Environmental Health* 11 (September 1965), 350.

15. Warren, *Brush with Death*, 210–11

16. Warren, *Brush with Death*, 307, fn. 4.

17. Quoted in Warren, *Brush with Death*, 212.

18. Lead Education and Abatement Design Group, <http://www.lead.org.au/fs/fst3.html> (February 11, 2002).

19. Warren, *Brush with Death*, 214, suggests that Kehoe took this position if for no other reason than to make room for a detailed critique of Patterson and to undermine his credentials.

20. Warren, *Brush with Death*, 216–17.

21. Ibid., 218–19. Indeed, Patterson's challenge to prevailing ideas about environmental lead was extending beyond the scientific and technical communities by the late 1960s. Saul Bellow modeled Albert Corde, his central character in his book *The Dean's December* on Patterson. Saul Bellow, *The Dean's December* (New York: Harper and Row, 1982).

22. Robert A. Kehoe, "Under What Circumstances Is Ingestion of Lead Dangerous?" in U.S. Public Health Service, *Symposium on Environmental Lead Contamination* (Washington: GPO, March 1966), 54.

23. Harriet Hardy, "Lead," in U.S. Public Health Service, *Symposium on Environmental Lead Contamination* (Washington: GPO, March 1966), 74–82.

24. Melvin W. First, "Possibilities of Removal of Sources of Lead Contamination in the Environment," *Symposium on Environmental Lead Contamination*, Public Health Service, (December 13–15, 1965), 91.

25. Ibid., 92.

26. Roy O. McCaldin, "Estimation of Sources of Atmospheric Lead and Measured Atmospheric Lead Levels," in U.S. Public Health Service, *Symposium on Environmental Lead Contamination* (Washington: GPO, March 1966), 8.

27. Harry Heimann in Discussion of Harry Heimann, "Risk of Exposure and Absorption of Lead," in U.S. Public Health Service, *Symposium on Environmental Lead Contamination* (Washington: GPO, March 1966), 147.

28. Robert Kehoe to Harriet Hardy (December 23, 1965), LIA Papers.

29. Robert Kehoe to John R. Goldsmith (November 16, 1959), LIA Papers. See also Kehoe to John Goldsmith (November 28, 1966), LIA Papers, in which Kehoe reiterates his worries that the profession questions his integrity. His concern is that people believe that his work "has been tilted toward the benefit of those who have provided the funds in support of our work."

30. Discussion of Harry Heimann, "Risk of Exposure and Absorption of Lead," in U.S. Public Health Service, *Symposium on Environmental Lead Contamination* (Washington: GPO, March 1966), 151.

31. LIA, "Minutes of Special Committee on Health and Safety" (January 14, 1966), Wormser MSS, American Heritage Center, University of Wyoming, Cheyenne. Included on the committee were S. D. Strauss, chairman, American Smelting and Refining Company; A. H. Drewes, National Lead Company; John

Englehorn, St. Joseph Lead Company; and Burt Goss and Carl Thompson, Hill & Knowlton.

32. LIA, "No Public Hazard from Lead Seen, Muskie Sub-Committee on Pollution Told," Press Release (June 9, 1966), Wormser MSS.

33. Senate, Committee on Public Works, Subcommittee on Air and Water Pollution, *Air Pollution—1966*, 89th Cong. 2nd Sess. (1966), 205.

34. Joseph C. Robert, *Ethyl: A History of the Corporation and the People Who Made It* (Charlottesville: University Press of Virginia, 1983), 294.

35. Senate Committee on Public Works, *Air Pollution—1966*, 205.

36. LIA, "Opinion Research Corp. Caravan Survey on Lead: Summary Report," in J. L. Kimberly to Board of Directors (March 7, 1967). LIA Papers. The summary report was prepared by Hill & Knowlton, Inc., LIA's public relations counsel."

37. Don G. Fowler, Director, and James C. Roumas, Assistant Director, *Health and Safety Report 1967*, LIA Annual Meeting (April 17–18, 1967), LIA Papers.

38. David M. Borcina, Secretary-Treasurer, LIA, to Members of the LIA (January 18, 1968), LIA Papers.

39. LIA, "Facts about Lead and the Atmosphere" (1968), LIA Papers.

40. LIA, Meeting of Board of Directors, Minutes (December 3, 1969), LIA Papers; LIA, Meeting of Board of Directors, Minutes (April 14, 1969), LIA Papers. In a 1972 letter to the editor of the *Washington Post*, the LIA maintained that "there was not a shred of evidence" to link "lead usage in gasoline with pediatric lead poisoning." The LIA argued that all pediatric lead poisoning was due to lead paint "now chipping and flaking in sub-standard housing." J. F. Cole, Director, Environmental Health, LIA, to Editor, *Washington Post* (June 30, 1972), LIA Papers.

41. Warren, *Brush with Death*, 220.

42. Robert, *Ethyl*, 295–96.

43. Warren, *Brush with Death*, 220.

44. Kehoe to Charles L. Goodacre (April 28, 1971), LIA Papers.

45. Warren, *Brush with Death*, 220–21.

46. Jerome F. Cole to Editor, *New York Times* (August 23, 1982), A-16.

47. Warren, *Brush with Death*, 222–23.

48. LIA [Secretary-Treasurer Robert Ziegfield], *Annual Report for the Year 1957* (1957) LIA Papers.

49. For a summary of the issues that OSHA was considering, see Department of Labor, Occupational Safety and Health Administration, "Proposed Standard for Exposure to Lead," *Federal Register* 42, 2 (January 4, 1977), 808–12.

50. For an extensive although incomplete list of more than one hundred occupations, see: Thomas D. Matte, Philip J. Landrigan, and Edward L. Baker, "Occupational Lead Exposure," in Herbert L. Needleman, ed., *Human Lead Exposure* (Boca Raton: CRC Press), 159.

51. "Post-Hearing Brief of United Steelworkers of America, AFL-CIO-CLC on Standard for Inorganic Lead" (June 20, 1977), Lead Docket H 004, Exhibit 343, Department of Labor Docket Office, Washington, DC.

52. Frank Nix, "Testimony on OSHA's Proposed Standard for Occupational Exposure to Lead" (April 1977), Lead Docket, H 004B, Exhibit 178, Department of Labor Docket Office.

53. "Post-Hearing Brief of United Steelworkers of America, AFL-CIO-CLC on Standard for Inorganic Lead" (June 20, 1977), Lead Docket, H 004, Exhibit 343, Department of Labor Docket Office.

54. Louis S. Beliczky, *Special Report to the International President* (June 22, 1976), Lead Docket H 004B, Exhibit 115B, Department of Labor Docket Office.

55. "Post-Hearing Brief of United Steelworkers of America, AFL-CIO-CLC on Standard for Inorganic Lead" (June 20, 1977), Lead Docket, H 004, Exhibit 343, Department of Labor Docket Office.

56. Ibid.

57. Ibid.

58. David P. McCaffrey, *OSHA and the Politics of Health Regulation* (New York: Plenum Press, 1982), 118–19; "Post-Hearing Brief of United Steelworkers of America, AFL-CIO-CLC on Standard for Inorganic Lead" (June 20, 1977), Lead Docket, H 004, Exhibit 343, Department of Labor Docket Office.

59. Charles Noble, *Liberalism at Work: The Rise and Fall of OSHA* (Philadelphia: Temple University Press, 1986), 190.

60. Sheldon Samuels, "Statement on Behalf of Peter Bommarito, President, United Rubber Workers" (March 1977), Lead Docket, H 004B, Exhibit 149, Department of Labor Docket Office.

61. "Post-Hearing Brief of United Steelworkers of America, AFL-CIO-CLC on Standard for Inorganic Lead" (June 20, 1977), Lead Docket, H 004, Exhibit 343, Department of Labor Docket Office.

62. Ibid.

63. Ibid.

64. Ibid.

65. Ibid.

66. Herbert Needleman, "Statement before the Department of Labor Public Hearing on Occupational Lead Standard" (March 1977), Lead Docket, H 004B, Exhibit 69, Department of Labor Docket Office.

67. See Warren, *Brush with Death*, 250–53, for a discussion of this issue.

68. Andrea M. Hricko, "Testimony on Reproductive Effects of Lead Exposure: Scientific Evidence and Policy Issues," Lead Docket, H 004B, Exhibit 60-A-2, Department of Labor Docket Office.

69. Ibid.

70. Ibid.

71. Vilma R. Hunt, "Testimony" (n.d.), Lead Docket, H 004B, Exhibit 59, Department of Labor Docket Office.

72. Jeanne M. Stellman, "Testimony on the Proposed OSHA Lead Exposure Standard" (March 1977), Lead Docket, H 004B, Exhibit 61, Department of Labor Docket Office.

73. Ibid. See also in Docket H 004B the statements by Camille Kozlowski, National Organization for Women, Exhibit 110; William M. Rom, University of Utah, College of Medicine, Exhibit 233; Madeline Janover, NOW Labor Task Force, Exhibit 109; Congresswoman Patricia Schroeder, Exhibit 71A; Olga Madar, president, Coalition of Labor Union Women (CLUW), Exhibit 71; Florence Simons, worker at Globe Union Co., Exhibit 73; and Jane Culbreth, National Federation of Business and Professional Women, Exhibit 226. See also Wendy Chavkin to Docket Officer, OSHA (May 29, 1981), Lead Docket, H 004E, Exhibit 527-51, Department of Labor Docket Office.

74. Samuel S. Epstein with Herbert Needleman and Donald Johnson, "AFL-CIO Proposed OSHA Lead Standard: Its Biological and Environmental Bases" (March 21, 1977), Lead Docket, H 004B, Exhibit 68, Department of Labor Docket Office.

75. Ibid.

76. Odessa Komer, "Foreword," in Jeanne Mager Stellman, *Women's Work, Women's Health: Myths and Realities* (New York: Pantheon Books, 1977), xvii.

77. United Auto Workers, "Supporting Materials for Testimony: Proposed Standard for Occupational Exposure to Lead" (March 7, 1977), Lead Docket, H 004B, Exhibit 232, 7, Department of Labor Docket Office.

78. Ibid.

79. Claudia Miller, "Testimony . . . on Behalf of the United Auto Workers of America" (April 11, 1977), Lead Docket, H 004B, Exhibit 155A, Department of Labor Docket Office.

80. Anne M. Trebilcock, "OSHA and Equal Employment Opportunity Laws for Women," *Preventive Medicine* 7 (September 1978), 372. See also Kenneth Bridbord, "Occupational Lead Exposure and Women," *Preventive Medicine* 7 (September 1978), 311–21.

81. Stellman, *Women's Work, Women's Health*, 178.

82. See Ruth Heifetz, "Women, Lead, and Reproductive Hazards: Defining a New Risk," in David Rosner and Gerald Markowitz, *Dying for Work: Workers' Safety and Health in Twentieth-Century America* (Bloomington: Indiana University Press, 1987), 162–63.

83. Stellman, *Women's Work, Women's Health*, 186.

84. Ibid.

85. "Post-Hearing Brief of United Steelworkers of America, AFL-CIO-CLC on Standard for Inorganic Lead" (June 20, 1977), Lead Docket, H 004, Exhibit 343, Department of Labor Docket Office.

86. Andrea M. Hricko, "Testimony on Reproductive Effects of Lead Exposure: Scientific Evidence and Policy Issues," Lead Docket, H 004B, Exhibit 60-A-2, Department of Labor Docket Office.

87. "Post-Hearing Brief of United Steelworkers of America, AFL-CIO-CLC on Standard for Inorganic Lead" (June 20, 1977), 54, Lead Docket, H 004, Exhibit 343, Department of Labor Docket Office.

88. Sheldon Samuels, "Statement on Behalf of Peter Bommarito, President, United Rubber Workers" (March 1977), Lead Docket, H 004B, Exhibit 149, Department of Labor Docket Office.

89. Ibid.

90. "Post-Hearing Brief of United Steelworkers of America, AFL-CIO-CLC on Standard for Inorganic Lead" (June 20, 1977), 54, Lead Docket, H 004, Exhibit 343, Department of Labor Docket Office.

91. Ibid., 59–65.

92. Jerome F. Cole to Max Allen, Canadian Broadcasting Company (January 18, 1974), Lead Docket, H 004, Exhibit 125, Department of Labor Docket Office.

93. Debevoise, Plimpton, Lyons, & Gates, Attorneys for LIA, Inc., "Post-Hearing Comments by the Lead Industries Association, Inc. Concerning the Proposed Standard for Exposure to Lead" (June 16, 1977), 2–4, Lead Docket, H 004B, Exhibit 335, Department of Labor Docket Office.

94. Ibid., 5–7.

95. Ibid.

96. Ibid., 18–19.

97. Ibid., 20–22.

98. Ibid., 30–34.

99. Ibid., 38–40.

100. Warren, *Brush with Death*, 249.

101. Ellen Silbergeld, Philip Landrigan, John Froines, and Richard Pfeffer, "The Occupational Lead Standard: A Goal Unachieved, a Process in Need of Repair," in Charles Levenstein and John Wooding, eds., *Work, Health, and Environment: Old Problems, New Solutions* (New York: Guilford Press, 1997), 133.

102. Noble, *Liberalism at Work*, 193.

103. Warren, *Brush with Death*, 250.

104. Silbergeld, Landrigan, Froines, and Pfeffer, 132.

105. Ibid., 133–134.

106. Ibid., 134.

107. Warren, *Brush with Death*, 229.

108. Quoted in Warren, *Brush with Death*, 229.

109. Herbert Needleman and David Bellinger, "Developmental Consequences of Childhood Exposures to Lead," *Advances in Clinical Child Psychology*, vol. 7, ed. by Benjamin Lahey and Alan Kazdin (New York: Plenum Press, 1984), 195.

110. Stephen Burd, "Scientists See Big Business on the Offensive," *The Chronicle of Higher Education* (December 14, 1994), A-27.

111. Thomas A. Lewis, "The Difficult Quest of Herbert Needleman," *National Wildlife* (April–May 1995), 24.

112. Bruce Lanphear, Kim Dietrich, Peggy Auinger, and Christopher Cox, "Cognitive Deficits Associated with Blood Lead Concentrations < 10 *mg*/dL in U.S. Children and Adolescents," *Public Health Reports* 115 (November–

December 2000), 521–29; John Rosen and Paul Mushak, "Primary Prevention of Childhood Lead Poisoning—the Only Solution," *NEJM* 344 (May 10, 2001), 1470–71; David C. Bellinger, "Interpreting the Literature on Lead and Child Development: The Neglected Role of the 'Experimental System,'" *Neurotoxicology and Teratology* 17 (1995), 201–12; John F. Rosen and Joel G. Pounds, "'Severe Chronic Lead Insult That Maintains Body Burdens of Lead Related to Those in the Skeleton': Observations of Dr. Clair Patterson Conclusively Demonstrated," *Environmental Research, Section A* 78 (1998), 140–51; Joel Schwartz, "Societal Benefits of Reducing Lead Exposure," *Environmental Research* 66 (1994), 105–24; David Salkever, "Updated Estimates of Earnings Benefits from Reduced Exposure of Children to Environmental Lead," *Environmental Research* 70 (1995), 1–6; Joel Schwartz, "Beyond LOEL's, p Values, and Vote Counting: Methods for Looking at the Shapes and Strengths of Associations," *NeuroToxicology* 14 (1993), 237–46; Joel Schwartz, "Low-Level Lead Exposure and Children's IQ: A Meta-analysis and Search for a Threshold," *Environmental Research* 65 (1994), 42–55.

113. Philip J. Landrigan, "Pediatric Lead Poisoning: Is There a Threshold?" *Public Health Reports* 115 (November/December 2000), 530–31.

114. See Philip Landrigan, interview transcript with Bill Moyers, "Trade Secrets," <www.pbs.org/tradesecrets/trans/intero3.html>; Environmental Working Group, Chemical Industry Archives, <http://www.chemicalindustryarchives.org/factfiction/facts/3.asp>.

115. Daland R. Juburg, *Lead and Human Health: An Update*, 2nd ed. (New York: American Council on Science and Health, 2000), 21.

116. Ibid., 6.

117. See Kaye Kilburn, "A Paradigm for Environmental Epidemiology: Why Are Effects of Environmental Exposures Different from Occupational Effects?" *Archives of Environmental Health* 55 (September–October 2000), 295–96.

118. "Update: Blood Lead Levels—United States, 1991–1994," *Morbidity and Mortality Weekly Reports* 46 (1997), 141–46, cited in Philip J. Landrigan, "Pediatric Lead Poisoning: Is There a Threshold?" *Public Health Reports* 115 (November–December 2000), 530–31.

119. Interview with Anthony Bale (June 20, 2001), New York.

CHAPTER 5. BETTER LIVING THROUGH CHEMISTRY?

1. Two industry spokespeople decried "the attitude of smugness which associates atmospheric pollution with industrial prosperity and ignores the desirability of its reduction." W. C. L. Hemeon, and T. F. Hatch, "Atmospheric Pollution," *Industrial and Engineering Chemistry* 39 (May 1947), 568. See also Robert E. Swain, "Smoke and Fume Investigations, a Historical Review," *Industrial and Engineering Chemistry* 41 (November 1949), 2384–88.

2. W. Michael McCabe, "Donora Disaster Was Crucible for Clean Air," <www.dep.state.pa.us/dep/Rachel_Carson/crucible.htm> (August 23, 2001).

See, for the most comprehensive analyses of the Donora disaster: Lynne Page Snyder, "The 'Death-Dealing Smog' over Donora, Pennsylvania: Industrial Air Pollution, Public Health Policy, and the Politics of Expertise, 1948–1949," *Environmental History Review* 18 (Spring 1994), 117–39; and Lynne Page Snyder, "'The Death-Dealing Smog over Donora, Pennslyvania':, Industrial Air Pollution, Public Health, and Federal Policy, 1915–1963," Ph.D. dissertation, University of Pennslyvania, 1994.

3. Lynn Glover, "Donora's Killer Smog Noted at 50," <www.dep.state .pa.us/dep/Rachel_Carson/killersmog.htm>. In London in 1952, more than one thousand people died as a result of another smog crisis, leading to worldwide attention to the issue. The first air pollution research bill was enacted in the United States in 1955.

4. MCA Statement, OSHA Vinyl Chloride Hearing, first draft (February 7, 1974), 1, Papers of the Manufacturing Chemists Association (later the Chemical Manufacturers Association) at Baggett, McCall, Burgess and Watson, Lake Charles, LA (hereafter referred to as MCA Papers).

5. MCA, Air Pollution Abatement Committee, "Minutes of Meeting" (January 11, 1950), MCA Papers.

6. "Air Pollution . . . How to Solve This Industrial Puzzler," *Modern Industry* 18 (September 15, 1949), 46–50. The article stated that California had already passed an air pollution law and that Pennsylvania was about to pass one. See also R. L. Ireland, "City Smog—A Dilemma of Public Hygiene," *National Safety News* (August 1949), 38, 39, 86–90: "The American Chemical Society devoted a two-day symposium to atmospheric contamination during its 1949 convention." "Federal Research, Local Control Urged for Air Pollution Problem," *Chemical & Engineering News* 28 (May 15, 1950), 1642–43; "Air Clean-up Still Going Full Blast," *Modern Industry* 20 (November 1950), 68: "Increasingly stringent laws, plus realization that polluted air is one of the quickest ways to lose the backing of the industrial community, are bringing increased attention to control of air pollution." H. H. Shrenk, "Air Pollution," *Chemical & Engineering News* 29 (April 23, 1951), 1640–42; "Chemical Industry Can Solve Its Own Air Pollution Problems," *Chemical & Engineering News* 31 (March 9, 1953), 995–96: Tone of the conference was set by R. H. Boundy of Dow, who suggested a five-point program for waging enlarged war on air pollution and William I. Burt of B. F. Goodrich "stated that the MCA Air Pollution Abatement Manual . . . is rapidly approaching 'completion.'"

7. MCA, Air Pollution Abatement Committee, "Minutes of Meeting" (January 11, 1950), MCA Papers.

8. MCA, Air Pollution Abatement Committee, "Minutes of Meeting" (September 13, 1950), MCA Papers.

9. MCA, Air Pollution Abatement Committee, "Minutes of Meeting" (October 22, 1952), MCA Papers. In 1952, the MCA established the Texas Chemical Manufacturers Council.

10. Paul L. Magill, "The Los Angeles Smog Problem," *Industrial and Engineering Chemistry* 41 (November 1949), 2476–86.

11. Robert T. Reinhardt, "West Coast: Smog Ceases to Be a Joke to Industrialists Spending Millions of $ for Control of Waste Gases," *Iron Age* 163 (April 14, 1949), 104.

12. MCA, Air Pollution Abatement Committee, "Minutes of Meeting" (April 21, 1954), MCA Papers.

13. MCA, Air Pollution Abatement Committee, "Minutes of Meeting" (February 9, 1955), MCA Papers.

14. "Production: It's Up to Industry Now," *Chemical Week* (March 1, 1952), 48; "Production . . ." *Chemical Week* (March 14, 1953), 69–76. The MCA in particular aggressively defended the industry from criticism by government officials. "MCA Protests Pollution Stand: Health, Education and Welfare Statements on Lack of Research and Information Challenged," *Chemical & Engineering News* 32 (August 23, 1954), 3361; "Industry's Air Pollution Includes . . . Carrying the Battle to Washington," *Steel* 135 (October 11, 1954), 70.

15. R. D. Scott, B. F. Goodrich Chemical Company, "Louisville Air Pollution Study," in MCA, Air Pollution Abatement Committee, "Minutes of Meeting" (May 22, 1956), MCA Papers.

16. MCA, Air Pollution Abatement Committee, "Minutes of Meeting" (September 14, 1960), MCA Papers.

17. MCA, Medical Advisory Committee, "Minutes of Meeting" (October 5, 1960), MCA Papers.

18. Ibid.

19. John C. Ruddock, "Proceedings," Meeting of the Sub Committee on Atmospheric Pollutants, Medical Advisory Committee, American Petroleum Institute (September 23, 1959), NARG 90 (Public Health Service), Air Pollution Medical Branch, Project Records, 1955–60, 241.5, Box 6. See also Leon O. Emik, Chief, Laboratory Investigations, Air Pollution Medical Program, to Chief, Air Pollution Medical Program, "Visit with Dr. John C. Ruddock, May 15, 1958" (May 29, 1958), NARG 90 (Public Health Service), Air Pollution Medical Branch, Project Records, 1955–60, 241.5, Box 6; John C. Ruddock, "Statement by Chairman, Sub Committee on Atmospheric Pollutants" (June 22, 1959), NARG 90 (Public Health Service), Air Pollution Medical Branch, Project Records, 1955–60, 241.5, Box 6.

20. MCA, Public Relations Advisory Committee, "Report of Glen Perry, Chairman," in "Minutes of the 115th Meeting of the Directors of the MCA" (February 13, 1962), MCA Papers.

21. MCA, Air Pollution Abatement Committee, "Minutes of Meeting" (February 7–8, 1962), MCA Papers.

22. Hal K. Rothman, *The Greening of a Nation? Environmentalism in the United States since 1945* (Fort Worth: Harcourt Brace College Publishers, 1998), 115.

23. Linda Lear, *Rachel Carson: Witness for Nature* (New York: Henry Holt, 1997), 429.

24. Ibid., 431.

25. MCA, "Meeting of the MCA Board of Directors" (September 11, 1962), MCA Papers. The board's actions were based on suggestions of its constituent committees. See, for example, MCA, Air Pollution Abatement Committee, "Minutes of Meeting" (May 9, 1962), MCA Papers.

26. General Hull, "The MCA Program: A Review," in "Meeting of MCA Board of Directors" (October 10, 1962), MCA Papers.

27. MCA, "Meeting of the MCA Board of Directors" (January 8, 1963), MCA Papers.

28. MCA, "Meeting of the MCA Board of Directors" (April 9, 1963), MCA Papers.

29. MCA, Ad Hoc Planning Committee on Environmental Health, Minutes (June 24–25, 1963), 2, MCA Papers.

30. Ibid., "Appendix 1, Draft 6/25/63, Environmental Health and the Chemical Industry" 2. See also MCA, "Recommendations of the Ad-Hoc Planning Committee on Environmental Health" draft (August 13, 1963), Appendix 1, MCA Papers, where it is stated that the "environment is hostile" and that "perfect environment and perfect well-being are not attainable."

31. MCA, Ad Hoc Planning Committee on Environmental Health, Minutes (June 24–25, 1963), "Appendix 1, Draft 6/25/63, Environmental Health and the Chemical Industry," 2, MCA Papers.

32. Ibid. See also MCA, "Recommendations of the Ad-Hoc Planning Committee on Environmental Health" draft, (August 13, 1963), Appendix 1."

33. General George H. Decker, "MCA Staff Report," in "Meeting of the MCA Board of Directors" (April 14, 1964), MCA Papers, Exhibit A. General George H. Decker, "MCA Staff Report," in "Meeting of the MCA Board of Directors" (May 12, 1964), MCA Papers, Exhibit H.

34. MCA, "Meeting of the MCA Board of Directors" (November 25, 1963), MCA Papers.

35. John O. Logan, Vice Chairman, "Report to the Board of Directors of the Manufacturing Chemists' Association, Environmental Health Committee" (March 9, 1965), MCA Papers.

36. MCA, "Recommendations of the Ad-Hoc Planning Committee on Environmental Health draft, 8/13/63, Appendix 1," 3. By April 1964, the MCA had replaced the ad hoc group with the Environmental Health Advisory Committee, composed of public relations experts, scientists, and managers from the member companies. Its mandate was to extend "industry interest and responsibility in environmental health to the ultimate use of chemicals." Further, the group was aimed at extending the gaze of the MCA beyond the plant or at the "moment and point of use." Now, the chemical industry decided that it had to "consider such matters in terms of appropriateness in the environment." See MCA, Minutes, Environmental Health Advisory Committee (April 9, 1963), MCA Papers.

37. MCA, "Recommendations of the Ad-Hoc Planning Committee on Environmental Health draft (August 13, 1963), Appendix 1," 3, MCA Papers.

38. MCA, Environmental Health Council, Minutes "Chart of Proposed Organization," v, vi, attached to MCA, "Recommendations of the Ad-Hoc Planning Committee on Environmental Health" draft (August 13, 1963).

39. MCA, Cleveland Lane, "Appendix No. 4, Report to the Environmental Health Advisory Committee MCA, on Public Relations Committee Activities" (May 1964), MCA Papers.

40. Ibid.

41. Ibid.

42. MCA, Environmental Health Advisory Committee (EHAC), Minutes (June 2, 1964), MCA Papers.

43. MCA, EHAC, "A Chemical Industry Policy for Legislative Action on Environmental Health," draft, (January 7, 1965), Appendix 2, MCA Papers.

44. MCA, EHAC, Minutes, draft (December 31, 1964), "Position Statement on Legislative Regulation of Industry in Regard to Environmental Health" (ca. January 7, 1965), MCA Papers.

45. MCA, EHAC, Minutes (June 2, 1964), MCA Papers.

46. MCA, EHAC, Minutes (January 7, 1965), MCA Papers, in "Supporting Addendum for a Chemical Industry Policy for Legislative Action on Environmental Health, Appendix 2" (approved January 7, 1965), "Position Statement on Legislative Regulation of Industry in Regard to Environmental Health."

47. MCA, EHAC, Minutes (June 2, 1964), MCA Papers.

48. MCA, EHAC, Minutes (January 7, 1965), in "Supporting Addendum for a Chemical Industry Policy for Legislative Action on Environmental Health, Appendix 2" (approved January 7, 1965), "Position Statement on Legislative Regulation of Industry in Regard to Environmental Health." MCA Papers.

49. See David Rosner and Gerald Markowitz, *Deadly Dust: Silicosis and the Politics of Occupational Disease in Twentieth Century America* (Princeton: Princeton University Press, 1991).

50. MCA, "Over-All Environmental Health Program as Recommended by the Environmental Health Advisory Committee" (March 1, 1966), MCA Papers.

51. Stanley Humphrey, Vice President, Booz, Allen, to Environmental Health Advisory Committee, MCA (March 1, 1965); MCA, Minutes, EHAC (June 22, 1965), MCA Papers.

52. MCA, EHAC, Minutes (August 5, 1965). See also MCA, EHAC, Minutes (October 8, 1965), MCA Papers.

53. MCA, EHAC, Minutes (November 11, 1965), MCA Papers.

54. MCA, EHAC, Minutes (March 1, 1966), MCA Papers.

55. MCA, "Over-All Environmental Health Program as Recommended by the Environmental Health Advisory Committee" (March 1, 1966), MCA Papers.

56. James Sterner, M.D., Chair, Environmental Health Advisory Committee, "Report to the Board of Directors of the Manufacturing Chemists' Association, Inc." (March 14, 1967), MCA Papers.

57. Ibid.

58. Ibid.

59. MCA, EHAC Minutes (ca. 1968), MCA Papers.

60. W. F. Bixby to MCA Air Quality Committee (January 25, 1967), Appendix 1 to MCA, Air Quality Committee, "Minutes of Meeting" (January 25–26, 1967), MCA Papers.

61. MCA, Air Quality Committee, "Minutes of Meeting" (February 18–19, 1969), MCA Papers.

62. J. S. Whitaker to Environmental Health Advisory Committee (December 9, 1969), MCA Papers.

63. J. Brooks Flippen, *Nixon and the Environment* (Albuquerque: University of New Mexico Press, 2000), 25.

64. George Best to Environmental Health Committee (January 20, 1970), MCA Papers.

65. Flippen, *Nixon and the Environment*, 46.

66. Ibid., 85.

67. Ibid., 86–88.

68. See David Vogel, *Fluctuating Fortunes: The Political Power of Business in America* (New York: Basic Books, 1989), 69.

69. Flippen, *Nixon and the Environment*, 88.

70. Ibid., 5.

71. Riley E. Dunlap, "Trends in Public Opinion Toward Environmental Issues: 1965–1990," in *American Environmentalism: The U.S. Environmental Movement, 1970–1990*, ed. by Riley E. Dunlap and Angela G. Mertig (Philadelphia: Taylor & Francis, 1992), 92.

72. Robert Gottlieb, *Forcing the Spring: The Transformation of the American Environmental Movement* (Washington: Island Press, 1993), 96.

73. See Vogel, *Fluctuating Fortunes*, 96.

74. Flippen, *Nixon and the Environment*, 5. David Vogel points out that between 1966 and 1968 eight significant pieces of consumer legislation were enacted, including the Truth in Lending Act, the Flammable Fabrics Act, the Fair Packaging and Labeling Act, and the Child Protection Act. See Vogel, *Fluctuating Fortunes*, 38. Samuel Hays, *Beauty, Health, and Permanence: Environmental Politics in the United States, 1955–1985* (Cambridge: Cambridge University Press, 1987); Martin V. Melosi, "Lyndon Johnson and Environmental Policy," in *The Johnson Years, Volume Two: Vietnam, The Environment, and Science* (Lawrence: University Press of Kansas, 1987), 115–17; Rothman, *The Greening of a Nation?*, 101–03.

75. Hays, *Beauty, Health, and Permanence*; Melosi, "Lyndon Johnson and Environmental Policy," 115–17.

76. Charles Noble, *Liberalism at Work: The Rise and Fall of OSHA* (Philadelphia: Temple University Press, 1986), 70. Coal miners working with the Black Lung Association and physicians such as Lorin Kerr also demanded improvements in working conditions. Compensation was perhaps the most important action involving safety and health in the decade.

77. Ibid.

78. Interview with Anthony Mazzocchi (January 26, 2001).

79. Ibid.

80. Tony Mazzocchi, "Introduction," in *A Collection of Documents from the OCAW Struggle for Worker Health and Safety* (Washington: Alice Hamilton College, 1998).

81. Interview with Tony Mazzocchi (January 26, 2001).

82. Tony Mazzocchi, "Crossing Paths: Science and the Working Class," *New Solutions* 8 (1998), 30.

83. Interview with Tony Mazzocchi (January 26, 2001), New York City.

84. Tony Mazzocchi, "Foreword," in "Proceedings," *Hazards of the Industrial Environment*, a conference sponsored by District 8 Council, Oil, Chemical and Atomic Workers International Union, Holiday Inn, Kenilworth, NJ (March 29, 1969), 2.

85. Ibid.

86. Interview with Tony Mazzocchi (January 26, 2001), New York City.

87. Tony Mazzocchi, in "Proceedings," *Hazards of the Industrial Environment*, a conference sponsored by District 7, Oil, Chemical and Atomic Workers International Union, Sheraton, Fort Wayne Motor Hotel, Fort Wayne, Indiana (October 24–26, 1969), 2.

88. Tony Mazzocchi, in "Proceedings," *Hazards of the Industrial Environment*, a conference sponsored by District 7, Oil, Chemical and Atomic Workers International Union, Rice Hotel, Houston, Texas (February 20–21, 1970), 55.

89. Interview with Tony Mazzocchi (January 26, 2001), New York City. In 1969, before the passage of the OSHAct, the Labor Department made the ACGIH standards for about 400 substances compulsory under the Walsh-Healey Act for companies doing business under federal contract.

90. Tony Mazzocchi, in "Proceedings," *Hazards of the Industrial Environment*, a conference sponsored by District 7, Oil, Chemical and Atomic Workers International Union, Sheraton, Fort Wayne Motor Hotel, Fort Wayne, Indiana (October 24–26, 1969), 1.

91. Tony Mazzocchi, in "Proceedings," *Hazards of the Industrial Environment*, a conference sponsored by District 8 Council, Oil, Chemical and Atomic Workers International Union, Holiday Inn, Kenilworth, NJ (March 29, 1969), 2.

92. Tony Mazzocchi, in "Proceedings," *Hazards of the Industrial Environment*, a conference sponsored by District 7, Oil, Chemical and Atomic Workers International Union, Sheraton, Fort Wayne Motor Hotel, Fort Wayne, Indiana (October 24–26, 1969), 31.

93. Tony Mazzocchi, in "Proceedings," *Hazards of the Industrial Environment*, a conference sponsored by District 8 Council, Oil, Chemical and Atomic Workers International Union, Holiday Inn, Kenilworth, NJ (March 29, 1969), 2. Mazzocchi underestimated the number of deaths at Gauley Bridge. See Martin Cherniack, *The Hawk's Nest Incident: America's Worst Industrial Disaster* (New Haven: Yale University Press, 1986).

94. Tony Mazzocchi, in "Proceedings," *Hazards of the Industrial Environment*, a conference sponsored by District 8 Council, Oil, Chemical and Atomic Workers International Union, Holiday Inn, Kenilworth, NJ (March 29, 1969), 13.

95. Tony Mazzocchi, "Foreword," in "Proceedings," *Hazards of the Industrial Environment*, a conference sponsored by District 8 Council, Oil, Chemical and Atomic Workers International Union, Holiday Inn, Kenilworth, NJ (March 29, 1969), 6.

96. Ray Davidson, *Peril on the Job: A Study of Hazards in the Chemical Industries* (Washington: Public Affairs Press, 1970), 184–85.

97. Tony Mazzocchi, in "Proceedings," *Hazards of the Industrial Environment*, a conference sponsored by District 5 Council, Oil, Chemical and Atomic Workers International Union, Mayo Hotel, Tulsa, Oklahoma (November 1–2, 1969), 1.

98. Tony Mazzocchi, in "Proceedings," *Hazards of the Industrial Environment*, a conference sponsored by District 7 Council, Oil, Chemical and Atomic Workers International Union, Sheraton, Fort Wayne Motor Hotel, Fort Wayne, Indiana (October 24–26,1969), 2.

99. Glenn Paulson in "Proceedings," *Hazards of the Industrial Environment*, a conference sponsored by District 8 Council, Oil, Chemical and Atomic Workers International Union, Holiday Inn, Kenilworth, NJ (March 29, 1969), 12.

100. Ibid.

101. Robert L. Marsh, in "Proceedings," *Hazards of the Industrial Environment*, a conference sponsored by District 8 Council, Oil, Chemical and Atomic Workers International Union, District 2 Council, Ramada Inn, Salt Lake City, Utah (May 21–23, 1970), 26.

102. John Dacey, in "Proceedings," *Hazards of the Industrial Environment*, a conference sponsored by District 8 Council, Oil, Chemical and Atomic Workers International Union, Holiday Inn, Kenilworth, NJ (March 29, 1969), 29.

103. Peter Mac Intyre, in "Proceedings," *Hazards of the Industrial Environment*, a conference sponsored by District 8 Council, Oil, Chemical and Atomic Workers International Union, Holiday Inn, Kenilworth, NJ (March 29, 1969), 33–38.

104. James Orth, in "Proceedings," *Hazards of the Industrial Environment*, a conference sponsored by District 8 Council, Oil, Chemical and Atomic Workers International Union, Holiday Inn, Baltimore, Maryland (June 14, 1969), 16.

105. Harold Smith, Local 8-447, Woodbridge [New Jersey] Chemical Corporation, in "Proceedings," *Hazards of the Industrial Environment*, a conference sponsored by District 8 Council, Oil, Chemical and Atomic Workers International Union, Holiday Inn, Kenilworth, NJ (March 29, 1969), 59.

106. Noble, *Liberalism at Work*, 85.

107. Ibid., 93–96.

108. Interview with Anthony Mazzocchi (January 26, 2001), New York City.

109. Ibid.

110. See Vogel, *Fluctuating Fortunes*, 86.

111. Noble, *Liberalism at Work*, 93–96.

112. Susan Mazzocchi, "The First Complaint Filed and the First Citation Issued under the Occupational Safety and Health Act of 1970 (OSHA)" (1978), in *A Collection of Documents from the OCAW Struggle for Worker Health and Safety* (Washington: Alice Hamilton College, 1998), 1–2, courtesy of Tony Mazzocchi.

113. Ibid., 4.

114. Ibid., 5–6.

115. Ibid., 18.

116. Ibid., 21.

117. Ibid., 30.

118. Stuart Auerbach, "The First Strike over Potential Hazards to Health," *San Francisco Examiner* (March 4, 1973), 21.

119. See Open Letter, "The Shell Strike for Workers' Health and Safety," in *A Collection of Documents from the OCAW Struggle for Worker Health and Safety* (Washington: Alice Hamilton College, 1998), n.p.

120. Auerbach, "The First Strike over Potential Hazards to Health"; "Oil Strikers Win Sierra Club Help," *San Francisco Examiner* (March 4, 1973); John A. Grimes, "Environmental Strike," Washington, DC, *Sunday Star and Daily News* (April 1, 1973), C-2.

121. "Giving Shell Some Gas: Environmental Issues Reach the Bargaining Table," *Environmental Action* (March 3, 1973), 3–4.

CHAPTER 6. EVIDENCE OF AN ILLEGAL CONSPIRACY BY INDUSTRY

1. John Kent, "Plastics in Your Future," *Science Digest* (February 1954), 53; "Chemical Field Expands Vastly," *New York Times* (January 5, 1956), 90. For the most part, this section depends upon David D. Doniger, *The Law and Policy of Toxic Substances Control: A Case Study of Vinyl Chloride* (Baltimore: Johns Hopkins University Press, ca. 1979); Peter Spitz, "The Rise of Petrochemicals," *Chemical Week* 151 (August 2, 1989), 24.

2. "Union Carbide Corporation Chronology of PVC Activities," in R. N. Wheeler Jr., "Literature Survey and Engineering Options," *Peterson vs. Union Carbide Corporation* (October 1989), 43; Mansel G. Blackford and K. Austin Kerr, *B. F. Goodrich: Tradition and Transformation, 1870–1995* (Columbus: Ohio State University Press, 1996), 239. Ralph L. Harding Jr., president, Society of the Plastics Industry, says first production was in 1939, but he was probably referring to Dow Chemical's entering into the field in Midland, Michigan. See Ralph L. Harding Jr., Testimony at OSHA Hearings, "Official Report of Proceedings before the Occupational Safety and Health Administration of the

Department of Labor in the Matter of a Proposed Permanent Standard for Occupational Exposure to Vinyl Chloride" (June 26, 1974), 330–331. See also Statement by V. K. Rowe before the U.S. Department of Labor, Occupational Safety and Health Administration (hereafter DOL, OSHA), "Transcript of Informal Fact-Finding Hearing on Possible Hazards of Vinyl Chloride Manufacture and Use" (February 15, 1974), 162.

3. Peter Spitz, "The Rise of Petrochemicals," *Chemical Week* 151 (August 2, 1989), 24; Barry Commoner, "The Promise and Peril of Petrochemicals," *New York Times Magazine* (September 25, 1977), 70.

4. Ralph L. Harding Jr., president, Society of the Plastics Industry, Testimony at OSHA Hearings, "Official Report of Proceedings before the Occupational Safety and Health Administration of the Department of Labor in the Matter of a Proposed Permanent Standard for Occupational Exposure to Vinyl Chloride (June 26, 1974), 330–31.

5. Ralph L. Harding Jr., president, SPI, U.S. Congress, Senate, Committee on Commerce, Sub-Committee on the Environment, *Hearing on the Dangers of Vinyl Chloride,* 93rd Cong., 2nd Sess. (Aug. 21, 1974), Serial No. 93-110.

6. David D. Doniger, *The Law and Policy of Toxic Substances Control,* 23; Blackford and Kerr, *B. F. Goodrich,* 239.

7. Joe Thornton, *Pandora's Poison: Chlorine, Health and a New Environmental Strategy* (Cambridge: MIT Press, 2000), 3.

8. Doniger, *The Law and Policy of Toxic Substances Control,* 26. By the 1970s there were ten companies producing vinyl chloride monomer in fifteen plants throughout the nation. Shell, Dow, and Goodrich together controlled approximately 56 percent of vinyl chloride monomer production. About twenty-three companies, operating thirty-seven plants nationwide, controlled the production of PVC. Finally, there were about eight thousand companies of a wide variety of sizes using PVC in the fabrication of consumer goods. David Doniger explains that the highly concentrated VCM and PVC industry "has made it easy for the industries to speak with one voice in regulatory proceedings regarding the limits of their technological and economic capabilities to control VC exposures" (25–26).

9. Doniger, *The Law and Policy of Toxic Substances Control,* 26.

10. Ashish Arora and Nathan Rosenberg, "Chemicals: A U.S. Success Story," in *Chemicals and Long-Term Economic Growth: Insights from the Chemical Industry,* ed. by Ashish Arora, Ralph Landau, and Nathan Rosenberg (New York: John Wiley and Sons, 1998), 95.

11. K. B. Lehmann, "Experimentelle Studien uber den Einfluss Tecnisch und Hygienisch Wichtiger Gase und Dampfe auf den Organismus," cited in Barry Castleman, *Asbestos: Medical and Legal Aspects,* 3rd ed. (Englewood Cliffs, NJ: Prentice-Hall, 1990), 224.

12. Manfred Bowditch et al., "Code for Safe Concentrations of Certain Common Toxic Substances Used in Industry," cited in Castleman, *Asbestos,* 225.

13. Gerald Markowitz and David Rosner, "The Limits of Thresholds: Silica and the Politics of Science, 1935–1990," *American Journal of Public Health* 85 (February 1995), 253–62.

14. MCA, Chemical Safety Data Sheet, SD-56, "Vinyl Chloride," 2.3.1., MCA Papers.

15. Henry F. Smyth Jr. to T. W. Nale, "attn: Weidlein" (November 24, 1959), MCA Papers.

16. V. K. Rowe to W. E. McCormick (May 12, 1959), MCA Papers.

17. Statement of V. K. Rowe, Testimony at OSHA Hearings, "Official Report of Proceedings Before the Occupational Safety and Health Administration of the Department of Labor in the Matter of a Proposed Permanent Standard for Occupational Exposure to Vinyl Chloride (July 28, 1974), 862.

18. V. K. Rowe to W. E. McCormick (May 12, 1959), MCA Papers.

19. Henry F. Smyth Jr. to T. W. Nale, "attn: Weidlein" (November 24, 1959), MCA Papers.

20. T. R. Torkelson, F. Oyen, and V. K. Rowe, "The Toxicity of Vinyl Chloride as Determined by Repeated Exposure of Laboratory Animals," *American Industrial Hygiene Association Journal* 22 (1961), 354–61.

21. Deposition of John Creech, M.D., *In the Matter of: Daniel J. Ross, et ux v. Conoco, Inc., et al.* (June 12, 2000), 49, 53, (June 13, 2000), 12, 17, 37–39, 191, MCA Papers. Solvay, the European producer, seems to have "discovered some cases of acroosteolysis in 1963." See Kenneth S. Lane, Assistant Medical Director, Union Carbide, "Meeting with Professor Maltoni, Arranged by Ethyl Corporation, and Held at International Hotel, Kennedy Airport, New York City, on June 5, 1974," MCA Papers.

22. W. E. McCormick, Goodrich, to R. Emmet Kelly et al. (June 10, 1966), MCA Papers.

23. W. E. McCormick to Robert Kehoe (October 16, 1964); Kehoe to R. Emmet Kelly, Monsanto (July 7, 1965), MCA Papers.

24. Kehoe to R. Emmet Kelly (February 2, 1965), MCA Papers.

25. Rex H. Wilson, M.D., to Dr. J. Newman, "Confidential" (November 12, 1964), MCA Papers.

26. R. Emmet Kelly to A. G. Erdman, Springfield, "PVC Exposure" (January 7, 1966), MCA Papers.

27. Ibid.

28. J. V. Wagoner to Proc Avon, "Confidential" (January 6, 1966), MCA Papers. Goodrich's Rex Wilson went to Brussels to see if he could stop the publication of the paper. R. Emmet Kelly to A. G. Erdman, Springfield, "PVC Exposure" (January 7, 1966), MCA Papers.

29. W. E. McCormick to Kelly (May 10, 1966), MCA Papers; McCormick to Kelly et al. (June 10, 1966), MCA Papers.

30. J. A. Bourque Jr. and P W. Townsend, "Confidential," "MCA Medical Advisory Committee Meeting re: PVC" (October 17, 1966), MCA Papers.

31. Ibid.

32. R. N. Wheeler, "Meeting PVC Resin Producers at Cleveland Engineering Society under the Sponsorship of MCA and B. F. Goodrich Chemical Company, October 6, 1966" (October 7, 1966), MCA Papers.

33. Ibid.

34. R. N. Wheeler to A. R. Anderson et al., "Subject: MCA Occupational Health Committee Meeting, Oct 6, 1966" (October 24, 1966), MCA Papers.

35. R. N. Wheeler Jr., "Career," in R. N. Wheeler Jr., *Peterson vs. Union Carbide Corporation*, Literature Survey and Engineering Opinions" (October 1989), 8, MCA Papers.

36. Wheeler, Memorandum, "Meeting at Ann Arbor, Michigan, MCA Occupational Health Committee" (January 24, 1967), MCA Papers.

37. William E. Nessell, M.D. [Monsanto], "MCA Meeting, Ann Arbor, Mich.: 1/24/67" (January 26, 1967), MCA Papers.

38. Ibid.

39. Ibid.

40. Rex Wilson, William McCormick, et al., "Occupational Acroosteolysis" *Journal of the American Medical Association* 201 (August 21, 1967), 577–81.

41. Deposition of John Creech, 78. Although listed as an author, Creech did not actually write the piece. Creech believes it was written primarily by Rex Wilson.

42. Rex Wilson, William McCormick, et al., "Occupational Acroosteolysis," 577–81.

43. A. Vittone Jr. to T. B. Nantz et al. (August 25, 1967), MCA Papers.

44. Institute of Industrial Health, University of Michigan, *Epidemiological Investigation of the Polyvinyl Chloride Industry in Reference to Occupational Acroosteolysis*, "Confidential Report to the Medical Advisory Committee, Manufacturing Chemists Association" (February 1969), 104, MCA Papers.

45. George Ingle, Monsanto, to W. E. Nessell (May 8, 1969), MCA Papers; MCA, Occupational Health Committee, Minutes of Meeting (April 30, 1969), MCA Papers.

46. Frank Carman, "Report of Meeting," PVC Resin Producers Representatives (May 6, 1969), MCA Papers.

47. Warren A. Cook, Paul Giever, et al., "Occupational Acroosteolysis: II. An Industrial Hygiene Study," *Archives of Environmental Health* 22 (January 1971), 79.

48. MCA, Occupational Health Committee, Minutes of Meeting (November 6, 1969), MCA Papers; MCA Plastics Committee, Minutes of Meeting (June 4, 1970), MCA Papers. The Michigan study was published as Bertram H. D. Dinman, Warren A. Cook, et al., "Occupational Acroosteolysis: I. An Occupational Study," "II. An Industrial Hygiene Study," and "III. A Clinical Study," *Archives of Environmental Health* 22 (January 1971), 61–91.

49. MCA, Plastics Committee, Minutes of Meeting (May 6, 1971), MCA Papers.

50. Bertram Dinman to Dr. N. V. Hendricks, Medical Department, Standard Oil (July 20, 1971), MCA Papers.

51. Kenneth Johnson, Assistant Technical Director, Occupational Health Programs, MCA, to Company Contacts, "Re: University of Michigan Acroosteolysis Project" (August 9, 1971), MCA Papers.

52. In December 1973, the MCA wrote to its member companies that there was virtually universal agreement that the AOL registry at the University of Michigan, which had been limping along for a few years, should be terminated. Thus, the largest database of people exposed to vinyl chloride was abandoned. A. C. Clark, MCA, to Designated Representatives of Companies, Subject: "Termination of Acroosteolysis Registry Project" (December 12, 1973), MCA Papers.

53. MCA, Environmental Health Advisory Committee, Minutes of Meeting (November 16, 1967), MCA Papers.

54. James S. Turner, "The Delaney Anticancer Clause: A Model Environmental Protection Law," *Vanderbilt Law Review* 24 (October 1971), 889–93.

55. Ibid., 894–95.

56. American Council on Science and Health, *Of Mice and Mandates: Animal Experiments, Human Cancer Risk and Regulatory Policies* (New York: ACSH, 1997), 27.

57. See Nicholas Wade, "Delaney Anti-Cancer Clause: Scientists Debate on Article of Faith," *Science* n.s. 177 (August 18, 1972), 588–91, for a discussion of the history and controversy surrounding the clause circa the early 1970s.

58. This paragraph is based upon Charles H. Blank, "The Delaney Clause: Technical Naivete and Scientific Advocacy in the Formulation of Public Health Policies," *California Law Review* 62 (1974), 1084–20.

59. Wade, "Delaney Anti-Cancer Clause," 588–591.

60. [Walter D. Harris], Handwritten Notes, "Given to R.J.O.[D]?, 5/17/76," MCA Papers. It is unclear from the documentation whether Dr. Viola actually delivered this paper. See George Roush to Richard Henderson (June 24, 1970), MCA Papers.

61. See P. Viola, A. Bigotti, and A. Caputo, "Oncogenic Response of Rats, Skin, Lungs, and Bones to Vinyl Chloride," *Cancer Research* 31 (May 1971), 516–22.

62. MCA, Occupational Health Committee, Minutes of Meeting (May 6, 1971), MCA Papers.

63. Ibid.

64. MCA, Occupational Health Committee, Minutes of Meeting (September 20, 1971), MCA Papers.

65. Pierluigi Viola to Kenneth D. Johnson (October 29, 1971), MCA Papers.

66. Union Carbide, Memorandum, "Manufacturers Chemists Association Occupational Health Committee VC Conference" (November 23, 1971), MCA Papers; S. F. Pitts to D. O. Popovac, CONOCO Interoffice Communication, "On MCA VCM Toxicity Subcommittee" (November 18, 1971), MCA Papers.

67. Pierluigi Viola to Kenneth D. Johnson (October 29, 1971), MCA Papers.

68. Robert Wheeler to Dernehl, Eisenhous, Steele, et al., Union Carbide, Memorandum, "Manufacturing Chemists Association Occupational Health Committee VC Conference" (November 23, 1971), MCA Papers.

69. Blackford and Kerr, *B. F. Goodrich*, 321, 324.

70. See Imperial Chemical Industries to MCA (August 16, 1972); George Best to Prospective Sponsors of Research (September 1, 1972); George Best to Lindsell, ICI (September 20, 1972), MCA Papers; Myron A. Mehlman, "In Memoriam: Professor Cesare Maltoni (1930–2001)," *Environmental Health Perspectives* 109 (May 2001), A201.

71. W. A. Knapp to J. C. Fedoruk and A. P. McGuire, Allied Chemical Corporation, Memorandum (November 20, 1972), MCA Papers.

72. Kenneth Johnson to Technical Task Force on Vinyl Chloride Research (October 19, 1972), MCA Papers.

73. D. A. Rausch, Dow, Inorganic Chemicals, "Confidential Treatment of European Study on Vinyl Chloride" (December 15, 1972), MCA Papers.

74. Walter Harris to George Best (October 20, 1972), MCA Papers.

75. W. Mayo Smith, Air Products and Chemicals (February 6, 1974): "This writer made a memo to file with no copies of the meeting in Washington at the MCA 14 November 1972."

76. Ibid. See also W. A. Knapp to J. C. Fedoruk and A. P. McGuire, Allied Chemical Corporation, Memorandum (November 20, 1972); Shell, "Private and Confidential, Memorandum of Discussion at MCA, Nov. 14" (November 17, 1972), MCA Papers.

77. "Notes from Meeting of Representatives of MCA" (Gasque (Olin), Kociba (Dow), Torkelson (Dow)), ICI, Montedison, Solvay et Cie, Rome-Progil, University of Bologna (Maltoni), "Conclusions from European Information" (January 17, 1973). See also MCA, Vinyl Chloride Research Coordinators, Minutes of Meeting (January 30, 1973), MCA Papers.

78. MCA, Ad Hoc Planning Group for Vinyl Chloride Research, Minutes of Meeting (December 14, 1971), MCA Papers.

79. Statement of Andrea Hricko and Bertram Cottine, Testimony at OSHA Hearings, "Official Report of Proceedings before the Occupational Safety and Health Administration of the Department of Labor in the Matter of a Proposed Permanent Standard for Occupational Exposure to Vinyl Chloride" (July 9, 1974), 1556.

80. Dow Chemical Company, Midland, Michigan, "Evaluation of Vinyl Chloride as a Propellant for Aerosols" (July 29, 1959), MCA Papers.

81. L. B. Crider to W. E. McCormick, Goodrich, Memorandum, "Some New Information on the Relative Toxicity of Vinyl Chloride Monomer" (March 24, 1969), MCA Papers.

82. W. A. Knapp, Allied Chemical, to W. S. Ferguson, Memorandum, "Vinyl Chloride Monomer" (March 1, 1973), MCA Papers.

83. R. N. Wheeler Jr. to Eisenhour et al., "Confidential" (February 13, 1973), MCA Papers.

84. Food, Drug, and Cosmetic Act, 409(c)(3) (A), 21 U.S.C. 348 (c)(3)(A) 1970.

85. Department of HEW, Food and Drug Administration, "Prior Sanctioned Poly Vinyl Chloride Resin," Notice of Proposed Rule Making, *Federal Register*, Vol. 38, No. 95 (May 17, 1973), 12931.

86. Ibid.

87. Health Services and Mental Health Administration, Occupational Safety and Health, "Request for Information on Certain Chemical and Physical Agents," *Federal Register* (January 30, 1973), 2782.

88. G. J. Williams to C. A. Gerstacker, Dow (March 5, 1973), MCA Papers.

89. George Best, MCA, to John D. Bryan, Conoco (March 26, 1973), MCA Papers.

90. Ibid.

91. In April 1973, Cesare Maltoni gave a paper at the Second International Cancer Conference in Bologna on occupational carcinogenesis. According to Sir Richard Doll, the paper included information on the carcinogenic properties of vinyl chloride. Deposition of William Richard Shaboe Doll, London, England, in *Carlin David Staples et al. vs. Dow Chemical* (January 26, 2000), 27. The data seemed to have little impact on an audience that was not aware of the significance of the information that low-level exposures could cause cancer. Surprisingly, with the exception of Doll, it appears that no one remembers hearing this information. One American, representing the National Cancer Institute, does not recall that the information was presented to the meeting. Indeed, at the time, the MCA never remarked on the incident, and subsequent events indicate that the MCA's members believed that the information was still secret in the United States. Testimony of Cesare Maltoni, Venice, Italy, Tape 1067 (1999), 2, transcript courtesy of Judith Helfand. Deposition of Umberto Saffiotti, Rockvelle, MD, in *Daniel J. Ross et al. vs. Conoco et al.* (April 10, 2000).

92. R. E. Sourwine to W. P. Lawrence, PPG, Confidential (March 30, 1973), MCA Papers; Vinyl Chloride Research Coordinators, Minutes of Meeting (April 4, 1973), MCA Papers.

93. "Industry's Latest Cancer Scare," *Business Week* (February 23, 1974), 100.

94. MCA, Vinyl Chloride Research Coordinators, Minutes of Meeting (May 21, 1973), MCA Papers.

95. Ibid.

96. Ibid.

97. R. N. Wheeler to Eisenhour et al. (May 31, 1973), MCA Papers.

98. Ibid.

99. Ibid.

100. Ibid.

101. "What's Next from OSHA? Keep an Eye on NIOSH," *Modern Plastics* (June 1973), 56.

102. D. P. Duffield, "Vinyl Chloride Toxicity—Meetings Held at MCA Headquarters, Washington, D.C. and National Institute of Occupational Safety

and Health, Rockville, Maryland, on 16th and 17th July 1973" (July 20, 1973), MCA Papers.

103. Kusnets, Shell, to Files, "Private and Confidential" (July 17, 1973), MCA Papers.

104. Ibid.

105. "Notes on Meeting between Representatives of MCA Technical Task Group on Vinyl Chloride Research and NIOSH" (July 17, 1973), MCA Papers; and R. N. Wheeler to Carvajal et al. (July 19, 1973), MCA Papers.

106. Richard B. James, untitled notes of NIOSH-MCA Meeting (July 17, 1973), in possession of Peter Infante. Keith Jacobson's handwritten notes also do not mention cancers at 250 ppm. See Keith Jacobson, handwritten notes (July 17, 1973), in possession of Peter Infante.

107. "Notes on Meeting between Representatives of MCA Technical Task Group on Vinyl Chloride Research and NIOSH" (July 17, 1973), MCA Papers; and R. N. Wheeler to Carvajal et al. (July 19, 1973), MCA Papers.

108. Doniger, *The Law and Policy of Toxic Substances Control*, 103, footnote 551. Doniger's analysis of the vinyl chloride story was published in 1978 and is revealing as a primary source of information not only because of its legislative and administrative history but also because it reflects the state of understanding of the crisis among informed persons of the time. Not having access to the MCA's records, Doniger incorrectly asserts that "there is no evidence that any company's cessation of VC use before the Goodrich disclosure in January 1974 was motivated by insider's information about the cancer hazard."

109. "Notes on Meeting between Representatives of MCA Technical Task Group on Vinyl Chloride Research and NIOSH" (July 17, 1973), MCA Papers.

110. R. N. Wheeler to Carvajal et al. (July 19, 1973), MCA Papers.

111. Flynt Kennedy, Conoco, to R. W. G. et al., "VCM" (July 19, 1973), MCA Papers.

112. R. N. Wheeler to Carvajal et al. (July 19, 1973), MCA Papers.

113. Flynt Kennedy, Conoco, to R. W. G. et al., "VCM" (July 19, 1973); George Best to Management Contacts of Companies (July 20, 1973), MCA Papers.

114. MCA to Technical Task Force on Vinyl Chloride Research, trans. by Dow (September 26, 1973), MCA Papers.

115. *Chemical Week* 137 (November 14, 1973), 19. See also NIOSH, "Health Hazard Evaluation Determination Report 72-58, City Foods, Seattle Washington" (September 1973), in Vinyl Chloride Docket, H-036, Exhibit 189G, Department of Labor Docket Office, Washington; Rudolph J. Jaeger and Ronald A. Hites, "Pyrolytic Evaporation of a Plasticizer from Polyvinyl Chloride Meat Wrapping Film," *Bulletin of Environmental Contamination and Toxicology* 11 (1974), 45–48.

116. Albert C. Clark, Vice President and Technical Director, MCA, to the Management Contacts of Companies Sponsoring the [Blacked-out], Confidential (December 7, 1973), MCA Papers.

117. Joe Klein, "The Plastic Coffin of Charlie Arthur," *Rolling Stone,* January 15, 1976. See also Paul Blanc, "The Tip of the Iceberg: A Living Newspaper Play" [mimeo] for an example of the ways that the broader public came to understand the crisis over vinyl chloride.

118. J. T. Barr, Air Products and Chemicals, to T. L. Carey, Interoffice Memorandum (January 29, 1974), MCA Papers.

119. Maurice N. Johnson, Testimony at OSHA Hearings, "Official Report of Proceedings before the Occupational Safety and Health Administration of the Department of Labor in the Matter of a Proposed Permanent Standard for Occupational Exposure to Vinyl Chloride, Washington (June 27, 1974), 552.

120. J. T. Barr, Air Products and Chemicals, to T. L. Carey, Interoffice Memorandum (January 29, 1974), MCA Papers.

121. Blackford and Kerr, *B. F. Goodrich,* 333.

122. J. T. Barr, Air Products and Chemicals, to T. L. Carey, Interoffice Memorandum (January 29, 1974), MCA Papers.

123. MCA, "Meeting of Technical Task Group on Vinyl Chloride Research" (January 25, 1974), MCA Papers.

124. Henry Falk, John Creech, et al., "Hepatic Disease among Workers at a Vinyl Chloride Polymerization Plant," *JAMA* 230 (October 7, 1974), 59–63.

125. "B. F. Goodrich (Louisville) [Seven Cases of Angiosarcomas]" (n.d.), Vinyl Chloride Docket, H-036, Ex. 189F, Department of Labor Docket Office.

126. Don A. Schanche, "Vinyl Chloride: Time Bomb on the Production Line," *Today's Health* 52 (September 1974), 19.

127. MCA, "Meeting of Technical Task Group on Vinyl Chloride Research" (January 25, 1974), MCA Papers; George Best to Marcus Key (January 25, 1974), MCA Papers.

128. Flynt Kennedy to Gamblin, Smith, and Tillson (January 31, 1974), MCA Papers. See also "Angiosarcoma of the Liver among Polyvinyl Chloride Workers—Kentucky" in Centers for Disease Control, *Morbidity and Mortality Weekly Report for Week Ending February 9, 1974* 23 (February 15, 1974), 49.

129. R. E. Laramy to Flynt Kennedy, "Subject: Trip to Attend Meeting of the Vinyl Chloride Safety Association" (February 11, 1974), MCA Papers.

130. Quoted in Blackford and Kerr, *B. F. Goodrich,* 333.

131. R. E. Laramy to Flynt Kennedy, "Subject: Trip to Attend Meeting of the Vinyl Chloride Safety Association" (February 11, 1974), MCA Papers.

132. "Smoke and Gas Producers Tested," *Science News* 95 (February 1, 1969), 116.

CHAPTER 7. DAMN LIARS

1. Occupational Safety and Health Act, 29 U.S.C. 651 et seq. (1970).

2. U.S. Department of Labor, Occupational Safety and Health Administration (hereafter DOL, OSHA), *Informal Fact-Finding Hearings on Possible*

Hazards of Vinyl Chloride Manufacture and Use (February 15, 1974), 20, MCA Papers.

3. "New Materials—and Perhaps Some Old Ones—Harbor New Dangers," *Medical World News* (May 3, 1974), 34.

4. Paul H. Weaver, "On the Horns of the Vinyl Chloride Dilemma," *Fortune* 90 (October 1974), 202.

5. DOL, OSHA, *Informal Fact-Finding Hearings on Possible Hazards of Vinyl Chloride Manufacture and Use* (February 15, 1974), 25–26, MCA Papers.

6. Ibid., 26. Selikoff cited acute animal toxicity reported in 1938 and chronic toxicity in 1961. "We didn't need the animal studies to warn us that workers could be harmed in VC-PVC manufacture."

7. Ibid., 26.

8. Ibid., 29.

9. Ibid., 30.

10. Ibid., 33.

11. Ibid., 34.

12. Ibid., 41.

13. Ibid.

14. Ibid., 125–26; Thomas F. Mancuso, "Cancer and Vinyl Chloride—Polymerization Implications, Problems and Needs" (February 1974), Vinyl Chloride Docket, H-036 Exhibit 3-11, Department of Labor Docket Office.

15. DOL, OSHA, *Informal Fact-Finding Hearings on Possible Hazards of Vinyl Chloride Manufacture and Use* (February 15, 1974), 126, MCA Papers. In a perceptive discussion of the new federal Occupational Safety and Health Act, Mancuso pointed out that the act called for a safe workplace that placed the "responsibility on industry to ensure that no harmful effects do occur as a result of exposures to the various chemicals and the work processes involved." Much better methods for ensuring safety were necessary. It was no longer sufficient to follow and document occupational disease in the work force in response to workers' compensation claims. "In the first place," he pointed out, "the worker doesn't even recognize an occupational disease when he sees one. In the second place, the general practitioner doesn't recognize it. Consequently, it doesn't come to a compensation claim." Mancuso, "Cancer and Vinyl Chloride, 155.

16. DOL, OSHA, *Informal Fact-Finding Hearings on Possible Hazards of Vinyl Chloride Manufacture and Use* (February 15, 1974), 66, MCA Papers.

17. MCA, Ad Hoc Planning Group for Vinyl Chloride Research, Minutes (December 14, 1971), MCA Papers.

18. DOL, OSHA, *Informal Fact-Finding Hearings on Possible Hazards of Vinyl Chloride Manufacture and Use* (February 15, 1974), 71, MCA Papers.

19. Ibid., passim.

20. Terry Yosie, interview transcript with Bill Moyers, "Trade Secrets" (March 26, 2001), PBS, <www.pbs.org/tradesecrets/trans/intero3.html>.

21. DOL, OSHA, *Informal Fact-Finding Hearings on Possible Hazards of Vinyl Chloride Manufacture and Use* (February 15, 1974), 179, MCA Papers.

22. "Battlelines Drawn on Vinyl Chloride Issue," *Chemical & Engineering News* (February 25, 1974), 16.

23. H. L. Kusnetz, Manager, Industrial Hygiene, Shell Head Office, Memorandum of Meeting of MCA Technical Task Group on Vinyl Chloride (February 26, 1974), MCA Papers. See also Jane Brody, "Rare Liver Cancer Discovered in 2 More at a Chemical Plant," *New York Times* (February 20, 1974), 23; Jane Brody, "Liver Cancer Case Found in 2nd Plastic Plant," *New York Times* (February 22, 1974), 35.

24. H. L. Kusnetz, Manager, Industrial Hygiene, Shell Head Office, Memorandum of Meeting of MCA Technical Task Group on Vinyl Chloride (February 26, 1974), MCA Papers. See also Jane Brody, "Rare Liver Cancer Discovered in 2 More at a Chemical Plant," *New York Times* (February 20, 1974), 23; Jane Brody, "Liver Cancer Case Found in 2nd Plastic Plant," *New York Times* (February 22, 1974), 35.

25. Lee B. Grant, Medical Director, PPG, to L. F. Sargert, Chemical Division General Office (March 7, 1974), MCA Papers.

26. William J. Driver, *Staff Report*, Attached to MCA, Board of Directors, Minutes, Del Monte Lodge, Pebble Beach, California (March 13, 1974), MCA Papers.

27. Zeb Bell, PPG, to Grant, M.D., and R. E. Sourwine (March 4, 1974), MCA Papers.

28. Zeb Bell to T. Z. Korsak (March 25, 1974), MCA Papers; Kenneth Johnson to Technical Task Group on Vinyl Chloride Research (March 11, 1974), MCA Papers.

29. "PVC Producers Gird for Battle against Cancer," *Chemical Week* 136 (April 3, 1974), 31.

30. R. L. Bourget, "Notes: Meeting of Vinyl Chloride Industry Management—MCA Headquarters—Washington DC 3/19/74" (March 21, 1974), MCA Papers.

31. MCA, Chronology (ca. July 1974), MCA Papers.

32. C. Maltoni and G. Lefemine, "The Potential of Experimental Tests in Predicting Environmental Oncogenic Hazards. An Example: Vinyl Chloride" (March 1974), MCA Papers [mimeo].

33. Albert C. Clark, MCA, "Vinyl Chloride and DDT: Environmental Effects," Letter to Editor, *Science* 189 (July 18, 1975), 174.

34. John T. Edsall, "Vinyl Chloride and DDT: Environmental Effects," Letter to Editor, *Science* 189 (July 18, 1975), 175.

35. "Cancer Experts at OSHA Session Find Insufficient Data to Set Firm Guidelines," *Occupational Safety and Health Reporter* 5 (1975), 835, 838.

36. Ibid., 839.

37. J. L. Creech and M. N. Johnson (B. F. Goodrich), "Angiosarcoma of the Liver in the Manufacture of Polyvinyl Chloride," *Journal of Occupational Medicine* 16 (March 1974), 150–51.

38. R. N. Wheeler to Technical Task Group on Vinyl Chloride Research, "Proposed Occupational Safety and Health Work Practice Standard for the

Manufacture of Synthetic Polymer Containing Vinyl Chloride" (May 13, 1974), MCA Papers.

39. "Cancer Experts at OSHA Session Find Insufficient Data to Set Firm Guidelines," *Occupational Safety and Health Reporter* 5 (1975), 839.

40. Daryl M. Freedman, "Reasonable Certainty of No Harm: Reviving the Safety Standard for Food Additives, Color Additives and Animal Drugs," *Ecology Law Journal* 7 (1978), 278.

41. *Federal Register*, Vol. 39, No. 194, part 2, OSHA, "Exposure to Vinyl Chloride, Occupational Safety and Health Standards" (October 4, 1974), 35890–98. On March 11, NIOSH had made its recommendation.

42. R. N. Wheeler Jr., Chairman, Subcommittee on Work Practices to Technical Task Group on Vinyl Chloride Research, MCA, "Proposed Occupational Safety and Health Work Practice Standard for the Manufacture of Synthetic Polymer Containing Vinyl Chloride" (March 7, 1974), in Wheeler to Technical Task Force on Vinyl Chloride Research (April 8, 1974), MCA Papers.

43. Thomas J. McGrath, Society of the Plastics Industry, to Members of Vinyl Monomers and PVC Producers Ad Hoc Committee (May 6, 1974), MCA Papers.

44. R. N. Wheeler to Technical Task Group on Vinyl Chloride Research, "Proposed Occupational Safety and Health Work Practice Standard for the Manufacture of Synthetic Polymer Containing Vinyl Chloride" (May 13, 1974), MCA Papers.

45. MCA, Chronology (ca. July 1974), MCA Papers.

46. H. L. Kusnetz, Manager, Industrial Hygiene, Shell Head Office, "VCM Meeting—April 15, 1974" (April 16, 1974), MCA Papers.

47. MCA Executive Committee, "Minutes of Meeting" (April 8, 1974), MCA Papers.

48. Wheeler, Union Carbide, Internal Correspondence, "Confidential" (April 17, 1974), MCA Papers.

49. H. L. Kusnetz, Manager, Industrial Hygiene, Shell Head Office, on VCM Meeting (April 15 and 16, 1974), MCA Papers.

50. Wheeler, Union Carbide, Internal Correspondence, "Confidential" (April 17, 1974), MCA Papers.

51. A. B. Steele, Union Carbide, to SPI Industry Contacts, "Formation of the VCM/PVC Industry Management Committee within the Society of the Plastics Industry" (April 19, 1974), MCA Papers. The Steering Committee consisted of Anton Vittone of Goodrich, Harry Connors of Diamond Shamrock, A. R. Adams of Air Products, G. J. Williams of Dow, and Ralph Harding of SPI.

52. Chemical Manufacturers Association (CMA), Special Programs Advisory Group, "Record of Meeting" (April 21, 1981), MCA Papers.

53. A. B. Steele, Union Carbide, to SPI Industry Contacts, "Formation of the VCM/PVC Industry Management Committee within the Society of the Plastics Industry" (April 19, 1974), MCA Papers.

54. Senate, Committee on Commerce, Subcommittee on the Environment, *Hearing on Dangers of Vinyl Chloride*, 93rd Cong. 2nd Sess. (August 21, 1974), Serial No. 93-110, 94.

55. A. B. Steele, Union Carbide to SPI Industry Contacts, "Formation of the VCM/PVC Industry Management Committee within the Society of the Plastics Industry" (April 19, 1974), MCA Papers.

56. A. C. Clark and George Best, MCA, to Management Contact of Companies Supporting the Vinyl Chloride Research Program (May 3, 1974), MCA Papers. On April 22, 1974, *Chemical & Engineering News* reported that IBT lab findings tended to confirm those of Maltoni, even at 50 ppm in mice, but not in rats and hamsters. See also "Unsafe at Any Level?" *Chemical Week* 136 (April 17, 1974), 15.

57. "Toxicity of Vinyl Chloride-Polyvinyl Chloride," *Annals of the New York Academy of Sciences* 246 (January 31, 1975).

58. F. T. DeWoody, PPG, to M. Petruccelli, "On VCM Safety Association Meeting at Cleveland" (May 30, 1974), emphasis in original; see also G. A. Work to R. P. Lynch, "Meeting on Vinyl Chloride Safety Association" (May 28, 1974), MCA Papers.

59. William J. Driver, "Staff Report" (June 5, 1974), Exhibit H, in MCA, Board of Directors, "Minutes" (June 5, 1974), MCA Papers.

60. Statement of Andrea Hricko and Bertram Cottine, Testimony at OSHA Hearings, "Official Report of Proceedings before the Occupational Safety and Health Administration of the Department of Labor in the Matter of a Proposed Permanent Standard for Occupational Exposure to Vinyl Chloride" (July 9, 1974), 1556–57. See also Andrea Hricko and Sidney Wolfe to Russell Train, EPA (February 21, 1974), attachment to Vinyl Chloride Docket, H-036, Exhibit 3-23, Department of Labor Docket Office.

61. "Clairol Recalls Aerosol Sprays," *New York Times* (April 4, 1974), 11; "EPA Will Study the Effects of Vinyl Chloride Escape in Air," *New York Times* (April 5, 1974), 50; "Aerosol Sprays Recalled by FDA," *New York Times* (April 18, 1974), 49.

62. *Federal Register*, Vol. 39, No. 82 (April 26, 1974), 14753; amended, with a list of products, Vol. 39, No. 140 (July 19, 1974), 26480.

63. Statement of Andrea Hricko and Bertram Cottine, Testimony at OSHA Hearings, "Official Report of Proceedings before the Occupational Safety and Health Administration of the Department of Labor in the Matter of a Proposed Permanent Standard for Occupational Exposure to Vinyl Chloride" (July 9, 1974), 1556–57. See also Andrea Hricko and Sidney Wolfe to Russell Train, EPA (February 21, 1974), attachment to Vinyl Chloride Docket, H-036, Exhibit 3-23, Department of Labor Docket Office. Almost immediately, the Consumer Product Safety Commission issued a press release that announced that it had "banned as health hazards household aerosol sprays using vinyl chloride as a propellant." Consumer Product Safety Commission, Press Release (August 16, 1974), MCA Papers.

64. Office of the Scientific Coordinator for Environmental Carcinogenesis, National Cancer Institute, Transcript of Meeting of the Interagency Collaborative Group on Environmental Carcinogenesis, "Vinyl Chloride Exposure and Neoplastic and Non-Neoplastic Disease" (April 17, 1974), Vinyl Chloride Docket, H-036, Exhibit 7-I, Department of Labor Docket Office.

65. EPA, Press Release, "EPA Urges Prompt Steps by Chemical Industry to Reduce Vinyl Chloride Air Emissions," *Environmental News* (June 11, 1974), Vinyl Chloride Docket, H-036, Exhibit 7(L), Department of Labor Docket Office.

66. "EPA to Set Vinyl Chloride Emissions Standard," *Environmental News*, in K. Johnson, MCA, to F. Kennedy, Conoco (October 2, 1974), MCA Papers. See also Glenn E. Schweitzer, "Environmental Concerns beyond the Workplace" (May 11, 1974), Vinyl Chloride Docket, H-036, Exhibit 155, Department of Labor Docket Office.

67. "Ban Is Asked on Vinyl Chloride in Food Packages," *New York Times* (July 2, 1975), 18.

68. Unfortunately, because of understaffing of the EPA, much less than half of the one thousand new chemicals manufactured in the country each year are evaluated even in the most cursory way. See Philip Landrigan, interview transcript with Bill Moyers, "Trade Secrets," <www.pbs.org/tradesecrets /trans/intero.html>.

69. SPI, Minutes, VCM and PVC Producers Group (February 18, 1975), MCA Papers.

70. CMA, Special Programs Advisory Group, "Record of Meeting" (April 21, 1981), MCA Papers. In April 1981, the EPA was still considering lowering the ambient air standard for vinyl chloride.

71. "Recommendations for Public Affairs Program for SPI's Vinyl Chloride Committee, Phase 1: Preparation for OSHA Hearings," in Jim Moore, Hill & Knowlton, to John Spano, Monsanto (June 12, 1974), MCA Papers.

72. "New Yorker Cites On-Job Hazards," *United Rubber Workers* journal (n.d.), in Vinyl Chloride Docket, H-036, Exhibit 3-13, Department of Labor Docket Office.

73. Lee Grant, MD [to V. A. Sarni, VP Industrial Chemical Division?] (July 12, 1974), re letter to John Stendor on Proposed Permanent Standards on VCM dated July 1, 1974, MCA Papers.

74. Ibid.

75. "ACS for Strict Vinyl Chloride Limits," *Chemical & Engineering News* 4 (July 15, 1974), MCA Papers.

76. A. B. Steele, Union Carbide Corporation, to Robert W. Cairns, Executive Director, American Chemical Society (July 18, 1974), MCA Papers.

77. Marcus Key, letter to editor of *Chemical & Engineering News* (June 10, 1974).

78. See J. T. Barr, Air Products, to R. Fleming, Air Products (July 16, 1974), MCA Papers.

79. J. William Lloyd to A. W. Barnes (July 19, 1974), in possession of Peter Infante. In August, appearing before the Senate subcommittee on the environment in a hearing about the "dangers of vinyl chloride," Key reiterated his charges of deception and laid out the fateful consequence of the industry's actions. "I would like to reemphasize that no information about liver cancers was given," he maintained. "If there had been, I think we would have taken an entirely different course of action in view of the widespread use of this material." Despite NIOSH's call in the *Federal Register* "for information on potential hazards associated with occupational exposure to vinyl chloride . . . from its 1972 Priority List" for "developing criteria documents," the industry had misled him and his agency. See Senate, Committee on Commerce, Subcommittee on the Environment, *Hearing on Dangers of Vinyl Chloride* 93rd Cong. 2nd Sess. (August 21, 1974), Serial No. 93-110, 40. Privately, the industry acknowledged the truthfulness of Key's statement while trying to qualify the fabrication it had promoted. "It is certain that the MCA group plus Dr. Duffield of ICI informed NIOSH that Maltoni had observed tumors at 250 ppm without specifying that they were angiosarcomas of the liver." See Zeb Bell to R. E. Widing, PPG Interoffice Correspondence (August 26, 1974), MCA Papers.

80. A. W. Barnes to J. W. Lloyd (October 9, 1974), in possession of Peter Infante.

81. Ibid.

82. At hearings held in June and July 1974, a docket of over four thousand pages was created from testimony provided by over two hundred organizations and individuals and in six hundred written statements. Labor and consumer groups strongly supported the "no detectable level" standard while industry opposed it. See Michael S. Brown, "Setting Occupational Health Standards: The Vinyl Chloride Case," in Dorothy Nelkin, ed., *Controversy: Politics of Technical Decisions,* 3rd edition (London: Sage Publications, 1992), 137.

83. Statement of Jerome Heckman, General Counsel, SPI, Testimony at OSHA Hearings, "Official Report of Proceedings before the Occupational Safety and Health Administration of the Department of Labor in the Matter of a Proposed Permanent Standard for Occupational Exposure to Vinyl Chloride" (June 26, 1974), 335–40, Vinyl Chloride Docket, H-036, Department of Labor Docket Office.

84. Statement by Raymond J. Abramowitz, Hooker Chemical and Plastics Corporation, (July 10, 1974), Vinyl Chloride Docket, H-036, Exhibit 55, Department of Labor Docket Office.

85. Paul H. Weaver, "On the Horns of the Vinyl Chloride Dilemma," *Fortune* 90 (October 1974), 203.

86. Ibid.

87. "Tighter Controls on Toxics Testing," *Chemical Week* 145 (August 24, 1983), 32–39.

88. Lucille C. Henschel, Acting Project Manager, Vinyl Chloride Research, MCA, to Vinyl Chloride Audit Task Group (January 11, 1979), MCA Papers.

89. CMA, Record of Meeting, Vinyl Chloride Audit Task Group (May 1–2, 1979), MCA Papers.

90. Bob West, Associates, Inc., "Confidential and Privileged Review and Audit of IBT" (May 10, 1980); VCM Technical Panel Meeting (May 14, 1980), MCA Papers.

91. "Tighter Controls on Toxics Testing," *Chemical Week* 145 (August 24, 1983), 32–39.

92. Statement of Peter Bommarito, President, United Rubber Workers, Testimony at OSHA Hearings, "Official Report of Proceedings before the Occupational Safety and Health Administration of the Department of Labor in the Matter of a Proposed Permanent Standard for Occupational Exposure to Vinyl Chloride" (June 25, 1974), 141.

93. Statement by Rudy Kaelin, President, Local 72, United Rubber Workers (ca. July–August 1974), Vinyl Chloride Docket, H-036, Exhibit 50, Department of Labor Docket Office.

94. Statement of Vern Jensen, President of Local 891, OCAW, Testimony at OSHA Hearings, "Official Report of Proceedings before the Occupational Safety and Health Administration of the Department of Labor in the Matter of a Proposed Permanent Standard for Occupational Exposure to Vinyl Chloride" (July 9, 1974), 1416, Vinyl Chloride Docket, H-036, Department of Labor Docket Office.

95. Statement of Anthony Mazzocchi, Testimony at OSHA Hearings, "Official Report of Proceedings before the Occupational Safety and Health Administration of the Department of Labor in the Matter of a Proposed Permanent Standard for Occupational Exposure to Vinyl Chloride" (July 9, 1974), 1413, 1436–37, Department of Labor Docket Office, H-036.

96. Sheldon Samuels, Director of Health, Safety, and Environment, Industrial Union Department, AFL-CIO, "Statement to OSHA" (August 23, 1974), Vinyl Chloride Docket, H-036, Exhibit 159, Department of Labor Docket Office.

97. Statement of Andrea Hricko and Bertram Cottine, Testimony at OSHA Hearings, "Official Report of Proceedings before the Occupational Safety and Health Administration of the Department of Labor in the Matter of a Proposed Permanent Standard for Occupational Exposure to Vinyl Chloride" (July 9, 1974), 1547–48, Vinyl Chloride Docket, H-036, Department of Labor Docket Office.

98. Ibid., 1555. Similarly, the American Public Health Association supported the "no detectable limit," effectively turning industry's argument on its head. Industry had argued that since there was no firm evidence of what level of VCM exposure caused cancer, government should take no precipitous action that would unduly burden industry. The APHA argued that since "a safe level of exposure cannot be determined . . . the proposed regulation that no detectable level be allowed is warranted and should be adopted." The association further argued that because of current technical limitations the proposed

standard was equating one part per million with no detectable level. With technological improvements, they maintained, this one part per million should ultimately be reduced to virtually zero exposure. See William H. McBeath to Docket Officer (July 11, 1974), Vinyl Chloride Docket, H-036, Exhibit 4-617, Department of Labor Docket Office.

99. Statement of Irving J. Selikoff, Testimony at OSHA Hearings, "Official Report of Proceedings before the Occupational Safety and Health Administration of the Department of Labor in the Matter of a Proposed Permanent Standard for Occupational Exposure to Vinyl Chloride" (June 25, 1974), 214, Vinyl Chloride Docket, H-036, Department of Labor Docket Office.

100. Statement of Andrea Hricko and Bertram Cottine, Testimony at OSHA Hearings, "Official Report of Proceedings before the Occupational Safety and Health Administration of the Department of Labor in the Matter of a Proposed Permanent Standard for Occupational Exposure to Vinyl Chloride" (July 9, 1974), 1555, Vinyl Chloride Docket, H-036, Department of Labor Docket Office.

101. Francis P. Grimes, United Steel Workers of America (June 25, 1974), Vinyl Chloride Docket H-036, Exhibit 60; Statement of Ralph Quattrocchi, Safety Director for Amalgamated Meat Cutters, Retail Food Store Employees Union, Local 342 (June 25, 1974), Vinyl Chloride Docket, H-036, Exhibit 80, Department of Labor Docket Office.

102. Senate, Committee on Commerce, Subcommittee on the Environment, *Hearing on Dangers of Vinyl Chloride*, 93rd Cong., 2nd Sess. (Aug. 21, 1974), 24, Serial No. 93-110, 1094.

103. Paul H. Weaver, "On the Horns of the Vinyl Chloride Dilemma," *Fortune* 90 (October 1974), 150.

104. Ibid., 150, 153.

105. Ibid., 150.

106. Ibid., 203.

107. Barry Kramer, "Vinyl-Chloride Scare Points Up Dangers of Other Chemicals," *Wall Street Journal* (October 7, 1974), 19.

108. Quoted in Kramer, "Vinyl-Chloride Scare Points Up Dangers of Other Chemicals."

109. Ibid.

110. DOL, OSHA, "Exposure to Vinyl Chloride, Occupational Safety and Health Standards," *Federal Register*, Vol. 39, No. 194, part 2 (October 4, 1974), 35890–98.

111. Ibid.

112. Ibid.

113. Michael S. Brown, "Setting Occupational Health Standards: The Vinyl Chloride Case," in Dorothy Nelkin, ed., *Controversy: Politics of Technical Decision* (London: Sage Publications, 1992), 142.

114. Ibid.

115. Zeb Bell et al., "OSHA Standards for VC" (October 9, 1974), MCA Papers.

116. Society of the Plastics Industry, VCM and PVC Producers Group, Minutes (October 11, 1974), MCA Papers.

117. Doniger, *The Law and Policy of Toxic Substances Control*, 27–28.

118. Joseph Fath, Testimony at OSHA Hearings, "Official Report of Proceedings before the Occupational Safety and Health Administration of the Department of Labor in the Matter of a Proposed Permanent Standard for Occupational Exposure to Vinyl Chloride" (June 27, 1974), 686, Vinyl Chloride Docket, H-036, Department of Labor Docket Office.

119. Joseph Fath, Vice President, Tenneco Chemicals, to John Lawrence, SPI (October 23, 1974), MCA Papers.

120. Public Affairs Committee to Steering Committee (of SPI) (November 22, 1974), MCA Papers.

121. Society of Plastics Industries, VCM and PVC Producers Group, Minutes (December 6, 1974), MCA Papers.

122. *SPI, Hooker, Union Carbide, B. F. Goodrich, Firestone, Uniroyal, General Dynamic, Diamond Shamrock vs. OSHA, 509 Federal Reporter, 2nd Series (1975)*, 1301–311. Oral arguments were made December 13, 1974; the date of decision was January 31, 1975.

123. Ibid.

124. SPI, VCM and PVC Producers Group, Minutes (February 18, 1975); Manufacturing Chemists' Association to Technical Task Group on Vinyl Chloride Research, Title 29, Labor Chapter XVII, Occupational Safety and Health Administration, Department of Labor, Part 1910, Occupational Safety and Health Standards, Standard for Exposure to Vinyl Chloride; [Fr Doc. 75-7727, Filed 3-24-75; 8:45 AM], *Federal Register*, Vol. 40, No. 58 (March 25, 1975), 13211, MCA Papers.

125. Steven Rattner, "Did Industry Cry Wolf?" *New York Times* (December 28, 1975), Section 3, 1, 5.

126. Ibid.

127. Mary Williams Walsh, "Keeping Workers Safe, but at What Cost?" *New York Times* (December 20, 2000), Section G, 1. Data in this article were drawn from OSHA and the Office of Technology Assessment.

128. Barry Kramer, "Vinyl-Chloride Scare Points Up Dangers of Other Chemicals," *Wall Street Journal* (October 7, 1974), 19.

129. Peter Infante, "Oncogenic and Mutagenic Risks in Communities with Polyvinyl Chloride Production Facilities," in "Abstracts of Papers on VCM Presented at the New York Academy of Sciences" (March 24–27, 1975), MCA Papers.

130. Barry Kramer, "Vinyl Chloride Tied to Higher Incidence of Miscarriages," *Wall Street Journal* (February 5, 1976); see also "Injury to Fetuses Is Traced in Study to Vinyl Chloride," *New York Times* (February 4, 1976), 23; "Second Region Studied for Birth Defects: Vinyl Chloride Is Suspected in Genetic Damage in West Virginia Area," *New York Times* (March 5, 1976), 49.

131. H. B. Lovejoy, M.D., to Frank Ludden, PPG (February 22, 1978), MCA Papers.

132. "Studies Update Vinyl Chloride Hazards," *Chemical & Engineering News* (April 7, 1980), 28.

133. Joseph Wagoner, "Toxicity of Vinyl Chloride and Poly(vinyl Chloride): A Critical Review," *Environmental Health Perspectives* 52 (1983), 65.

134. Paul H. Weaver, "On the Horns of the Vinyl Chloride Dilemma," *Fortune* 90 (October 1974), 202. See Jim Morris, "In Strictest Confidence: The Chemical Industry's Secrets," *Houston Chronicle* (September 27, October 25, November 29, 1998), a series that details the vinyl story of the 1990s.

135. David P. McCaffrey, *OSHA and the Politics of Health Regulation* (New York: Plenum Press, 1982), 132–37.

136. Philip J. Landrigan and William J. Nicholson, "Benzene," in *Environmental and Occupational Medicine*, 3rd edition, ed. by William N. Rom (Philadelphia: Lippincott-Raven, 1998), 1112.

137. McCaffrey, *OSHA and the Politics of Health Regulation*, 132–37.

138. Tabershaw-Cooper Associates, "Epidemiological Study of Vinyl Chloride Workers," "Final Report" crossed out and "DRAFT" put on every page (April 15, 1974), MCA Papers.

139. Tabershaw-Cooper Associates to MCA, "Epidemiological Study of Vinyl Chloride Workers," Final Report (Berkeley: May 3, 1974), MCA Papers.

140. Tabershaw-Cooper Associates, "Epidemiological Study of Vinyl Chloride Workers," Final Report (May 3, 1974), Vinyl Chloride Docket, H-036, Exhibit 107[n], Department of Labor Docket Office.

141. "Study Shows Death Rate Average for VC Workers," *MCA News* (May 1974), 1.

142. Testimony of Dr. J. William Lloyd, OSHA Hearings, "Official Report of Proceedings before the Occupational Safety and Health Administration of the Department of Labor in the Matter of a Proposed Permanent Standard for Occupational Exposure to Vinyl Chloride," OSHA Hearings Transcript (June 25, 1974), 108–09, MCA Papers.

143. Irving R. Tabershaw and William R. Gaffey, "Mortality Study of Workers in the Manufacture of Vinyl Chloride and Its Polymers," *Journal of Occupational Medicine* 16 (August 1974), 509–18.

144. DOL, OSHA, "Exposure to Vinyl Chloride, Occupational Safety and Health Standards," *Federal Register*, Vol. 39, No. 194, part 2 (October 4, 1974), 35890–98.

145. Senate, Committee on Commerce, Subcommittee on the Environment, *Hearing on Dangers of Vinyl Chloride*, 93rd Cong., 2nd Sess. (August 21, 1974), Serial No. 93-110, 42.

146. Ibid. Recent analysis by Richard Lemen also indicts the report's findings that vinyl chloride workers had lower disease rates for all but cancers. He points out that the comparison groups to which vinyl workers were compared were grossly inappropriate because average death rates for all Americans

included the elderly and those too ill or disabled to work. Hence, the vinyl workers, most of whom would be younger and more fit than those unable to work, looked healthier. He termed this misuse of the data the "healthy workers" effect. See Richard Lemen, Deposition of Richard A. Lemen, Ph.D. (June 11–13, 2001), taken in *McKinley et al. vs. Gencorp, Inc., et al.*, in the Court of Common Pleas for Ashtabula County, Ohio; No. 98-CV-00797.

147. Senate, Committee on Commerce, Subcommittee on the Environment, *Hearing on Dangers of Vinyl Chloride*, 93rd Cong., 2nd Sess. (August 21, 1974), Serial No. 93-110, 42, 50.

148. Ibid. See also Torkelson to Johnson, MCA (November 12, 1974), MCA Papers.

149. "Supplementary Epidemiological Study of Vinyl Chloride Workers, I," Submitted to MCA (Berkeley: Tabershaw-Cooper Associates, May 30, 1975), MCA Papers.

150. Richard J. Waxweiler, William Stringer, Joseph K. Wagoner, and James Jones, "Neoplastic Risk among Workers Exposed to Vinyl Chloride," *Annals of the New York Academy of Sciences* 271 (1976), 47.

151. "U.S. Checking to See if Deaths of Workers Linked to Chemical," *Houston Post* (February 16, 1979), MCA Papers.

152. Robert Wheeler to Dr. John Stanford (March 5, 1979), MCA Papers.

153. MCA, Vinyl Chloride Research Coordinators, "Record of Meeting" (March 21, 1979), MCA Papers.

154. D. A. Kuhn to Plant Managers, Conoco Interoffice Communication, "Confidential" (March 7, 1979), MCA Papers.

155. F. C. Dehn to B. C. Brennan and R. E. Stack (March 14, 1979), MCA Papers.

156. R. Gary Wilson to I. C. Klimas, PPG Interoffice Communication (March 26, 1979), MCA Papers.

157. "Studies Update Vinyl Chloride Hazards," *Chemical & Engineering News* (April 7, 1980), 27.

158. Zeb Bell to F. C. Dehn (September 26, 1980), MCA Papers.

159. Environmental Health Associates, "Draft Epidemiological Study, of Vinyl Chloride Workers" (August 5, 1986), MCA Papers. Its final report was similar. See Environmental Health Associates, "Final Report: An Update of an Epidemiological Study of Vinyl Chloride Workers, 1942–1982" (October 17, 1986), MCA Papers.

160. Ellen Kessler and Paul W. Brandt-Rauf, "Occupational Cancers of the Nervous System," *Seminar in Occupational Medicine* 2 (December 1987), 311–14.

161. W. D. Broddle to M. K. Pita, Legal, Conoco Interoffice Communication (March 17, 1989), MCA Papers.

162. Otto Wong et al., "An Industry-Wide Epidemiologic Study of Vinyl Chloride Workers, 1942–1982," *American Journal of Industrial Medicine* 30 (1991), 317–34.

163. Robert K. Hinderer, Manager, Health and Toxicology Environment, Health and Safety Management Systems, Goodrich, to Roy T. Gottesman, Vinyl Institute (October 21, 1991), MCA Papers.

164. Hasmukh C. Shah, CMA, Letter to the Editor, "Diagnostic Bias in Occupational Epidemiologic Studies," *American Journal of Industrial Medicine* 24 (1993), 249–50; Otto Wong and M. Donald Whorton, Letter to the Editor, "Diagnostic Bias in Occupational Epidemiologic Studies: An Example Based on the Vinyl Chloride Literature," *American Journal of Industrial Medicine* 24 (1993), 251–56.

165. See Philip Landrigan, interview transcript with Bill Moyers, "Trade Secrets" (March 26, 2001), PBS, <www.pbs.org/tradesecrets/trans/intero3 .html>.

166. Chris Bozman and Joe Ledvina to Paul Carrico, Vista Interoffice Communication (April 9, 1991), MCA Papers.

167. "Transcribed Notes from 4/1-2 LCVCM Employee Focus Groups," Attached to Chris Bozman and Joe Ledvina to Paul Carrico, Vista Interoffice Communication (April 9, 1991), MCA Papers.

168. "Now You Know," *The Source*, Lake Charles, Louisiana (August 1995), 3.

169. Weaver, "On the Horns of the Vinyl Chloride Dilemma," 153.

170. See David Vogel, *Fluctuating Fortunes: The Political Power of Business in America* (New York: Basic Books, 1989), 225.

171. MCA, Government Relations Committee Report to the Board of Directors, Don A. Goodall, Chairman (February 8, 1977), Exhibit F, Board of Directors, Minutes, MCA Papers.

172. Ibid.

173. Quoted in Vogel, *Fluctuating Fortunes*, 196.

174. "The Fallen Giant," *Fortune* 138 (December 8, 1997), 156.

CHAPTER 8. OL' MAN RIVER OR CANCER ALLEY?

1. Edwin Adams Davis, *The Story of Louisiana*, Vol. 1 (New Orleans: J. F. Hyer Publishing Co., 1960), 297–98.

2. Ibid., 353; William McGinty Garney, *A History of Louisiana* (New York: Exposition Press, 1951), ch. 21, p. 270.

3. Peter Spitz, "The Rise of Petrochemicals," *Chemical Week* (August 2, 1989), 26.

4. "Petrochemicals: A Bright Star in the Lone Star Economy," *Journal of Commerce* (November 15, 1988), 8-B.

5. T. Harry Williams, *Huey Long* (New York: Alfred A. Knopf, 1969), 308.

6. Ibid., 354.

7. Alan Brinkley, *Voices of Protest: Huey Long, Father Coughlin and the Great Depression* (New York: Vintage Books, 1982), 25.

8. Williams, *Huey Long*, 365.

9. Brinkley, *Voices of Protest,* 30.

10 Davis, *The Story of Louisiana,* 347; "Louisiana's Economy," *The Economist* (June 24, 1989), 26.

11. John Robert Moore, "The New Deal in Louisiana," in John Braeman, Robert H. Bremner, and David Brody, *The New Deal, Vol. 2, The State and Local Levels,* (Columbus: Ohio State University Press, 1975), 140–41.

12. Brinkley, *Voices of Protest,* 31.

13. Davis, *The Story of Louisiana,* 347–48.

14. Ibid.

15. Peter Gwynne, "SOS from a Salt Dome," *Newsweek* (February 16, 1981), 88. "Formed over millions of years as salt pushed its way up through heavier rocks, the domes are resistant to fracturing and able to withstand heat better than rock. They can be hollowed out by pumping in water, which dissolves the salt; when the hollow is large enough, a saturated solution of brine keeps it open without eroding more salt. Then oil or gas can be pumped into what is literally a bargain basement: oilmen say it would cost 20 times as much to store ethylene gas in surface tanks as it does underground, and an area of land that could store 200 million barrels of oil underground could hold only 3 million on its surface."

16. *Green Fields: Two Hundred Years of Louisiana Sugar (A Catalogue Complementing the Pictorial Exhibit)* (Lafayette: University of Southwestern Louisiana, 1980), 84.

17. National Agricultural Workers Union, Research and Education Department, *The Louisiana Sugar Cane Plantation Workers vs. The Sugar Corporations, U.S. Department of Agriculture, et al.: An Account of Human Relations on Corporation-Owned Sugar Cane Plantations in Louisiana under the Operation of the U.S. Sugar Program, 1937–1953* (Washington: Inter-American Educational Association, Inc., 1954), 129.

18. Susan Reed, "His Family Ravaged by Cancer, an Angry Louisiana Man Wages War on the Very Air That He Breathes: Work of A. Favorite in Ascension Parish," *People Weekly* 35 (March 1991), 42–44.

19. National Agricultural Workers Union, Research and Education Department, *The Louisiana Sugar Cane Plantation Workers vs. The Sugar Corporations,* 25.

20. Ibid.

21. Ibid., 152.

22. Harnett T. Kane, "Land of Louisiana Sugar Kings," *National Geographic* (April 1958), 565.

23. Davis, *The Story of Louisiana,* 354–55.

24. "Plant Contract Is Let: Catalytic Construction Company to Build Facility for Ethyl," *New York Times* (May 18, 1956), 35; "Grace Gets License to Radiate Plastic," *New York Times* (October 17, 1965), 52.

25. Ernest Obadele-Starks, *Black Unionism in the Industrial South* (College Station: Texas A&M University Press, 2000).

26. E. N. Brandt, *Growth Company: Dow Chemical's First Century* (East Lansing: Michigan State University Press, 1997), 285.

27. Ibid, 285.

28. Ibid.; Mary Ann Sternberg, *Along the River Road, Past and Present on Louisiana's Historic Byway* (Baton Rouge: Louisiana State University Press, 1996), 209.

29. Brandt, *Growth Company*, 285.

30. Adam Fairclough, *Race and Democracy: The Civil Rights Struggle in Louisiana, 1915–1972* (Athens: University of Georgia Press, 1995), 210, 216.

31. Ibid., 297.

32. Ibid., 301–02.

33. Jerry Purvis Sanson, *Louisiana during World War II: Politics and Society, 1939–1945* (Baton Rouge: Louisiana State University Press, 1999), 268.

34. Fairclough, *Race and Democracy*, 328–30.

35. "Plaquemine Peace Holds after Riots," Baton Rouge *Advocate* (September 3, 1963), A-1, A-4. See also Larry Stringer and Gibbs Adams, "Plaquemine Council Refuses Requests of CORE Leaders," Baton Rouge *Advocate* (August 30, 1963), A-1, A-3; "CORE Asks Court Order Be Lifted," Baton Rouge *Advocate* (August 25, 1963), A-1, A-8.

36. James O'Byrne, "The Death of a Town: A Chemical Plant Closes In," New Orleans *Times-Picayune* (February 20, 1991), A-12.

37. Jon Bowermaster, "A Town Called Morrisonville," *Audubon* 95 (July–August 1993), 42–51. See also Linda Villanosa, "Showdown at Sunrise," *Essence* 22 (July 1991), 55, 61, 109–11; and "Before and After the Bull-Doze," <www.kittner.com/reve.html> for Reveilletown, Louisiana.

38. Bowermaster, "A Town Called Morrisonville"; Villanosa, "Showdown at Sunrise"; "Before and after the Bull-Doze," <www.kittner.com/reve.html>; O'Byrne, "The Death of a Town."

39. Bowermaster, "A Town Called Morrisonville."

40. O'Byrne, "The Death of a Town."

41. Keith Schneider, "Chemical Plants Buy Up Neighbors for Safety Zone," *New York Times* (November 28, 1990), A-1.

42. Emily Kern, "Grand Jury to Look into Drinking Water Contamination," Advocate Online (January 12, 2002), <http://br.theadvocate.com/news/story.asp?StoryID=27078> (February 15, 2002).

43. Pat Bryant, "A Lily-White Achilles' Heel," *Environmental Action* 21 (January/February 1990), 28–29.

44. Greenpeace, "PVC—The Poison Plastic," <www.greenlink.org/affinity/82297/plastic.html>; Monique Harden, "Letter to Editor," Baton Rouge *Advocate* (July 31, 1997), 8-B.

45. Schneider, "Chemical Plants Buy Up Neighbors for Safety Zone," A-1.

46. Ibid.

47. Ibid.

48. Gwynne, "SOS from a Salt Dome."

49. Interview with Beth Zilbert (March 18, 1998), New York City.

50 Marvin A. Schneiderman, "The Links between the Environment and Health," in *Proceedings of the National Conference on the Environment and Health Care Costs,* House of Representatives Caucus Room, Washington, DC (August 15, 1978), 42.

51. David R. Goldfield, *Promised Land: The South since 1945* (Arlington Heights, Ill.: Harlan-Davidson, 1987), 203–04. Japanese industries may have been particularly sensitive to the environmental effects of their industries given Minamata and a crisis regarding PCBs mixed into cooking oil that had resulted in a variety of symptoms in Kyushu in 1968. See Kim N. Dietrich, "Environmental Neurotoxicants and Psychological Development," in G. Taylor, K. O. Yeates, and M. D. Ris, eds., *Pediatric Neuropsychology: Research Theory and Practice* (New York: Guilford Press, 1999), 217.

52. "Louisiana's Petrochemical Corridor," Baton Rouge *Advocate* (September 12, 1999), 49.

53. David Zwick and Marcy Benstock, *Water Wasteland: Ralph Nader's Study Group Report on Water Pollution* (New York: Grossman Publishers, 1971), 20.

54. Interview with Ruth Heifetz (June 14, 2001), Berkeley, California.

55. Hans W. Maull, "Japan's Global Environmental Policies," in Andrew Hurrell and Benedict Kingsbury, eds., *The International Politics of the Environment* (Oxford: Oxford University Press, 1992), 358.

56. "Water from Mississippi River Linked to Cancer Death Trends," *New York Times* (November 8, 1974), 29.

57. Donald Jansen, "Jersey Hunts Dumpers of Toxins," *New York Times* (January 30, 1978), A-1. Under pressure from the federal government, which threatened to withhold over $500,000, Dale Givens, the chief of Louisiana's Water Pollution Control Division, announced in 1982 that he would for the first time seek to determine which industries were dumping wastes into the river. See "La. to Toughen on Mississippi River Dumpers," *Platt's Oilgram News* 60 (January 13, 1982), 4.

58. Reginald Stewart, "Derailment Still Keeps 1,500 Away from Town," *New York Times* (October 11, 1982), A-12.

59. Nan Powers, "Expansion to Prevent Another Livingston," Baton Rouge *Advocate* (April 24, 1988), G-1.

60. Stewart, "Derailment Still Keeps 1,500 Away from Town."

61. Powers, "Expansion to Prevent Another Livingston."

62. Russell Robbinson, President, Local 4-620, Geismar, Louisiana, in "Proceedings," *Hazards in the Industrial Environment,* a conference sponsored by District 4 Council, Oil, Chemical and Atomic Workers International Union, Rice Hotel, Houston, Texas (February 20–21, 1970), 43–44.

63. Robert Gottlieb, *Forcing the Spring: The Transformation of the Environmental Movement* (Washington: Island Press, 1993), 296.

64. Ibid.

65. Interview with Tony Mazzocchi (January 26, 2001), New York, New York.

66. Gottlieb, *Forcing the Spring*, 297.

67. Peter Fairley, "Louisiana Plants Find Pride in Performance," *Chemical Week* (July 1/8, 1998), 45–48; Matt Witt, "Labor's New Leverage: Unions Are Forging Alliances That Corporations May Regret," *Washington Post* (May 10, 1987), B-5; Frank Swoboda, "5½ Year Labor Lockout Ends," *Washington Post* (December 16, 1989), A-20; "Louisiana's Petrochemical Corridor," Baton Rouge *Advocate* (September 12, 1999), 49.

68. Oil, Chemical and Atomic Workers Union, *Locked Out*, video produced about the BASF strike (1984).

69. "OCAW/NTC Hire Organizer: A Labor/Environmental Alliance," *LEAN News* 4 (August 1990), 9, 16.

70. Eric Silver, "Indian Gas Disaster Leaves 410 Dead," London, *The Guardian* (December 4, 1984).

71. Robert D. Bullard and Beverly H. Wright, "The Quest for Environmental Equity: Mobilizing the African-American Community for Social Change," in Riley E. Dunlop and Angela G. Mertig, eds., *American Environmentalism: The U.S. Environmental Movement, 1970–1990* (Washington: Taylor and Francis, 1992), 45.

72. Rae Tyson and Julie Morris, "The Chemicals Next Door: A First Peak 'Behind the Plant Gates,'" *USA Today* (July 31, 1989), 1-A.

73. Ibid.

74. Peter Fairley, "Louisiana Plants Find Pride in Performance," *Chemical Week* (July 1/8, 1998), 45.

75. Ibid.

76. Ibid.

77. *Oprah* television show (May 22, 1989), quoted in Elizabeth Whelan, *Toxic Terror: The Truth behind the Cancer Scares* (Buffalo: Prometheus Books, 1993), 42.

78. "Protesters Plug Up Waste Pipe," Baton Rouge *Advocate* (November 4, 1988), B-8.

79. "Great Louisiana Toxics March Sets the Pace for the Movement," *Rachel's Environment and Health Weekly* 101 (October 31, 1988) <http://www.monitor.net/rachel/r101.html>.

80. Ibid. See also Michael Brown, *The Toxic Cloud* (New York: Harper & Row, 1987), 151–54; Michael Brown, *Laying Waste: The Poisoning of America by Toxic Chemicals* (New York: Pantheon, 1979), 157–64.

81. "Great Louisiana Toxics March Sets the Pace for the Movement," *Rachel's Environment and Health Weekly* 101 (October 31, 1988), <http://www.monitor.net/rachel/r101.html>.

82. "Historic Toxic March Brings Attention to Cancer Alley," *LEAN News* 3 (March 1989), 1, 4, 8, 12, 15.

83. Ron Faucheau, "How a Populist Conservative Came out of Nowhere to Capture the Governor's Mansion in One of America's Toughest Political Battlegrounds," *Campaigns and Elections* (December 1995/January 1996), 36.

84. Interview with Paul Templet (November 2, 2000), Baton Rouge.

85. Ibid.

86. "Interview: Paul Templet Named DEQ Secretary," *LEAN News* 2 (April 1988), 3; Interview with Paul Templet (November 2, 2000), Baton Rouge.

87. David Hunter, "Louisiana Works Hard for a New Status," *Chemical Week* (May 22, 1991), 32.

88. Mary Buckner Powers, "Delta State Rises to Face Growing Pollution Crisis," *Engineering News-Record* (June 28, 1990), 71.

89. Interview with Paul Templet (November 2, 2000), Baton Rouge.

90. Ibid.

91. Barbara Koppel, "Cancer Alley, Louisiana," *The Nation* (November 8, 1999), 22.

92. Interview with Paul Templet (November 2, 2000), Baton Rouge.

93. Ibid.

94. Koppel, "Cancer Alley, Louisiana."

95. Interview with Paul Templet (November 2, 2000), Baton Rouge; Koppel, "Cancer Alley, Louisiana."

96. Hunter, "Louisiana Works Hard for a New Status."

97. Powers, "Delta State Rises to Face Growing Pollution Crisis."

98. Fairley, "Louisiana Plants Find Pride in Performance."

99. Hunter, "Louisiana Works Hard for a New Status."

100. Ibid.

101. Ibid.

102. Gregory Morris, "Back on the Bayou: The Chemical Sector Enjoys Renewed Support," *Chemical Week* (May 26, 1993), 33.

103. Richard Baudouin Jr., "Decline and Fall of the Roemer Empire," *The New Democrat* (September 1991), 15.

104. Ibid.

105. Edwards, a Democrat, was first elected governor in 1971. He quickly established himself as a "wheeling and dealing, mabashed [sic] womanizing, and high-rolling Las Vegas gambling" populist. By the end of his second term in 1979, he benefited from an economic expansion that allowed him to raise taxes on oil and gas without alienating an industry flush from the oil boom that followed the OPEC oil crisis of the mid-1970s. Limited by state law to two terms, Edwards took a hiatus (during which time Dave Treen became the first Republican governor since Reconstruction), only to be reelected with 61 percent of the vote in 1983. The economic recession of the early Reagan years and a federal criminal indictment in 1985 undermined Edwards's popularity, and Buddy Roemer was elected. When Roemer's popularity slipped and he did not even make the Democratic primary runoff, Edwards and Duke squared off in a campaign

that attracted national and even international attention. Edwards, despite already having a reputation for corruption and sexual prowess, outwitted David Duke in the final runoff election after commenting that he, like Duke, "was a wizard under the sheets." He created what some considered a "bizarre coalition of blacks, Cajuns, and labor—his usual base—together with conservative business people and mainstream Republicans who dreaded the national implications of a Duke victory." See Ron Faucheau, "How a Populist Conservative Came out of Nowhere to Capture the Governor's Mansion in One of America's Toughest Political Battlegrounds," *Campaigns and Elections* (December 1995/January 1996), 36. In keeping with Louisiana's colorful political tradition, the choice was summed up in one popular bumper sticker: "Vote for the Crook, It's Important." Also, interview with Paul Templet (November 2, 2000), Baton Rouge.

106. Gregory Morris, "A Controversial Appointment in Louisiana,"*Chemical Week* (January 1–8, 1992), 7.

107. Morris, "Back on the Bayou."

108. "Louisiana Scales Back Protections," *Engineering News-Record* (January 27, 1992), 10; Barbara Koppel, "Cancer Alley, Louisiana."

109. "Louisiana Scales Back Protections," *Engineering News-Record* (January 27, 1992), 10; Koppel, "Cancer Alley, Louisiana."

110. Gregory Morris, "Louisiana to Repeal Environmental Scorecard," *Chemical Week* (March 4, 1992), 9.

111. Gregory Morris, "Louisiana: Bullish on Chemicals Business," *Chemical Week* (May 27/June 3, 1992), 36.

112. Gregory Morris, "Taxes, Torts, and Trade Top Gulf Coast Challenges," *Chemical Week* (May 18, 1994), 38.

113. Ibid., 40.

114. Tim Cornitius, "Gulf Coast Flourishes; Louisiana, Texas Lead Resurgence," *Chemical Week* (May 17, 1995), 37.

115. Morris, "Louisiana: Bullish on Chemicals Business."

116. Interview with Paul Templet (June 14, 2001), Berkeley, California.

117. Morris, "Louisiana: Bullish on Chemicals Business."

118. J. Michael Kennedy, "'Chemical Corridor' by 'Old Man River,' New Health Fear," *Los Angeles Times* (May 9, 1989), 1. See also "Miscarriage Study Proceeds," *LEAN News* 2 (1988), 10.

119. James O'Byrne, "State Analyzes Miscarry Rates," Baton Rouge *Advocate* (November 27, 1988), B-1.

120. Kathy Yates, "Vinyl Chloride's Effects in St. Gabriel Investigated," Plaquemine *Post South* (August 6, 1987), 1-A, 2-A, attached to Roy Gottesman, Vinyl Institute, to "The VI Health, Safety and Environment Committee" (August 13, 1987), MCA Papers.

121. Kennedy, "'Chemical Corridor' by 'Old Man River,' New Health Fear."

122. Vickie Ferstel, "Studies Make No Concrete Cancer-Pollution Link," Baton Rouge *Advocate* (June 24, 1998), 1-A.

123. O'Byrne, "State Analyzes Miscarry Rates."

124. Ferstel, "Studies Make No Concrete Cancer-Pollution Link."

125. "St. Gabriel Study Rigged against Community, Women Say," *LEAN News* 4 (August 1990), 6. Former DEQ chief Paul Templet says that the miscarriage rates were 18 percent higher among white women, but African American women would not talk to investigators about miscarriages. That reduced the overall number of miscarriages per capita, lowering the statistical significance of the findings below the commonly accepted 95 percent significance level. It was later revealed that the plant produced ethylene oxide, a reproductive toxin. Interview with Paul Templet (June 14, 2001), Berkeley, California.

126. Ferstel, "Studies Make No Concrete Cancer-Pollution Link."

127. "Environmental Racism Exists in Louisiana," National Public Radio, *Weekend Edition/Saturday* (May 15, 1993).

128. Ferstel, "Studies Make No Concrete Cancer-Pollution Link."

129. Ben Goldman et al., *Mortality and Toxics along the Mississippi River* (Washington, 1988), and Pat Costner, Joe Thornton, et al., *We All Live Downstream: The Mississippi River and the National Toxics Crisis* (Washington: Greenpeace, 1989), cited in "Munching Peanut Butter in Cancer Alley," *Rachel's Hazardous Waste News* 168 (February 13, 1990), electronic edition, <http://www.ejnet.org/rachel/rhwn168.htm>.

130. Ibid.

131. Vivien W. Chen et al., "Cancer Incidence in the Industrial Corridor: An Update," *Journal of the Louisiana State Medical Society* 150 (1998), <http://www.lsms.org/journal/98cancer.html>. See also Chen et al., "Highlights of Cancer Incidence in Louisiana, 1988–1992," *Journal of the Louisiana State Medical Society* 149 (April 1997), 119–24; F. D. Groves, P. A. Andrews, V. W. Chen, E. T. Fonthan, and P. Correa, "Is There a 'Cancer Corridor' in Louisiana?" *Journal of the Louisiana State Medical Society* 148 (April 1996), 155–65. See also special issues on cancer in Louisiana in *Journal of the Louisiana State Medical Society* in 1992, 1993, and 1995.

132. Louisiana Chemical Association, press release (July 7, 1989), MCA Papers.

133. Chen et al., "Cancer Incidence in the Industrial Corridor: An Update"; See also Chen et al., "Highlights of Cancer Incidence in Louisiana, 1988–1992"; Groves, Andrews, Chen, Fonthan, and Correa, "Is There a 'Cancer Corridor' in Louisiana?"; special issues on cancer in Louisiana in *Journal of the Louisiana State Medical Society* in 1992, 1993, and 1995.

134. Elizabeth Kirschner, "Louisiana Is No 'Cancer Alley,'" *Chemical Week* (June 16, 1993), 21.

135. Louisiana Chemical Association, "Facts and Myths about Cancer in Louisiana," <http://www.lca.org/health.html>.

136. Michael Gough (Cato Institute), "Does Environmentalism Kill?" *EPA Watch* (March 10, 1999), cited in National Center for Policy Analysis, "Louisiana: Below Average Incidence, Above Average Mortality," <http://www.ncpa.org/pi/enviro/pd033199h.html>.

137. Robert Kuehn to Michael Mattheisen, Mary O'Lone, and Marsha Moncrieffe, "Re: Additional Information on Title VI Complaint against Louisiana Department of Environmental Quality for Shintech Plant Permitting" (December 23, 1997), in Tulane Environmental Law Clinic (TELC) Papers, New Orleans.

138. Richard P. Ieyoub to Vivien Chen (November 17, 1997), enclosed in Robert Kuehn to Michael Mattheisen, Mary O'Lone and Marsha Moncrieffe, "Re: Additional Information on Title VI Complaint against Louisiana Department of Environmental Quality for Shintech Plant Permitting" (December 23, 1997), TELC Papers.

139. James J. Cox to Vivien W. Chen (October 20, 1997), TELC Papers.

140. Interview with Paul Templet (November 2, 2000), Baton Rouge.

141. Robert Bullard, *Dumping in Dixie: Race, Class, and Environmental Quality* (Boulder: Westview Press, 1990, 1994), 97.

CHAPTER 9. A HAZY MIXTURE

1. "The History of the Community of Convent," citing Interview with Emelda West in "Shintech Environmental Justice Comments Attachments," mimeo (ca. 1997). See also "Convent" in Claire D'Artois Leeper, *Louisiana Places: A Collection of the Columns from the Baton Rouge Sunday Advocate* (Baton Rouge: Legacy Publishing Company, 1976), 68.

2. Shintech application, "Advanced Notification, Office of Commerce and Industry" (1996), Tulane Environmental Law Clinic Papers, New Orleans (hereafter TELC Papers).

3. Dennis Cauchun, "Racial, Economic Divide in La.," *USA Today* (September 9, 1997), A-3.

4. U.S. Environmental Protection Agency (hereafter EPA), "Title VI Administrative Complaint, re: Louisiana Department of Environmental Quality/Permit for Proposed Shintech Facility" (draft revised demographic information) (April 1998), 20.

5. Environmental Health Center, "1,2-Dichloroethane ($C_2H_4Cl_2$) Chemical Backgrounder, Attachment 25, p. 2 to EPA, "Title VI Administrative Complaint, re: Louisiana." See also Marc Schleifstein, "Louisiana Ranks Second in Toxic Waste Disposal; EPA Reports Numbers Up Slightly in 97," New Orleans *Times-Picayune* (May 14, 1999), A-2.

6. Bill Dawson, "Texas Leads Nation in Toxic Pollution—and In Reducing It," *Houston Chronicle* (May 15, 1999), A-37. According to Louisiana's own Department of Environmental Quality, 7.5 million pounds of toxic material was spewed into the air of tiny St. James Parish alone in 1995. See Louisiana Department of Environmental Quality home page, <www.deq.state.la.us/osec/tri95/tri_9.htm>, "Top Ten Parishes with Largest Toxics Released to Air."

7. U.S. EPA, "Title VI Administrative Complaint, re: Louisiana Department of Environmental Quality/Permit for Proposed Shintech Facility," 13. See also

John C. Pine, "Proximity of Minority Block Groups and TRI Sites in Louisiana" (March 22, 1996), Attachment 13 to the previously cited EPA complaint, which points out that 84 percent of Louisiana TRI sites "are located within two miles of minority population as measured by block groups with 40% or greater black population."

8. Beverly Wright, *Convent, Louisiana—A Historical and Toxicological Review*, mimeo (New Orleans: Xavier University, Deep South Center for Environmental Justice).

9. Ibid. See also Beverly Wright, "Endangered Communities: The Struggle for Environmental Justice in the Louisiana Chemical Corridor," *Journal of Public Management and Social Policy* 4 (1998), 181–91.

10. "St. James Parish TRI Emissions into the Air with and without Shintech," in "The Story of St. James' Citizens for Jobs and the Environment and Their Struggle for Environmental Justice," attached to "Summary of the Meeting of the National Environmental Justice Advisory Council," a federal advisory committee, Indian Springs Lodge and Conference Center, Wbeno, Wisconsin (May 13–15, 1997); Marsha Shuler, "Official Defends Makeup of Task Force," Baton Rouge *Advocate* (January 21, 1998).

11. "The Myth of Shintech Jobs: Selling False Hopes to Local Residents," Louisiana Environmental Action Network, mimeo (1997).

12. David D. Duncan, "Environmental Justice and Permitting: Cases Applying EPA's Guidance and Regulations," *Environmental Regulation and Permitting* 8 (Summer 1999), 109.

13. Hal Rothman, *The Greening of a Nation? Environmentalism in the United States since 1945* (Fort Worth: Harcourt Brace College Publishers, 1998), 159.

14. Riley E. Dunlap, "Trends in Public Opinion toward Environmental Issues: 1965–1990," in *American Environmentalism: The U.S. Environmental Movement, 1970–1990*, ed. by Riley E. Dunlap and Angela G. Mertig (Philadelphia: Taylor & Francis, 1992), 106. See also Riley E. Dunlap, "Public Opinion and Environmental Policy," in *Environmental Politics and Policy* ed. by J. P. Lester (Durham: Duke University Press), 87–134.

15. Dunlap, "Trends in Public Opinion toward Environmental Issues: 1965-1990," 106. See also Dunlap, "Public Opinion and Environmental Policy," 87–134.

16. Whitney Young, quoted in Robert Gottlieb, *Forcing the Spring: The Transformation of the American Environmental Movement* (Washington: Island Press, 1993), 254.

17. Gottlieb, *Forcing the Spring*, 254–60. See also Eileen Maura McGurty, "From NIMBY to Civil Rights: The Origins of the Environmental Justice Movement," *Environmental History* 2 (July 1997), 303–05.

18. "Environmental Justice Highlights," *Detroit Free Press* (June 28, 1998), A12.

19. Benjamin F. Chavis Jr. and Charles Lee, *Toxic Wastes and Race in the United States* (New York: Commission for Racial Justice, United Church of

Christ, 1987); Ronald Begley and Elisabeth Kirshner, "The Demand for Environmental Justice," *Chemical Week* (September 15, 1993), 27; Robert D. Bul-lard, ed., *Unequal Protection: Environmental Justice in Communities of Color* (San Francisco: Sierra Club Books, 1994); Robert D. Bullard, *Dumping in Dixie: Race, Class and Environmental Quality* (Boulder: Westview Press, 1990); McGurty, "From NIMBY to Civil Rights," 303–05. Also see Jim Schwab, *Deeper Shades of Green: The Rise of Blue-Collar and Minority Environmentalism in America* (San Francisco: Sierra Club Books, 1994).

20. Chavis and Lee, *Toxic Wastes and Race in the United States*; Ronald Begley and Elisabeth Kirshner, "The Demand for Environmental Justice," *Chemical Week* (September 15, 1993), 27; Bullard, *Unequal Protection*; Bullard, *Dumping in Dixie*.

21. Bullard, *Dumping in Dixie*.

22. Harris, DeVille & Associates, Inc., "Environmental Equity Chronology," mimeo (April 27, 1993).

23. Robert Bullard, "Environmental Justice for All," in Bullard, ed., *Unequal Protection*, 7.

24. For people below the poverty line, the figures were 181 percent above the national average and 22 percent above the state average. "Louisiana: Global Toxic Hot Spot," Greenpeace Media Center, <http://www.greenpeaceusa.org/media/factsheets/hotspottext.htm>.

25. Beverly H. Wright, Pat Bryant, and Robert D. Bullard, "Coping with Poisons in Cancer Alley," in Bullard, ed., *Unequal Protection*, 114–15.

26. Gottlieb, *Forcing the Spring*, 188.

27. Environmental Racism Exists in Louisiana," National Public Radio, *Weekend Edition/Saturday* (May 15, 1993).

28. "A Testimony of Florence T. Robinson before the House Energy Subcommittee, Subcommittee on Transportation and Hazardous Waste, Hearing on Public Involvement in Superfund Program" (Washington: Federal Document Clearing House, October 14, 1993).

29. "Environmental Racism Exists in Louisiana," National Public Radio, *Weekend Edition/Saturday* (May 15, 1993).

30. Ibid.

31. Jerome Balter, "The EPA Needs a Workable Environmental Justice Protocol," *Tulane Environmental Law Journal* 12 (Spring 1999), 360.

32. Harris, DeVille & Associates, Inc., "Environmental Equity Chronology," mimeo (April 27, 1993).

33. Balter, "The EPA Needs a Workable Environmental Justice Protocol," 360–61.

34. Editorial, *Oil & Gas Journal* 95 (September 22, 1997), 21.

35. Ibid.

36. Gregory Morris, "Taxes, Torts, and Trade Top Gulf Coast Challenges," *Chemical Week* (May 18, 1994), 41.

37. Ibid.

38. Ron Faucheau, "How a Populist Conservative Came Out of Nowhere to Capture the Governor's Mansion in One of America's Toughest Political Battlegrounds," *Campaigns and Elections* (December 1995/January 1996), 36.

39. "Louisiana: Swimming with Sharks," *The Economist* (March 23, 1996), 26.

40. Carl Redman, "Foster Says Maybe Buying Duke's List Was 'Bad Judgment'" Baton Rouge *Advocate Online*, <http://www.theadvocate.com/news/story.asp?StoryID=6701> (May 28, 1999).

41. "Louisiana: Swimming with Sharks," *The Economist* (March 23, 1996), 26.

42. "State Regulation Louisiana DEQ Chief to Step Down," *Chemical Week* (December 20/December 27, 1995), 10.

43. Tim Cornitius, "Louisiana Lures Investors with Business Reforms," *Chemical Week* (April 9, 1997), 25.

44. Larry Terry, "Gulf Coast Fishing: Luring Firms with State Incentives," *Chemical Week* (May 13, 1998), 27–37.

45. Cornitius, "Louisiana Lures Investors with Business Reforms."

46. Don Richards, "Louisiana Is Counting on Chemical Industry for Economic Growth," *Chemical Market Reporter* (November 25, 1996), 3.

47. "House Appropriations Chairman Stresses State's Need for Diversified Economy," Baton Rouge *Advocate Online*, http://www.theadvocate.com/archive/story.asp?StoryID=11110 (May 12, 1998).

48. Ken Silverstein and Alexander Cockburn, "The Chemical Plant That Could Break Tulane," *Counterpunch* (July 16–31, 1997), 4.

49. "Soft Environmental Penalties Troubling," Baton Rouge *Advocate* (June 15, 1998), 6-B.

50. Foster no longer required ongoing environmental assessments for new facilities, only for "major" industrial sites. He gave the authority to designate "major" sites to his Department of Environmental Quality secretary, who seemed less concerned with problems of pollution than with the benefits of economic development. Barbara Koppel, "Cancer Alley, Louisiana," *The Nation* (November 8, 1999), 22.

51. "Pollution Record Source of Shame," Baton Rouge *Advocate* (June 28, 1998), 16-B.

52. Koppel, "Cancer Alley, Louisiana."

53. "Pollution Record Source of Shame," Baton Rouge *Advocate* (June 28, 1998), 16-B.

54. Peter Fairley, "Louisiana Plants Find Pride in Performance," *Chemical Week* (July 1/8, 1998), 47.

55. Robert Westervelt, "Shintech Building Major Complex on Gulf Coast," *Chemical Week* (January 3/January 10, 1996), 9.

56. Kevin P. Reilly, Louisiana Department of Environmental Quality, to Richard Mason, Shintech (April 3, 1996), TELC Papers.

57. "Tax Breaks Available to Shintech's Proposed Plant," leaflet by Louisiana Coalition for Tax Justice (n.d.), TELC Papers.

58. Robert Westervelt, "Shintech Selects Louisiana Site for Chlor-Alkali Complex," *Chemical Week* (October 30, 1996), 17.

59. Bill Dawson, "Regional Case May Set Precedent for Environmental Justice," *Houston Chronicle* (September 1, 1997), 40. See also U.S. EPA, "Title VI Administrative Complaint, re: Louisiana Department of Environmental Quality/Permit for Proposed Shintech Facility" (draft revised demographic information) (April 1998), 14, for review of operating facilities, including IMC-Agrico Fostina and Uncle Sam Plant, Chevron Chemical, Air Products and Chemicals, Star Enterprise, Occidental Chemical, and American/Gulf Coast, TELC Papers. In 1978 Goodrich and Bechtel created the Convent Chemical Company and in 1979 began construction of a $269 million chemical complex on a 675-acre site in Convent to produce PVC feedstocks. See Mansel G. Blackford and K. Austin Kerr, *B. F. Goodrich: Tradition and Transformation, 1870–1995* (Columbus: Ohio State University Press, 1996), 329–30; Westervelt, "Shintech Selects Louisiana Site for Chlor-Alkali Complex."

60. Louisiana Department of Environmental Quality, Office of Air Quality and Radiation Protection, "Record of Decision: Polyvinyl Chloride Manufacturing Complex Shintech Inc. and Its Affiliates Convent, St. James Parish, Louisiana" (May 23, 1997), TELC Papers.

61. Ibid., 28.

62. Ibid., 38.

63. Donald L. Bartlett and James B. Steele, "Paying a Price for Polluters: Many of America's Largest Companies Foul the Environment but Clean Up on Billions of Dollars in Tax Benefits," *Time* (November 23, 1998), 72.

64. Ibid.

65. David Firestone, "Economic Crisis Costly for Louisiana Governor," *New York Times* (June 25, 2000), A-12.

66. Elizabeth Teel, Tulane University Environmental Law Fellow, "This River Road Is a Museum without Walls," unpublished manuscript (1999), TELC Papers.

67. Bartlett and Steele, "Paying a Price for Polluters."

68. Paul H. Templet, "The Positive Relationship between Jobs, Environment and the Economy: An Empirical Analysis and Review," *Spectrum* (Spring 1995), 48. See also, "The Full Economic Costs of Louisiana's Oil/Gas and Petroleum Industries" (mimeo) in Paul Templet, coordinator, "People First: Developing Sustainable Communities" (March 1997), 2. The Institute for Environmental Studies, under Templet's direction, published a host of articles analyzing the economic effect of pollution.

69. "Job Hunt for Low-Trained Workers at Odds with Reality," Shreveport *Times* (September 20, 1998).

70. Ibid.

71. Bullard, *Unequal Protection*, 116–17.

72. Environmental Racism Exists in Louisiana," National Public Radio, *Weekend Edition/Saturday* (May 15, 1993).

73. Charles Lee and Damu Smith, *From Plantations to Plants: Report of the Emergency National Commission on Environmental and Economic Justice in St. James Parish, Louisiana* (Cleveland: United Church of Christ Commission for Racial Justice, September 15, 1998), 22–23. See also Roberta Stewart and Jennifer Lewis to Michael Mattheisen, Office of Civil Rights, EPA, et al. (Dec. 10, 1997), TELC Papers.

74. Environmental Racism Exists in Louisiana," National Public Radio, *Weekend Edition/Saturday* (May 15, 1993).

75. Bartlett and Steele, "Paying a Price for Polluters."

76. "Poor Residents in Louisiana Fight Plan for Chemical Site," *New York Times* (May 12, 1997), B-8.

77. We are indebted to Ms. West and Ms. Roberts for accompanying us on a tour of the area and sharing with us many hours of their time.

78. Duncan, "Environmental Justice and Permitting: Cases Applying EPA's Guidance and Regulation," 109. Organizers were well aware that the deadly chemical dioxin, produced by the burning of plastics and other industrial processes, caused a range of diseases, including cancers, and that accidental spills, leaks, and explosions often released a variety of toxic chemicals into the air and water. See "Shintech and Environmental Racism," *Corporate Watch*, <http://www.corpwatch.org/trac/japan/intl/jpn/shintech.html>.

79. Mary Green, "Letter to Editor," Baton Rouge *Advocate* (August 7, 1997), 8-B.

80. Lee and Smith, *From Plantations to Plants*, 17.

81. "Addis PVC Storage Tank Blows Top," Baton Rouge *Advocate* (December 26, 1997), B-1, quoted in Lee and Smith, *From Plantations to Plants*, 16.

82. "Louisiana Jury Award Spurs Call for Halt to PVC Production," *Reuters* (October 17, 1997), quoted in Lee and Smith, *From Plantations to Plants*, 20.

83. Maria Giorano, "Shintech Foes File Suit, Turn to EPA; St. James Group Suing the Parish," New Orleans *Times-Picayune* (June 14, 1997), 1.

84. Richard B. Schmitt, "Louisiana Shackles Law-School Clinics," *Wall Street Journal* (October 29, 1998), B-1.

85. Giorano, "Shintech Foes File Suit, Turn to EPA."

86. "EPA to Set Vinyl Chloride Emissions Standard," *Environmental News*, in K. Johnson, MCA, to F. Kennedy, Conoco, (October 2, 1974), MCA Papers.

87. "Vinyl Chloride Statement by the Administrator [Russell E. Train]," attached to "EPA to Set Vinyl Chloride Emissions Standard," *Environmental News*, in K. Johnson, MCA, to F. Kennedy, Conoco, (October 2, 1974), MCA Papers.

88. "EPA to Set Vinyl Chloride Emissions Standard," *Environmental News*.

89. David D. Doniger, *The Law and Policy of Toxic Substances Control: A Case Study of Vinyl Chloride* (Baltimore: Johns Hopkins University Press, ca. 1979), 78, 81. "National Emission Standards for Hazardous Air Pollutants: Standard for Vinyl Chloride," *Federal Register* 41 (October 21, 1976), 46560.

90. Dawson, "Regional Case May Set Precedent for Environmental Justice."

91. Robert Westervelt, "EPA's Decision on Shintech Plant May Set a Precedent," *Chemical Week*, (July 16, 1997), 7.

92. Ibid.

93. Quote from Patricia Melancon in Westervelt, "EPA's Decision on Shintech Plant May Set a Precedent."

94. Rafael DeLeon to J. Dale Givens (August 8, 1997), TELC Papers.

95. Lisa Lavie to Carol Browner (August 27, 1997), TELC Papers.

96. "Civil Rights Not the Role of the EPA," Baton Rouge *Advocate* (September 23, 1997), 6-B.

97. "Louisiana Is Counting on Chemical Industry for Economic Growth," *Chemical Market Report* 250 (November 25, 1996), 3.

98. "Governor's Threats on Aid Criticized," Baton Rouge *Advocate* (July 22, 1997), 1-A. See also Katherine S. Mangan, "La. Governor Threatens to End Tax Breaks for Tulane U. in Dispute over Law Clinic," *Chronicle of Higher Education* (September 5, 1997), A-55, in which he is quoted as calling the law clinic "a bunch of modern day vigilantes who are just making up reasons to run business out of the state."

99. John McMillan, "State Official Attacks Tulane Clinic," Baton Rouge *Advocate* (August 14, 1997), 4-B.

100. "Foster: Threat Against Tulane Is Appropriate," Baton Rouge *Advocate* (July 24, 1997), 1-A.

101. Mangan, "La. Governor Threatens to End Tax Breaks for Tulane U. in Dispute over Law Clinic."

102. "New Legal Help for Environmentalists," *LEAN News* 3 (September 1989), 5.

103. Ibid.

104. "Tulane Law Clinic Guards State's Interest," New Orleans *Times-Picayune* (September 1, 1997), B-6.

105. Marcia Coyle, "Governor V. Students in $700M Plant Case," *National Law Journal* (September 8, 1997), A-1, A-26.

106. Robert H. Gayle Jr. to Chief Justice Pascal F. Calagero Jr. (July 8, 1997), TELC Papers.

107. "TU Law Clinic: DEQ Staff Pro Shintech," New Orleans *Times-Picayune* (December 23, 1997), A-2; "High Court Reviewing Rules over Law Clinics," Baton Rouge *Advocate* (December 31, 1997), 7-B. See also Sheila Kaplan and Zoe Davidson, "The Buying of the Bench," *The Nation* (January 26, 1998), 11–18; and Gerald Markowitz and David Rosner, "Pollute the Poor," *The Nation* (July 6, 1998), 8–9.

108. James Gill, "Putting the Judiciary on the Spot," New Orleans *Times-Picayune* (April 22, 1998), B-7. See also James Gill, "Beleaguered Environmentalists," New Orleans *Times-Picayune* (June 13, 1997), B-7.

109. Susan Hansen, "Backlash on the Bayou," *American Lawyer* (January/February 1998), 54.

110. Sheila Kaplan and Zoe Davidson, "Louisiana: Polluters Target Top Court," MSNBC (January 1, 1998), <http://www.msnbc.com/news/135643.asp#body>.

111. Gill, "Putting the Judiciary on the Spot." See also Gill, "Beleaguered Environmentalists."

112. Gill, "Putting the Judiciary on the Spot."

113. Marc Schleifstein, "Professors to Protest Curbs on Law Clinics," New Orleans *Times-Picayune* (January 5, 1999), 3-A.

114. Joe Gyan Jr., "Demonstrators Assault Ruling," Baton Rouge *Advocate* (June 27, 1998), 2-B.

115. Eamon M. Kelly, "A Power Play against Environmental Justice," New Orleans *Times-Picayune* (June 25, 1998), B-6.

116. Quoted in "Law Clinics Say Rules Hurt Poor," Baton Rouge *Advocate* (June 18, 1998),1-A. See also Mark Schleifstein, "Foster, Clinics Face Off on Rules Legal Debate Goes beyond Shintech," New Orleans *Times-Picayune* (August 2, 1998), A-1.

117. James Gill, "High Court Target of Disgust," New Orleans *Times-Picayune* (June 28, 1998), B-11.

118. Marc Schleifstein, "Kennedy Defends Tulane's Law Clinic, Slams Governor," New Orleans *Times-Picayune* (November 3, 1998), A-4.

119. Marc Schleifstein, "Rules on Law Clinics Relaxed, But Fight Persists on Indigent Issue," New Orleans *Times-Picayune* (March 23, 1999), A-1.

120. Barbara Koppel, "Cancer Alley, Louisiana," *The Nation* (November 8, 1999), 21.

121. Ibid.

122. "Economic Chief Targets Groups; Reilly, Shintech, Compiled Files on Opponents," New Orleans *Times-Picayune* (November 6, 1997), A-2.

123. Marsha Shuler, "Johnson, Shintech, Big Loan," Baton Rouge *Sunday Advocate* (September 14, 1997), 1-A, 15-A.

124. "Foster Disputes Loan Report," Baton Rouge *Advocate* (September 16, 1997), 1-A; "1997 Was Year to Reflect and Forget," Baton Rouge *Sunday Advocate* (December 28, 1997), A-1; "Non-Profit Group Awarded Grant; Foster Sought Leader's Support," New Orleans *Times-Picayune* (October 13, 1997), A-1.

125. Ibid.

126. Terry Carter, "EPA Steps in to Clean the Air," *ABA Journal* (November 1997), 32: Carter paraphrases Robert Kuehn of the Tulane Environmental Law Clinic. See also Paul Hoversten, "EPA Puts Plant on Hold in Racism Case," *USA Today* (September 11, 1997), A-2; "Shintech Siting Dispute Awakens a Sleeping Giant," *Chemical Week* 159 (October 8, 1997), 45.

127. Bruce Alpert, "Environmental Justice Is a Delicate Balance between Jobs, Rights," *Houston Chronicle* (June 28, 1998), 2; "Shintech Loses Round in PVC Permit Battle," *Chemical Week* (September 17, 1997), 12.

128. "Environmental Justice," *Oil & Gas Journal* 95 (September 22, 1997), 21.

129. "EPA Guidance Draws Fire, but Details Await Shintech Decision," *Chemical Week* (February 25, 1998), 13.

130. "EPA Ruling on Environmental Justice Promises to Cast Long Shadow," *Chemical Market Reporter* (March 30, 1998), 19.

131. Alpert, "Environmental Justice Is a Delicate Balance between Jobs, Rights." See also Ivy Meeropol, "Environmental Racism: Dumping on Minorities in Rural America," *Paper* (June 1998), 38.

132. "Moving Shintech Plant Might Not End Racism Inquiry," Houma, Louisiana, *Daily Courier* (September 20, 1998), B-1, B-2. See also Frank Esposito, "Many Factors Lead Shintech to Alter Plans for PVC Plant," *Plastic News* (September 28, 1998), 6.

133. "Company Evades 'Environmental Racism' Test," *New York Times* (September 20, 1998), A-42.

134. "Moving Shintech Plant Might Not End Racism Inquiry," Houma, Louisiana, *Daily Courier* (September 20, 1998), B-1, B-2.

135. "USA: Major Civil Rights Victory—Shintech Pulls Out!" *Corporate Watch*, <http://www.corpwatch.org/trac/corner/worldnews/other/282.html>.

136. Patrick Courreges, "New Organization to Protest Shintech Plant," Baton Rouge *Advocate Online* (November 4, 1998), <http://www.theadvocate.com/story.asp?storyid=13437>.

137. Don Richards, "Collapse of Shintech Project Crimps Economy in Louisiana," *Chemical Market Reporter* (October 19, 1998), 5.

138. Chris Frank, "Fires at Dow's Plaquemine Plant Cause Release of Chlorine into Air," Baton Rouge *Advocate* (October 4, 1994), 1-B.

139. Frank, "Fires at Dow's Plaquemine Plant Cause Release of Chlorine into Air"; "No Injuries Reported in Chemical Release," Baton Rouge *Advocate* (December 12, 1994), 4-B; "Plant 'Explosion' Was Safety Release," Baton Rouge *Advocate* (March 20, 1995), 5-B; "Gas Leak Blamed on Pipe; No Injuries Reported in Dow Incident," Baton Rouge *Advocate* (April 29, 1995), 3-B–4-B; "Chemical Leak at Plant Closes La. 1," Baton Rouge *Advocate* (April 12, 1995), 3-B–4-B; "Toxic Chemical Spill Is Called No Threat," New Orleans *Times-Picayune* (December 21, 1993), B4.

140. Don Richards, "Shintech and Opponents Brace for Another Round," *Chemical Market Reporter*, (March 22, 1999), 7.

141. "Shintech Announces Proposed PVC Facility in Louisiana" (press release) (September 17, 1998), TELC Papers.

142. "Rally against Dioxin Emissions Planned at Dow, Shintech Units," Baton Rouge *Advocate Online* (January 27, 2000), <http://www.theadvocate.com/story.asp?StoryID=10538>; Gottlieb, *Forcing the Spring,* 274.

CHAPTER 10. SCIENCE AND PRUDENT PUBLIC POLICY

1. These included Nobel Prize winners George Wald, who was the Higginson professor of biology at Harvard University; Rene Dubos, a world-famous

microbiologist at Rockefeller University, Barry Commoner, an activist and academic from Washington University and now at Queens College of the City University of New York; and other noted professors from universities such as MIT and Stanford. Some important early monographs were written by Paul Ehrlich, *The Population Bomb* (New York: Ballantine Books, 1968); Barry Commoner, *Science and Survival* (New York: Viking Press, 1967); Rachel Carson, *Silent Spring* (Boston: Houghton Mifflin, 1962); and Supreme Court Justice William O. Douglas, *The Three Hundred Year War: A Chronicle of Ecological Disaster* (New York: Random House, 1972).

2. Edith Efron, *The Apocalyptics: Cancer and the Big Lie* (New York: Simon and Schuster, 1984), 21–123.

3. Elizabeth M. Whelan, *Toxic Terror* (Ottawa, Ill.: Jameson Books, 1985), 15–16. See also Elizabeth M. Whelan, *Toxic Terror: The Truth behind the Cancer Scares* (Buffalo: Prometheus Books, 1993), 35.

4. American Council on Science and Health, "About ACSH," <http://www.acsh.org/about/index.html>.

5. Sheldon Rampton and John Stauber, *Trust Us, We're Experts! How Industry Manipulates Science and Gambles with Your Future* (New York: Jeremy P. Tarcher/Putnam, 2001), 244–47, 259–66.

6. "The ACSH: Forefront of Science, or Just a Front?" *Consumer Reports* (May 1994), 319. See also Ernest W. Lefever, Raymond English, and Robert L. Schuettinger, *Scholars, Dollars and Public Policy: New Frontiers in Corporate Giving* (Washington: Ethics and Public Policy Center, 1983), 55.

7. Rampton and Stauber, *Trust Us, We're Experts!* Michael Fumento, in *Science under Siege*, also focuses on the need to base policy on sound science instead of on political considerations, but he then goes on to equate the alarm sounded by environmentalists with the Reign of Terror during the French Revolution. "What is needed is to end our reign of terror, to restore sanity and sound principles to our revolution . . . it is time to begin shaping policies on the basis of science, rather than shaping science to fit policies." Michael Fumento, *Science under Siege: Balancing Technology and the Environment* (New York: William Morrow, 1993), 372.

8. Christopher Foreman Jr., *The Promise and Peril of Environmental Justice* (Washington: Brookings Institute, 1998), 108.

9. Henry Payne, "Green Redlining, How Rules against 'Environmental Racism' Hurt Poor Minorities Most of All," *Reason* 30 (October 1998), 32.

10. Study by Southern University, in "Society and Politics—Environmental Justice: Poorest People Live Near Plants—Study," *National Journal's Greenwire* (May 26, 1999).

11. Stephen B. Huebner, "Storm Clouds Brewing on the Environmental Justice Horizon," *Regulation* (Winter 1998), 10–11.

12. Ibid.

13. "Environmental Justice," Editorial, *Oil & Gas Journal* (September 22, 1997), 21.

14. Julian Morris, "Introduction," in Julian Morris, ed., *Rethinking Risk and the Precautionary Principle* (Oxford: Butterworth Heinemann, 2000), viii.

15. Francis O. Adeola, "Environmental Injustice in the State of Louisiana? Hazardous Wastes and Environmental Illness in the Cancer Corridor," *Race, Gender & Class* 6 (1998), 103–04.

16. Sylvia Noble Tesh, *Uncertain Hazards: Environmental Activists and Scientific Proof* (Ithaca: Cornell University Press, 2000), 26–27.

17. Interview with Dr. Craig Zwerling (July 5, 2000), New York City. See also Phil Brown, "Popular Epidemiology and Toxic Waste Contamination: Lay and Professional Ways of Knowing," in Steve Kroll-Smith, Philip Brown, and Valerie Gunter, eds., *Illness and the Environment* (New York: New York University Press, 2000), 364–83.

18. Peter M. Van Doren, "The Effects of Exposure to 'Synthetic' Chemicals on Human Health: A Review," *Risk Analysis* 16 (1996), 367–76.

19. Richard A. Couto, "Failing Health and New Prescriptions: Community Based Approaches to Environmental Risks," in Carole E. Hill, ed., *Current Health Policy Issues and Alternatives: An Applied Social Science Perspective* (Athens: University of Georgia Press, 1986), 64.

20. Sylvia Noble Tesh, *Uncertain Hazards,* 33.

21. Tesh argues that "because health differences between exposed communities and unexposed communities are hard to detect, because in small communities the data are rarely statistically significant, and because it is nearly impossible to get reliable exposure information[,] few risk assessments, therefore, will be strong enough to support aggressive environmental policies." Tesh, *Uncertain Hazards,* 38. See also Daryl M. Freedman, "Reasonable Certainty of No Harm: Reviving the Safety Standard for Food Additives, Color Additives, and Animal Drugs," *Ecology Law Quarterly* 7 (1978), 245–84, for a discussion of the problem of applying traditional measures of risk to the new chemicals being added to Americans' food in the mid-1970s.

22. For a critique of reductionism in epidemiology, see Mervyn Susser and Ezra Susser, "Choosing a Future for Epidemiology: 2. From Black Box to Chinese Boxes and Eco-Epidemiology," *American Journal of Public Health* 86 (May 1996), 676.

23. James O'Byrne, "State Analyzes Miscarry Rates," Baton Rouge *Advocate* (November 27, 1988), B-1, B-8, B-10.

24. Science Advisory Board, EPA, *An SAB Report: Review of Disproportionate Impact Methodologies, a Review by the Integrated Human Exposure Committee (IHEC) of the Science Advisory Board (SAB),* EPA SAB–IHEC–99–007 (Washington: December 1998).

25. Peter T. Gregg, "Environmental Justice—Where Are We Now?" *For the Defense* 41 (May 1, 1999), 25.

26. Ibid. See also Richard J. Lazarus and Stephanie Tai, "Integrating Environmental Justice into EPA Permitting Authority," *Ecology Law Quarterly* 26 (1999), 617–78.

27. Science Advisory Board, EPA, *An SAB Report: Review of Disproportionate Impact Methodologies.*

28. Ibid.

29. Ibid., 16–17.

30. Ibid., 28.

31. Paul W. Brandt-Rauf, Jinn-Chyuan Luo, Tsun-Jen Cheng, Chung-Li Du, Jung-Der Wang, and Marie-Jeanne Marion, "Mutant Onconprotein Biomarkers of Vinyl Chloride Exposure: Applications to Risk Assessment, in *Human Monitoring after Environmental and Occupational Exposure to Chemical and Physical Agents*, ed. by D. Anderson, A. E. Karakaya, and R. J. Sram (Amsterdam: ILS Press, 2000). See also J. Keilhorn et al., "Vinyl Chloride: Still a Cause for Concern," *Environmental Health Perspectives* 108 (2000), 579–88.

32. Ann Carrns, "CDC Cites Chemical Levels in Humans," *Wall Street Journal* (March 22, 2001), B-17; Andrew C. Revkin, "Study of Chemicals in Americans Shows Encouraging Trends," *New York Times* (March 22, 2001), A-16.

33. Joe Thornton, *Pandora's Poison: Chlorine, Health, and a New Environmental Strategy* (Cambridge: MIT Press, 2000), 6; "Weed Killer Deforms Frogs in Sex Organs, Study Finds," *New York Times* (April 17, 2002), <http://www.nytimes.com/2002/04/17/science/17frog.html> (April 19, 2002).

34. National Research Council, Committee on Environmental Epidemiology, *Environmental Epidemiology, Vol. 1, Public Health and Hazardous Wastes* (Washington: National Academy Press, 1991), 1, 256.

35. Ibid., 267.

36. U.S. Environmental Protection Agency, 2001, TSCA Chemical Testing Policy. Office of Pollution Prevention and Toxics, <http://www.epa.gov/oppt-intr/chemtest/sct4main.htm> (January 27, 2002).

37. Linda Starke, ed., *State of the World 2000: A Worldwatch Institute Report on Progress toward a Sustainable Society* (New York: W. W. Norton, 2000), 178–79, 173.

38. Business Roundtable, "Rush to Judgment: A Primer on Global Climate Change" (September 11, 1996), <www.brtable.org/document.cfm/30>. (September 12, 2001).

39. National Research Council, Committee on Environmental Epidemiology, *Environmental Epidemiology*, 270.

CONCLUSION

1. See Philip Landrigan, interview transcript with Bill Moyers, "Trade Secrets," <www.pbs.org/tradesecrets/trans/intero3.html> (April 17, 2002).

Index

Page listings in *italics* refer to illustrations.

Compositor: Michael Bass & Associates
Text: 10/13 Aldus
Display: Bank Gothic Medium
Printer and binder: Malloy Lithographing, Inc.